FIRST RESPONDER

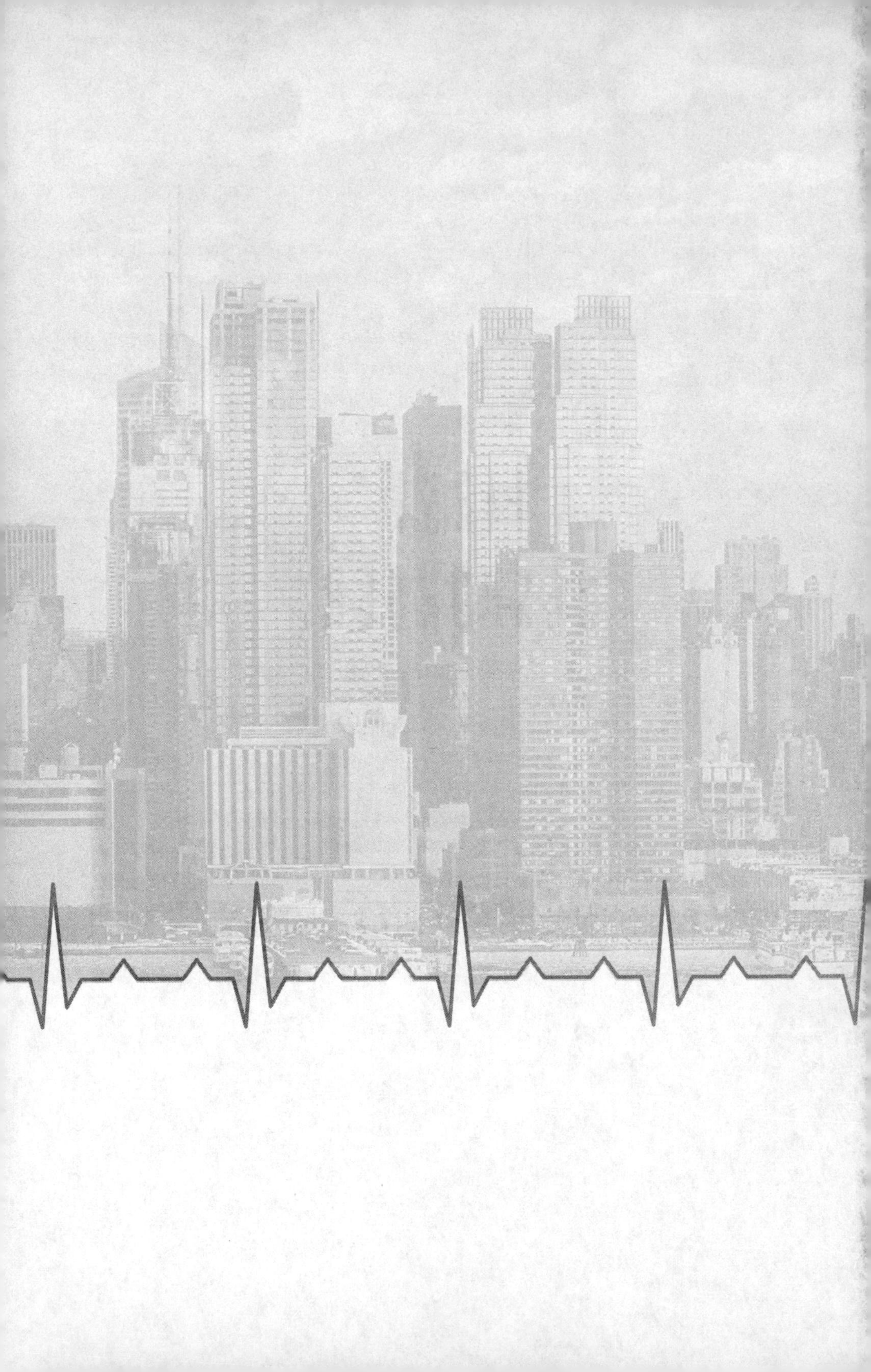

FIRST RESPONDER

A Memoir of Life, Death, and Love on New York City's Front Lines

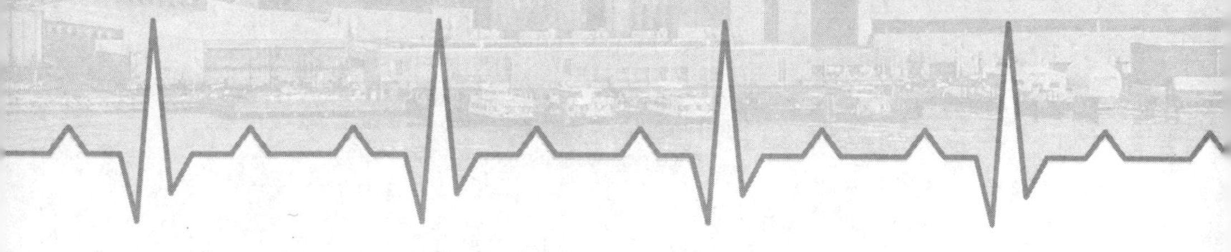

JENNIFER MURPHY

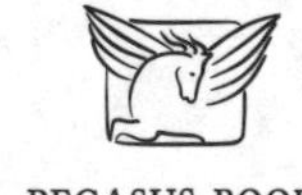

PEGASUS BOOKS
NEW YORK LONDON

FIRST RESPONDER

Pegasus Books, Ltd.
148 West 37th Street, 13th Floor
New York, NY 10018

First Pegasus Books cloth edition April 2021

Interior design by Timothy Shaner, NightandDayDesign.biz

ISBN: 978-1-64313-682-0

10 9 8 7 6 5 4 3 2 1

Printed in the United States of America
Distributed by Simon & Schuster
www.pegasusbooks.com

For Ylfa and Mike,

and forever and ever amen for Pat—

Thank you for saving my life

We, the unwilling, led by the unknowing, are doing
the impossible for the ungrateful. We have done
so much, for so long, with so little, we are now
qualified to do anything with nothing.

—Konstantin Josef Jireček

Heroes are rare.

—James Baldwin

CONTENTS

AUTHOR'S NOTE

In compliance with healthcare privacy laws, the locations, times, names, and identifying details of patients have been changed aside from race, as race plays a critical role in healthcare and medical outcomes. Similarly, details concerning investigations and crisis cases have been altered to protect client confidentiality. Any similarity with an actual case or patient is coincidental. With the exception of a handful 9/11 veteran first responders who specifically asked that their real names be used, the names and, where necessary, identifying details of active-duty first responders have been changed so that they could speak freely without fear of recrimination and to protect privacy. My memories of emergencies have been cross-checked with other first responders where possible, and differing accounts of what unfolded on scene are included for the reader's review. Dialogue has been recalled from memory, my memories substantiated by years of journals and notes. In the spirit of "nothing about us without us," stories from the personal lives of first responders have been included with their blessings and at their direction, with hope that the public might see us more clearly in the fullness of our humanity, and experience what it feels like to walk in our shoes.

PREFACE

The second you put on a uniform people forget you're a human being. They call you a hero. Endow you with superhuman qualities you may or may not possess.

Bravery. Strength. Resilience.

I'm not by nature a courageous woman. Bravery is a performance. It's something I had to practice in order to excel at on the street, where the stakes were unbelievably high. Before I could demonstrate valiance in the face of human catastrophe, I had to be hauled through the hellscape of failure.

Of the four Fs that comprise the body's survival responses to stress—fight, flight, freeze, and yes, fornicate—freezing was my least favorite to experience on scene. Yet there I stood one green summer afternoon in Brooklyn during the summer of 2018, a six-foot-one, redheaded emergency medical technician, a physically unmissable woman, concretized at the sight of a bleeding food delivery biker lying supine in the sunlit street, having just been struck by a car.

Holy shit, I thought. *This is an emergency.*

Now, I don't know about you, but when I see someone wearing an EMT uniform, I'm pretty sure they're supposed help out in this sort of situation.

But that didn't mean I could. I was glaciated by fear. I'd been an EMT at Park Slope Volunteer Ambulance Corps for a few months, and this was my first serious trauma job. While I'd opted to play the part of rescuer in the theater of pre-hospital emergency care in the streets—a choice that seemed dizzyingly stupid—my nervous system demanded I hide in plain sight. Anxiety rendered me useless.

It was a show, this accident. So many people on scene, the sidewalks spilling with onlookers. Where did they all come from? Didn't they have anything better to do on a beautiful Saturday afternoon in Brooklyn, the sun high and the sky blue? I usually worked nights, so I'd never had to face this kind of crowd in daylight. It was too bright out. I wanted to yank the sun out of the sky and kill the lights. The glare coming off a fire rig parked to the side was incredible. It made everything I looked at turn garish and red. There was a police car blocking the street, cops directing traffic, telling the gawking crowd to stand back. "Nothing to see here, folks. Nothing to see."

But there was everything to see. It was the only thing to see.

I understood now why they called war the theater. The emergency rendered me an actor frozen onstage, unable to remember my lines. Humiliated by my inability to move, I stood in the street clutching a stretcher whose brakes I couldn't get to work, sweating through my uniform before an audience of bystanders who'd gathered to watch the gruesome matinee, shocked to see how many people had taken out their phones to record videos of a stranger's pain. Not just the stranger's pain—mine. They were recording me, too. I wanted to run screaming offstage. If there were an eject button, I would have hit it.

There was so much happening all at once. Everyone in action but me, drowning in a sea of surreally slow time. There were voices all around me, but I couldn't tell where they were coming from. I heard only a high-pitched ringing in my ears. It wasn't just the guy laid out in the street with blood guttering from his forehead, darkening his face and spilling into his eyes, his legs twisted to the side as if he were running. It was the swarm of firefighters encircling him, then looking at me, waiting, expecting me to do something. Act!

Was this really happening? It was unreal. Too real. Another ambulance was parked up the block. Bystanders had flagged it down, but the EMTs couldn't take the downed biker because they already had a patient stretchered inside their truck. It was up to me. Us. Where was he? My partner?

There. Ship wasn't hard to spot on this affluent, mostly white block of brownstoned Park Slope. A burly Black rescuer and career EMT twenty years my junior, he stood a few inches taller than me. Ship had a serious disposition and gobs of experience in the field. Often when we arrived

xiv

together on scene people looked up at us in speechless shock at the sight of two towering rescuers sliding off the truck.

Ship worked with a fleet of turnout-geared firefighters to collar, backboard, stretcher, lift, and load the patient into the ambulance without any assistance from me. The audience scattered like thrown dice. Their show was over.

For us, it had just begun.

On the back of the bus, as we call ambulances in New York City, my hands shook terribly. I could barely grip my hot-pink stethoscope. The truck stank of blood and sweat and turned my stomach to liquid. My mouth went dry and tasted of chalk.

Ship hovered over the stretcher and assessed the biker for trauma, cutting off his pants and groping his legs, asking him questions about the location and severity of his pain, taking his vitals. I tried to ask the patient questions, too, but he spoke little English. He had no identification. No insurance. No problem. As one of the city's volunteer ambulance companies, we transported patients regardless of their ability to pay.

Words uttered by the critically injured and sick as well as those approaching death were always humbling and sacred to witness. Agonized men often cried out for their mothers. Others mumbled spiritual pleas to angels near and far. Undocumented workers frequently asked for their bosses.

"Call my boss," the patient kept saying. "Where's my bike? I need my bike."

A Fire Department lieutenant came up to our truck and asked for the patient's name, then assured the guy he would keep the bike at his firehouse. "We've got your bike, buddy. You can come get it once you're out of the hospital."

"Where's my bike?" the patient asked.

Concussed people repeat themselves. Getting them to understand what happened is like trying to eat soup with a fork.

Ship radioed a note to the nearest trauma-receiving hospital, letting them know we were three minutes out and what we were bringing their way. Then he jumped off the truck, shut the back doors, hopped in the front, and blared down the tree-lined blocks to the nearest ER.

There, minutes later, a chaos of nurses and doctors stood outside the trauma room when we rolled in. Ship bounded forward and gave them the lowdown on the situation, known as a triage report. Quickly the hospital staff transferred the patient off our stretcher and onto a bed, cut off his shirt, hooked him up to a vitals device, and began doing whatever it was doctors and nurses did. We stumbled out of the trauma room.

In the hallway, Ship handed me a bouquet of disinfectant wipes to decontaminate the stretcher. Then he looked at me and said, "We need to talk. That can never happen again."

I stood in sorrow and listened.

"First of all, do you remember your protocols for trauma?"

"Yes. I just couldn't remember them on scene. There were so many people."

"It's a show. You're always going to have a lot of people on scene for serious jobs, and on day tours everyone is out on the street. Next time when you get a job for a biker or pedestrian hit by a car, think bleeding control, collar, stretcher. Get them out of the street and away from people. Do you remember what you did next, on the ambulance?"

I had no memory of anything at all.

"You grabbed your stethoscope to take vitals. And that's good, that has to happen within five minutes, but first talk to the patient and assess them for physical trauma. You need to be asking them what hurts and how bad and where. Find out if they lost consciousness if you haven't done that already. Cut off their clothes and look at their injuries. Walk your hands up and down their legs and anything else that hurts. All of that has to happen immediately if the patient is stable. You understand?"

"Yes," I said. My eyes were wet. I felt destroyed.

"You OK?"

"Yeah, I'm good."

"I'm asking you because it looks like you're crying."

"I just need a minute," I said as tears raced down my cheeks. "I'm OK. I'm just disappointed in myself, that's all."

"Don't be. This was your first trauma, right? You got this. You'll get the next one."

But would I? Suddenly I worried I didn't have what it takes to save lives. That deciding to become an EMT was another one of my harebrained ideas. Maybe I wasn't built for this. Maybe I should give up. Quit. I prayed the rest of our tour would be quiet and dreaded the possibility of another job. I wanted only to go home and sob and tell Park Slope I was done. That would be all, thanks. Sorry. Job's not for me. I wasn't designed for this. It wasn't in me. I thought it was, but I was wrong.

Outside, in the hospital ambulance bay, we climbed on the truck and cleaned up the back. It looked like a battlefield after a war where all the soldiers died. Coagulated blood spattered on the gray floor. Ripped-open packets of trauma dressing and gauze thrown all about. Plastic wrapper from the collar. Blood pressure cuff that needed to be cleaned and put back inside the tech bag. My stethoscope abandoned on the blue bench where family members sometimes sat. I didn't realize I didn't have it on me anymore. I lassoed it around my neck.

For an hour, we sat on the ambulance in dead silence. Then, to my horror, we got another job. Injury major, this time in Prospect Park. My entire body felt like a squashed banana. This time it would be different, I told myself as Ship air-horned his way to the park. It had to be different. That could never happen again. *Bleeding. Collar. Stretcher.* We arrived in the park where the trees dropped the temperature and the air was cool and smelled sweetly of grass.

Before Ship fully parked the ambulance, I jumped out the passenger door and ran to a moaning biker who'd been pitched into the lacerating bramble. We were first on scene, mercifully alone. I asked the patient what happened, what hurt, if he'd lost consciousness or remembered the accident. He said he'd crashed into something and flew over his handlebars, landing on his side. His neck hurt.

Ship handed me a collar. I adjusted it to the biker's size and then clasped it around his neck. We lifted him onto the stretcher and loaded him into the ambulance as a fire engine pulled up. A lieutenant slid off the rig and came up to our bus. "We're good," I said. "You guys can go." And off they went.

Inside the ambulance, I cut off the patient's pants and put a cold pack on his swollen knee. Soon we were back in the ER, transferring our patient to nurses and decontaminating the bloody stretcher. This time as I cleaned it down with lemony disinfectant wipes, I thrummed with amazement at what had just transpired. I couldn't stop smiling. I'd never experienced this version of myself before. I'd never transformed so quickly, in a matter of hours, from a bystander paralyzed by fear into a useful participant in an emergency, into someone who could do something, who could help.

The lost dog of my confidence rushed back to me and gave birth to a new confidence that hadn't existed before.

The emergency shredded the unhelpful story I'd told myself for some time, that I was too fragile and sensitive to be a rescuer and I had no business on the street, replacing it with an image of myself as a calm, capable woman trained to stop bleeding and stabilize a spine. My writer's mind went to a line by Denis Johnson, one of my favorite authors. "I make the road. I draw the map. Nothing just happens to me. I'm the one happening." That was it exactly. I was happening. I was a first responder. It was an incredible feeling. I wanted it to last forever.

In the hospital, Ship put his hands on my shoulders and stepped toward me. He hugged me, applauding my performance in the park, telling me he knew I could do it.

"That's my girl! You flew off that truck! I'm proud of you!"

Lesson learned. Bring the body and the mind will follow. The way to unthaw a frozen mind was to get into action. Get out of myself. Get off the ambulance. Move.

That night when I got home, I showered and then sat alone in the dark for a long time, staring at the giant split leaves of the bird of paradise tree towering over my couch. I thought about the food delivery biker who'd been hit by that car and realized I hadn't written down the address of the firehouse where the lieutenant was storing his bike. There'd be no way for him to retrieve it when the hospital released him. His boss would be pissed. Maybe he'd be fired for losing it. It was my mistake, and one that may have resulted in the loss of his livelihood.

Then I remembered how humiliating it had felt to freeze on scene. How embarrassing to stand in the middle of that painfully bright street in front of staring bystanders and, worse, my first-responder colleagues, all of those firefighters and cops. I felt fraudulent and ashamed, undeserving of a uniform. Next tour, next week, would the rescuers from that job remember me from the accident? The statue on the street? Was that who I would be to them now, the EMT who froze? Would it happen again when I saw something I'd never seen before? What else would I see on the street? Would it leave marks? What kind; how deep; where? Was there a way to remove them, or were they permanent?

I asked myself these questions for weeks.

PREFACE

A friend once told me he prays every time he hears an ambulance scream down the street. I presumed he was praying for the sick, injured, or dying patient secured to the stretcher. Not for the EMT or paramedic tasked with driving the bus, or the unbelted rescuer teching in the back, responsible for keeping the patient alive en route to the hospital.

Who rescues the rescuers?

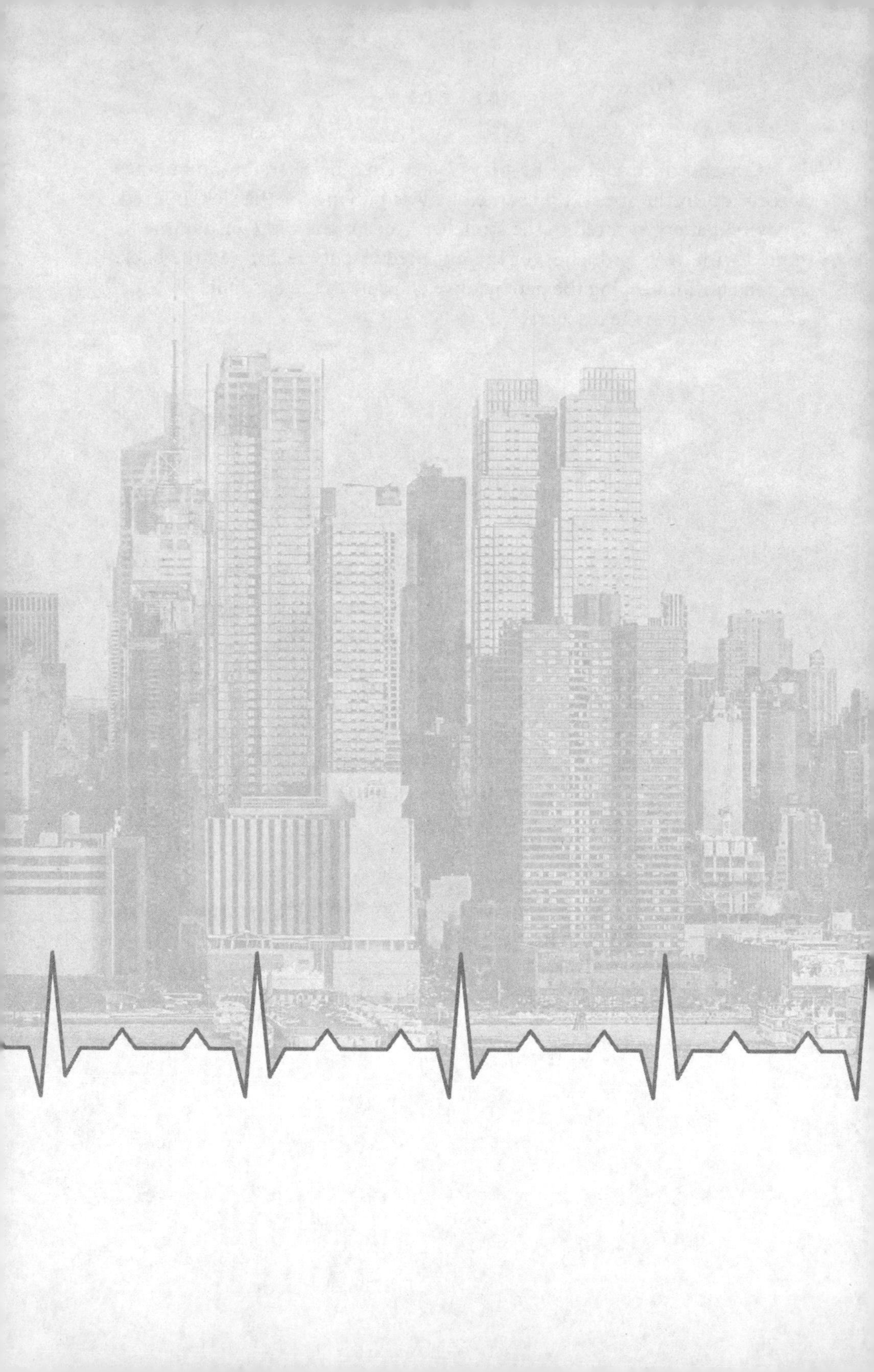

PART ONE

DECISIONS, DECISIONS

1

MINOR SURGERY, MAJOR EMERGENCY

Before you become an EMT it helps to know what it's like to be a patient in an emergency.

One night in December 2015, two years before I became a first responder, I had a medical disaster that resulted in me being stair-chaired and carried out of my apartment, strapped onto a stretcher, and loaded inside the back of an ambulance for the first time in my life.

My disaster started off pretty low-key, as many do. One day my ob-gyn called me into her office and announced I had an ovarian cyst that needed to be surgically removed.

"Is it cancer?" I asked.

I had melanoma in my twenties, so that was at the forefront of my mind. Having a medical history of cancer is like having a criminal record. It's a felony. No matter how many years you're in the clear—seven, ten, or in my case, fourteen—you're never truly off the hook. You hold your breath every time a physician says something the least bit disconcerting. Your doctors hold their breath, too. With melanoma, they always consider the possibility of metastasis to your lungs, bone, brain, and other internal organs.

"Ovarian cysts are very common," my ob-gyn said, feeding me some grade-A, organic medical drivel. In other words, she had no idea. "Because you have a history of melanoma that's always a risk. But cysts are very common."

I mean, if you have to say it twice.

The doctor referred me to a surgeon for laparoscopy. Easy breezy operation, she said. Minor procedure. No overnight hospital stay. No scars. Just a few tiny incisions to my stomach.

I went home crestfallen.

Early one morning a few weeks before my operation, I sat alone in the waiting room of a hospital in Manhattan, sipping coffee and answering an assault of morbidly depressing questions.

Did I have a will? A family member who could take care of me after surgery? Was I an organ donor?

There were many things I enjoyed being asked over coffee upon awakening. How did I sleep, for instance, or did I have any dreams? But whether or not I wanted to donate my eyeballs to science if I flatlined on the operating table was not among them.

I was working and going to grad school at the time, at NYU. I was an MFA student in their creative writing program for fiction, my dream degree as a writer. I'd intended to get this degree ages back, in my twenties. But some events got in the way that delayed my plan. I was now forty, and I didn't want anything to interrupt my creative happiness again. The surgery was calendared over winter break.

Some break. I felt like I couldn't catch one.

As far as having family to take care of me after surgery went, that was a no-go. I grew up in Bakersfield, a high-desert roadside city in Central California, a few hours northeast of LA. Bakersfield was a toilet-bowl-shaped basin of oilfields, orange groves, truck stops, neo-Nazis, country music, Basque sheepherders, and in recent years, the nation's most murderous police force.

Would you like to visit?

The air was so clotted with pollutants from cows and cars that particle matter could be found in the crumpled Kleenexes of everyone who sneezed. Summers, the Mojave sun ramped up to 110 degrees. As a child it fried my nice Irish skin. I'd grown up at a time when sunblock was a quaint idea, and spent the greater part of my childhood sunburned. Often, my skin peeled off in long, translucent strips.

I came from your typical dysfunctional Irish Catholic family. A service family. My great-grandfather was a police chief. My uncle was a sheriff on the bomb squad. Another was an ER doctor. Another, a prosecutor. One aunt was an ER nurse, and my other aunt clerked for a judge.

My dad was religious and angry. He'd grown up poor in Los Angeles. One of his first jobs was washing bricks. His parents drank too much, then bad things happened that went undiscussed, so he swore off "the devil's urine." He never drank. Rage was his beverage of choice.

When she wasn't at work or in the kitchen, my mom was dead in the bed on Valium. She suffered from debilitating migraines, and that's what doctors prescribed to unhappy women with migraines back then. What scraps of attention she had left went to my brother. He was five years older than me.

My brother suffered enormously when we were kids. He was mercilessly bullied. At night he used to bash his head against his headboard to knock himself out so he could sleep. That's how I went to bed each night, listening to my brother ram his head against his headboard.

So that was home.

I lived in New York City for a reason.

I loved New York, but the last few years it seemed like all I did outside of work and school was go to doctor's appointments. I had some ongoing medical issues that started before I matriculated at NYU.

A few years earlier I'd gone to an art opening and collapsed. I woke up on the floor of a gallery with a crowd of artistic-looking faces gazing down at me, my head in the lap of my future ex-boyfriend, the architect.

Should I tell you he was Black? I'm not sure it matters as it pertains to the subject at hand. Or maybe it does, since there aren't that many Black architects, and on account of that fact, my boyfriend felt like he had to work twice as hard as his white peers, and because he worked so hard, he had no time left for our relationship, so I more or less tapped out on neglect. So perhaps it does matter in this context.

Anyway, I asked my boyfriend what happened since I had no idea. I was exhausted beyond belief and couldn't think straight. My brain felt like a microwave that had blown up after someone stuck a metal bowl inside it. My boyfriend informed me I'd passed out and had a seizure.

Interesting, I thought from the floor. I'd never had a seizure in my life.

He helped me up and walked me outside, then took me home to rest. The fainting or seizures or whatever they were continued. Every three or four months I dropped like a swatted fly. Someone always caught me before I hit the ground, which was kind. I'm tall, so I fall from a great height.

I'd since broken up with that boyfriend and been priced out of Fort Greene, where we lived, moved east across Brooklyn to Stuyvesant Heights, a historic section of Bed-Stuy, into an apartment found for me by my friend Clara, who lived near my building, been accepted to NYU, and endured countless medical exams that more or less ruined my first year as a fiction-writing student.

I had blood draws. MRIs. Sleep-deprived EEGs. EKGs. CT scans with and without contrast. Physicians went hard with tests, worried the melanoma had metastasized to my brain. In the end all my test results came back normal. I was a medical mystery.

Baffled, one of my doctors asked if I'd experienced any significant trauma in my life. I shrugged and said, "Bits and bobs," and gave him some lowlights. His eyes widened as I talked. He suggested I might be experiencing something called psychogenic non-epileptic seizures. These were triggered by psychological events rather than epilepsy. Fascinating—unless it's happening to you. He urged me to secure a trauma-informed therapist who did EMDR.

I knew Eye Movement Desensitization and Reprocessing was a type of therapy designed to alleviate distress associated with traumatic memories and disturbing life experiences. I'd heard about it from my military veteran friends. Some of them said it really helped them. I thought that was very nice for them. They'd gone to war. But EMDR for me? That seemed a bit *large*.

That being said, the fainting was becoming a nuisance, so I followed my doctor's advice. A few weeks later I plopped down on a couch before a therapist who specialized in EMDR. She had a warm disposition and worked out of a windowed office that overlooked the Brooklyn skyscape. She asked why I was there. I said a doctor had suggested I see a trauma specialist after I had some unexplainable medical issues.

The therapist nodded. To begin, she asked me to tell her about my life from childhood up to the present moment

Ah, dear. That story?

I gave it to her straight. It took about an hour. When I finished talking, she looked like she'd been electrocuted.

She said I most certainly qualified for EMDR.

"Really?" I said. "Isn't it mostly for soldiers?"

"You qualify," she said.

I decided to trust her. That was a smart move, because too not long after I started doing EMDR, the fainting stopped. I felt like I got my life back. At last I could enjoy my time at NYU.

And then I got the cyst.

My friends were my family in New York. I needed one of them to look after me post-surgery.

My best friend, Felice, was my emergency contact on my medical forms. A poet, playwright, daughter of Guyanese immigrants, and watcher of trash reality television, like me, Felice and I met at the Nuyorican Poets Cafe in 1998. This was the New York City of *Village Voice* newspapers and rich, lacy pancakes at the Noho Star, Dan Savage's "Savage Love" sex column, and Lauryn Hill's first solo album crooning from every speaker in downtown Manhattan, before the city turned into a shopping mall with Citibanks and Starbucks on every corner, and the artistic soul of Manhattan fled to Brooklyn and other boroughs.

Early in our friendship Felice and I lost a mutual poet friend to cancer, one of Felice's dearest friends. The loss welded us together. A friendship flowered in time-lapse bloom. A sisterhood of poetry and grief. We spoke on the phone nearly every day for twenty years and called each other sister.

Because she was Black and I was white, Felice and I fielded endless questions about how we became sisters, and were constantly asked to write and speak about interracial friendship, a subject on which we were anthologized many times, since the world found it so crazy, so wildly unbelievable, that two women of such different backgrounds could be so close.

Felice took the day off from work to accompany me to the hospital. But then my surgery got rescheduled at the last minute and her boss wouldn't give her another day off.

Enter Natalie. I met her through Felice one summer years back, when Felice was teaching a class on Fire Island and everyone kept mistaking her for a nanny. She called for backup, and Natalie and I and our friend Kerri ferried out to assist.

Natalie was emotionally unflappable, a corporate attorney who looked after her extended Jamaican family while working full-time, while also getting a martial art belt of some important color. She was perfect for this job, and she'd saved me many times before. During the financial crisis of

2008, when I was living in Paris, I found myself suddenly out of work. Natalie flew to London on business, took the train to France, and, unprompted, paid my rent at a time when I was penniless.

She agreed to pick me up from the hospital post-op and stay the night at my place to watch over me. Now I just had to get through the next few weeks of school before winter break.

Surgery break.

In grad school those weeks before the operation, I tried to write about what was going on in my life medically, but it made me anxious to face things on the page. Every time my stories were up for discussion in workshop I sweated through my clothes.

I thought I would find my people in grad school, which on the one hand I did. Readers and writers. But on the same hand, I felt like the freak in the room.

Many of the stories produced by my peers at NYU were quiet and elegant. At the height of drama a cup of tea got poured and some of it splashed on the main character's pants. My stories contained massive amounts of violence. Horrible things happened to people in my fiction. In one novel in progress I killed all my characters in the first chapter.

"Jennifer, does this character have to boil to death at the end of the story?" my professor Nathan Englander asked me one day in workshop.

I could only be me.

I tried to stop killing my darlings, but it just kept happening. What obsessed me as a writer was somewhat of a self-driving car. Nathan told me not to worry about it. He said he was the freak in his grad program, too. He said the freak was the one who got published.

"Think Coen brothers," he said. "Think *Fargo.* If you need to keep the woodchipper, keep it."

Saturdays I volunteered with the NYU Veterans Writing Workshop, a group of military vets from various wars, and wow, did that room change me. Talk about the woodchipper. These writers penned characters who got blown up, fell sick with burn-pit cancer, and shot dogs every other page.

When my sister-in-arms Yael, a poet and cofacilitator, told us she was pregnant, one of the guys stared funereally at the table and said, "I guess this means no more dead-baby jokes." The second she waddled out of the room they let it rip. Dead-baby jokes galore.

I laughed at these jokes for months.

The vets called me Unicorn because I fit in with them. When a few of them wrote women characters who were saintly Madonnas, cheating whores, or suburban girlfriends who couldn't possibly understand how their swaggering military boyfriend characters felt when they returned from war, I redlined their work and insisted they round out their shakily drawn women.

I devoured war literature. In workshop I moaned about searching for myself in these books and never finding anyone resembling me.

Where were the alpha females? The women who endured violence and told the story? Several of us agreed the War on Terror was increasingly domestic, being battled-out online, some of the country's most pressing threats coming not from al-Qaeda hiding in the mountains of Afghanistan, but from far-right and neo-Nazi extremist groups radicalized at home, in the good ol' USA, weaponizing platforms like Facebook and YouTube, which refused to take a stand against hate. In my work life I was a player in these digital firefights. Where was the book about that?

The vets sighed. Some of them said they were waiting for a chick to write the next great book about war.

"I'm a chick, so I'll do it," I told them.

They chuckled because I was a civilian.

But in the end, that didn't matter. As stated, the War on Terror was increasingly domestic.

The vets did the same thing for my work in terms of critiquing my pages. One day, I brought in a story I'd written about a girl who grew up in the California desert. I assigned her a drunk, angry, military father who shot her in the head. I was terrified to get their feedback. But I respected them as writers and people, so I desperately wanted to hear what they had to say. I was so nervous the day my story was on the table I worried I might faint.

Creative writing workshops at NYU followed standard protocols for receiving feedback on your work. The writer sat in total silence and listened to people discuss their creation, taking notes. At the end you were allowed to ask questions. I never got used to this format. It felt like ripping your heart out of your chest, putting it on the table, and being muzzled and made to watch while your peers stabbed it to death.

That day, because of my story's content, I was especially afraid. Ten or so minutes into class my worst fear materialized.

One guy said he thought it was the best story submitted so far. But then others spoke. A lot of them. They unleashed torrents of outrage at me for drawing a veteran who was so cliché. Painting a character in that damaging stereotype of the angry, drunk, violent vet that plagued them in real life. They were massively disappointed in me. They thought I was an ally.

I got so turned around in the thunderstorm of their remarks that by the time they finished talking I wasn't sure where I was. My head hurt and I couldn't speak. I feared I might cry. When I finally found my voice, it was small and wobbly.

After a while I said, "So that was based on a true story. It's the most personal thing I've ever written. I made it fiction, because telling the story straight is too hard for me."

Silence entered the room. The vets looked at me.

"Tell us the real story," one of them said quietly.

"I don't know if I can do it without crying."

"That's OK," another said. "Tell us."

I took a deep breath and blew out the story, as much of it as I could bear telling the entire group. Other parts of it I revealed later to one or two of them, in more intimate settings, over coffee, or sitting on park benches, shoulder to shoulder.

My father wasn't military, like the guy in my story. He managed a moving company. I played volleyball in high school. I was a star athlete. One of the girls on my club team was this beautiful blonde girl named Heather. She was smart and kind and athletically talented, and I desperately wanted to be like her. Her life seemed charmed. One of her sisters played club, too, on the court a few feet away from ours. Heather's mom was nice and always at our games. If I met her father, I blacked that out.

One day when I was fifteen my parents came into my room and my dad told me something had happened. He said, "Your friend Heather's dead. Her father killed her and his whole family and himself. Dinner's ready."

I repeated that line to myself for years: Your friend Heather's dead. Her father killed her and his whole family and himself.

Dinner's ready.

My childhood ended that day. Suddenly I was fifty years old. I didn't understand what'd happened. And something about my dad's deadpan delivery scared me. The only death I'd experienced up to that point was that of my childhood cat, who got made into a frisbee by a car. When my cat died, my dad came running into the house to tell me, sobbing and heaving with fireworks of tears. But when Heather and her entire family were killed, he gave me the news like a weather report.

Up to that point my father's temper had always scared me. But never for a second had I considered he might kill me. I didn't know fathers could do that. This was in 1991, before groups of people were getting shot to death every month in white suburban America. Back then, a murder-suicide of five people was a pretty big deal. The Internet wasn't in use yet and no one told me the details of how Heather got killed, so I never knew the story. The not-knowing tortured me. I needed to know so I could understand.

One day after the massacre our volleyball coach sat us down and passed out felt hearts to iron on our uniforms, in memory of Heather and her sisters. That's what we got. Your friend just got shot to death by her father, here's an iron-on heart.

Therapy wasn't in circulation back then, so the tragedy was made worse by the times it took place in. To merit therapy you had to be a loser with some pretty loose screws. The way you handled things was you kept your mouth shut, never spoke about how you felt, never let anyone know what happened inside your house or that you suffered. You sucked it up and pressed on. That's what winners did. So I was a winner.

No one invited me to Heather's funeral or even told me there was one, so I didn't get a memorial service to grieve and help me out in terms of processing her death, either.

After the massacre my world pretty much fell apart. I started drinking, smoking, cutting school. My grades dropped. Prior to that I'd been a straight-A student. A good girl. Alcohol gave me courage and a voice, which I desperately needed and used in screaming matches against my father, since I was now newly and privately terrified he might snap one day and take my life. We fought constantly.

Then I started having panic attacks and hallucinations. Night terrors, only they happened in daylight, too. I imagined my dad chasing me down the street with a machete, trying to stab me to death. I told no one about this. I didn't know what was happening to me. I thought I was going crazy. I broke out in scaly rashes all over my body. The doctors said it was psoriasis.

Soon, I found it unbearable to be in my house. A year later, at sixteen, I had a blowout with my father over something minor, and I went to my bedroom and started packing. My mom came into my room to see what I was doing.

"I can't live here anymore," I told her. "I'm moving out. Don't try to stop me."

My mom nodded then said, "Meet me in the garage in five minutes. I'm going with you."

And my family split up.

Now, I did not intend to bring my mother with me when I extracted myself from the house. But there she was. For a while we stayed at my grandparents' house, until my mom found a condo she could afford.

Growing up, I thought we were rich. We lived in a big house. We had a pool and two cars in the garage. I never wanted for anything materially. But then one day my mom came into my grandma's sewing room and handed me a shoebox and a pair of scissors. I looked inside. Dozens of credit cards, all in my father's name.

"Cut them up," she said. "We have nothing."

For decades, I couldn't remember Heather's name. Then, a year before I wrote the story, when I was home one night reading one of my professor's books, Darin Strauss's memoir, *Half a Life*, I suddenly remembered it. Immediately I went online and searched for articles about the massacre and found out how Heather had been murdered. As I was reading the articles, I fainted for the third or fourth time.

"The news stories said Heather's dad was an Air Force veteran and later worked for NASA," I told the vets that day in workshop. "Since NASA is in the business of manufacturing heroes, that didn't seem like a reason for a man to kill his family. I needed a reason in my story, so I blamed it on the military. And I know that's unfair. But I honestly don't know how to tell this story. I'm struggling," I said, and now my face was hot and demolished with tears. "It's toxic. It's making me sick. I need help, and I didn't know what else to do except try to work on it here."

When I finished talking someone trotted out of the room and came back with tissues. I blew my nose and took some sips of air. The vets thanked me for telling them what happened. Yael suggested we take a little break. Almost everyone needed to step outside and smoke. One by one the vets stood up and came across the room and hugged me. They apologized profusely and sincerely. They said they'd do anything to help me tell the story, real or fiction, however they could, which meant the world to me.

It saved me, to know they were there and had my back.

Not long after that, a bunch of them brought in their service patches and pins and quietly handed them to me. Air Force, Army, Marines. Iraq. Afghanistan. Vietnam.

I knew from my day job that in the service world, patches and pins and coins were a fist bump, a hat tip to say, *Thank you for having skin in the game, you're one of us, you belong.* Their kindness and understanding filled me with incomprehensible gratitude. I'd wanted to belong to something all my life.

The laparoscopic surgery went smoothly. I'd been operated on before, back when I had cancer, and always enjoyed being put under. I was sober over ten years, so this was a freebie. A real treat to be transported back to that dreamy state. The only thing I loved more than being sober was being drunk. If drinking hadn't stopped working for me, I'd still be doing it.

I woke up after the operation in a hospital bed feeling groggy, with Natalie at my side and an extremely annoying nurse shaking me awake. Conversations with this nurse revolved around how to get me out of there as quickly as possible. I felt like a cow being shoved out of a meat processing plant.

Natalie was a dream. She'd brought me coffee. I sipped it and relaxed and felt no pain at all. I was still high on anesthesia. Wonderful stuff. At some point my surgeon floated by and told me everything went super. He wrote me a prescription for painkillers. One of the big boys. Oxycodone. Narcotic. High risk for addiction and dependence.

"For laparoscopic surgery?"

"You just had major surgery," he said.

I reminded him I was sober and asked him to hit me with some non-narcotics. Surgeries are tricky for us sober folks. Trips to the doctor and dentist with prescriptions for narcotics often strip people of long-term sobriety in one afternoon. And once you let go of the sober balloon string, you never know if you'll get it back. The first time you get sober is grace.

From what I've observed from relapsers over the years, the second time, if you get a second time, is hell on ice.

My doctor shut down my request and vanished.

I flagged down the grouchy nurse and told her I didn't want to take narcotics, since I was sober. She also gave me strong words about how I'd just had major surgery and needed to take the medication as prescribed. Advil wouldn't cut it.

Doctors! Nurses! Shaking my head. Before they slice you open like roast turkey, they tell you it's no big deal, your surgery. Then when you act like it's no big deal, they say you just had major surgery. Which one did I have? Minor or major? Make a decision, pals.

The nurse reappeared and handed me a cup, then made me hobble to the bathroom to fill it. She said she couldn't release me until I could urinate. She seemed in quite a rush. I took the specimen cup to the bathroom. My bladder failed to do its magic. A thimble of pee was all I could produce.

"Sorry," I said, handing her the empty cup.

She looked at it and said, "Good enough."

Natalie wheelchaired me out of the hospital and eased me into a cab. On the ride to Brooklyn I felt fantastic. The taxi driver pulled over when he heard me complain of being thirsty. He went to his trunk and came back with a bottle of water and handed it to me. I love New Yorkers. We get a bad rap for being assholes. But when you're hurting, New Yorkers will always help out.

The pain hit later, at home. The anesthesia wore off and my stomach felt like it had been munched on by the star of *Jaws*. I took a painkiller. It did nothing. My belly grew bigger as the hours passed. I tried to sleep but had sharp abdominal pain and a thickening sense of doom. By nightfall I was doubled over.

Natalie said it was because I'd just had major surgery—a phrase I was hearing a little too frequently for my taste—but that didn't feel right. Something seemed off. The pain worsened. It was now after midnight and I still couldn't produce more than a thimble of pee, and because of the pain I couldn't stop crying.

I told Natalie to call one of my former colleagues, a retired Italian cop named Nick who wore a thick gold chain around his neck and looked like he'd just flown in from Sicily. Cops were always awake. Ex-cops, too. I could call them day or night and they'd pick up the phone. Natalie gave Nick the lowdown and asked what we should do.

"Call 911 on speaker phone," he said, "so I can listen."

Natalie called 911. Minutes later, a twosome of EMTs were in my bedroom. I don't remember anything about them or what they did. Their visit was a blur. I was pretty sure they took my vitals. I signed something on a laptop. In my memory, I was begging them to take me to the hospital. But they left me at home.

"Jen, that's not what happened at all!" Natalie said when we went over that night. The way she told it, the EMTs took my vitals and they were normal. I asked them what they thought I should do and mentioned I'd only taken one painkiller because I was sober, so I was nervous to take more and get strung out on drugs. They said I should take another one, eat some soup, and try to sleep. I agreed. The EMTs departed.

I did what I was told. Took another painkiller. Ate soup. Went to bed. Two hours later I woke up in agony, my stomach looking like I was about to give birth to one of God's children. I was still unable to manifest a drop of urine. By now it was two or three o'clock in the morning.

"I need to go to the hospital," I told Natalie. "You have to call 911 again."

"Jen, no," she said. "The EMTs were just here. You don't need to go to the hospital. You're in pain because you just had major surgery. And you're fucked up because you're on narcotics. Trust me, you're OK. You're just panicking. And you're high."

I climbed in bed and got under the covers. Then I pulled the duvet over my head and snuck in another call to 911. I'd never called 911 in my life and this night I called twice.

"Jen!" Natalie screamed from the living room, overhearing me. "You don't need to go to the hospital!"

Sorry, I disagreed. So did the next pair of EMTs who appeared in my bedroom.

My next set of first responders were men. I couldn't walk so they loaded me onto what looked like a wheelchair and carried me down three flights of steps, sweating and grunting as they worked. I felt bad for them. I was light, but still.

Outside, a party of emergency vehicles was parked in front of my building. All this for me? You shouldn't have.

The EMTs loaded me into the ambulance. Natalie begged them to take me to Manhattan, back to the hospital where I'd had surgery. The EMTs radioed their dispatcher and got approval to transport me all the way into the city, which was about a forty-five-minute drive. Soon we were moving. It was a long, slow ride, and I was relieved and elated to be headed to the ER at last.

I'd never been on an ambulance before. One EMT drove and Natalie sat up front with him. The other rescuer sat in the back, on a long bench next to me. I handed him my driver's license and insurance card, and he typed my information into his laptop. When he asked for my medical history and I gave it to him all in one slug.

"Alcoholism, skin cancer, psychogenic non-epileptic seizures from PTSD, and freshly out of supposedly minor laparoscopic surgery to remove an ovarian cyst."

He didn't flinch. He took it like a champ.

I had a sudden urge to urinate but knew nothing substantial would come out. "I have to pee," I said. "I'm so sorry. I don't want to get your ambulance dirty, but I can't help it."

"Go for it," he said. "We work in Brownsville. You have no idea what kinds of fluids have been in the back of this truck. Pee all you want. We'll clean it up later."

God bless him. Saints, these EMTs.

"Do you think I'm overreacting?" I asked him after I released a pathetic trickle of urine. "Do you think my friend's right? I had surgery and I'm supposed to be in pain and really don't need to go to the hospital? I'm just panicking because I'm sober and on narcotics, so I'm out of my fucking mind?"

He looked at me and said in the softest, kindest voice, "Whenever you're in this much pain and your body can't resolve it, you're right to panic. Your body is doing what it should be doing. You need to go to the hospital."

I wept when he said that, I felt so relieved. I loved him right then. I loved him for believing me, and helping me, for treating and transporting me and being on my side. He was an angel. A stranger and an angel, a strangel. I wanted to be like him. I'd never felt so cared for by someone I didn't know.

* * *

At the hospital the EMTs transferred me onto a bed. I was so thankful for what they did I asked Natalie to get their shield numbers so I could write them a thank-you note.

Soon, a nurse chomping gum appeared and did an ultrasound on my stomach. "You need a catheter," she said.

She went away and came back and inserted one. I felt a pinch. Then a flood of urine rushed out of me. Sweet relief! It was phenomenal, bliss, better than all the drinks and drugs and sex I'd ever had in my life combined. I peed for what seemed like centuries, rivers of urine flowing into a plastic jug attached to the rail of my hospital bed. My God, I loved that catheter.

"Your bladder was still asleep from the surgery," the nurse said, cracking bubbles. "You should've come in much sooner, instead of waiting. Your bladder could have burst, then you would have gone into septic shock, and that's a real emergency."

Real emergency. Well, what the fuck was this?

The second she said that I looked at Natalie, since I knew this news would crush her. "Girl, I'm OK," I said. "I'm fine."

Natalie was standing by a curtain, staring morbidly at the floor. She wouldn't look at me.

"Nat! Natalie! Look at me. I'm totally fine. I feel fantastic."

We got home from the hospital around six o'clock in the morning and went to sleep. When I woke up later that afternoon, I opened my bedroom door and found Natalie lying on her side on my blue velvet couch, quietly weeping.

"Oh no!" I said. "What's wrong? Are you OK?"

"No," she said miserably. "Jen, I almost killed you. You could've died and it would've been my fault, because I told you not to go to the hospital."

"But I didn't die. I'm great. Look," I pointed at my catheter. "I'm peeing and I don't even feel it. I love this thing. They should make these to go in purses. No more waking up at night. No more walking all over the city looking for a bathroom. There's nowhere to pee in New York City. This thing's amazing."

"Jen," Natalie said, sitting up, still crying. "I love you so much, and I almost killed you."

"Yes, this is true. But you didn't kill me. It's like when a guy says he was so sad he almost cried. That means he didn't cry. No tears fell. I feel great, Nat. And I'm not dead. I'm alive."

Alive, and so inspired by the EMTs I met that night. Over the months, as I recovered, I wondered if maybe I could do what they did. Help someone like they'd helped me. Go from being a patient in the back of the ambulance to one of the rescuers up front.

I doubted it. I was a businesswoman and a writer. Neither of these jobs were tactical. I sat at a desk all day. But the idea wouldn't leave me, and the inspiration just kept coming.

A year or so after my surgery I got a text from a friend of Nick, the ex-cop Natalie had called the night of my emergency. The text arrived at five o'clock in the morning and said to give the guy a call. The time stamp told me something awful had happened. I was terrified. Loads of cops died of heart attacks, stroked out, or dropped dead from unknown causes (stress) after they retired. Around this time Nick was one of my closest friends.

I called the guy who'd texted me, and he said Nick'd had a heart attack, but he was alive. *Whew.* When we hung up, I cried tears of sorrow chased by relief.

I visited Nick in the hospital a week or so later. He'd been a boss in the NYPD, a cop's cop, one of those guys who said the rosary to Reagan, so the blue man's group went crazy for him. I couldn't take him anywhere without Jimmy or Mikey or Ricky Bobby coming out of the woodwork to shake his hand, pick up his lunch tab, and write him fraternal love notes on diner napkins.

I went to see him early in the morning to avoid the parade of cops who would inevitably swing by to pay their respects and kiss his Irish ass. I'd met Nick through work years back and we'd grown close, so I could just talk to him like a normal person. He liked that. But it also rankled him that I didn't fall into a salutary trance like everyone else. Nick called me Lioness because I roared at him a lot, mainly about politics, and he did the same on the shouting front with me. I called him Lion.

"You know, Lioness," he said in the hospital, when I gave him the eyeball roll about cops bowing at his feet day and night. "I was a pretty big deal in the NYPD."

I nodded and said, "And then what happened?"

"Fuck you!" he said, laughing. Then he had to stop because his chest hurt.

Some months later, over lunch, I told Nick about my simmering unicorn dream of becoming an EMT. He encouraged me to do it. We shared a reverence for service. But that wasn't the only thing nudging me toward the street.

After he had his heart attack, I couldn't relax around him without knowing what to do if, God forbid, he had another one. Suddenly it seemed irresponsible not to know how to do something as basic as CPR.

"It stresses me out to be around you now," I told him. "If you drop dead, I won't be able to bring you back."

"Thirty and two, thirty and two," he said, referring to the chest-compression-to-breath ratio of CPR.

Another day I shared my EMT dream with a buddy from the NYU Vets Writing Workshop. I asked if he thought I should do it.

"Hell yeah!" he said. "I loved learning medical shit in the Marines. It was really fun. I think you'd be good at it, too."

Like me, this guy abhorred cubicle life. We worked in the same field, and he wanted to quit his job and apply to get an MFA in fiction at NYU; he was only a weekender, he wasn't enrolled. But he didn't know if he should do it.

"Hell yeah!" I said. "If you get accepted and quit your job, I'll hire you. And I'll make sure you have of time to write."

Guess who got accepted to NYU's fiction writing program and matriculated the following fall. Guess who worked with me now. Guess who became an EMT.

As far as that surgery went, the cyst was a cyst, not cancer. My emergency was real, not panic. And judging by the bill the hospital slapped me with—around $83,000—I'm going to agree the surgery was major. If I hadn't been insured, it could have bankrupted me.

Years passed and I never got around to writing that thank-you note to the EMTs who saved me. So this urine-drenched chapter goes out to them, in Brownsville.

Thank you, gentlemen.

2

EMERGENCY CARE IN THE STREETS

First night of EMT school I was more excited than nervous. Classes took place in the evenings twice weekly at a senior facility in East New York, a few subway stops from my house. I had no idea if I'd enjoy the course or be able to handle it, but I had some hope. I was naïvely optimistic. That was in December 2017.

In the senior facility, a security guard directed me to a cafeteria turned into a makeshift classroom. The room stank of urine and forgotten old people. Sad red and green streamers I guessed were for Christmas hung from the light fixtures. I was the first student there. I was a neurotic early arriver, so that was typical. Soon, one of the instructors appeared and bounded up to me. He was a burly, unshaven middle-aged guy named Nate who looked like he hadn't slept in a week. We introduced ourselves.

"Basketball?" he said.

"Volleyball."

"Outdoor?"

"Indoor. College."

"Ever model?"

"For two weeks in my twenties."

"Why only two weeks?"

"I almost got a job playing Queen Elizabeth in a Parkay butter commercial, but when I didn't get the part my agent told me I needed to lose weight in my arms, so I quit."

"Lose weight!" Nate said. "You? What are you, 120?"

"Something like that."

Nate was a family man and career paramedic. He seemed amused by my presence in class and asked what I did for a living. I often asked myself the same question.

I told him I was a writer and investigator-slash-crisis-manager who specialized in electronic crimes, loosely defined as "things that went wrong on the Internet." In recent years, mass shootings had reached epidemic proportions, so much of my time was spent online, searching for kill threats by members of various hate groups. Men, mainly white men, boys, really, posting rancid manifestos on the Internet, saying they planned to shoot up a school, or parade, or hospital. Lighthearted stuff like that.

I didn't say all that to sound important. Telling people I was a private investigator was a trap. Thanks to TV and genre fiction, if I said I was a PI people assumed I was slinking down alleyways in a fedora and trench coat with a gun stuffed in my purse or crawling around parking lots sticking GPS trackers under the cars of philandering men. As the detective friend who convinced me to get into this grim field told me fifteen years ago, "You're a good writer and a horrible gossip, and that's all a private investigator is. But you'll never work surveillance."

"Interesting," Nate said when I finally stopped talking.

Interesting was what my mother said whenever I cooked something inedible, in lieu of spitting it out. I asked what he meant.

"I know your type. You're the type of woman who's never satisfied. You're smart. You like to learn. You like to be in school. I bet you have a few advanced degrees."

I blushed. I had that MFA along with a master's degree from the University of Chicago—where fun goes to die.

"I know who you are," Nate said. "I had a woman like you in my last class. She had a bunch of different degrees."

"Does she work on an ambulance now?"

"No. Never worked one day as an EMT."

"And you don't think I'll ever work on an ambulance?"

"No," he said, walking to the front of the classroom.

Men. They misread me.

Gradually, a dozen or so students shuffled into the cafeteria along with Nate's co-instructor, Carrie. She was a tall, soft-spoken EMT and former cop who'd retired early and disabled after being injured on the job. She got run down in the street by some drug dealers. When the car hit her, she came out of her shoes. I'd heard that happened to people who got hit by cars.

Most of the students were twenty years my junior, brown and Black and Asian, many of them first- or second-generation immigrants. Their collars were blue. I felt at home. I sat beside a guy who worked at a hardware store and in front of a cheerful woman whose wrists were licked with scars, which I wondered about. Two giggly, dark-haired sisters sat in the back, next to a pretty but exasperated-looking woman desperate to get out of her job at the US Postal Service.

Carrie cleared her throat and told us what books to buy. A go-to text in the field, optional for purchase, was Nancy Caroline's *Emergency Care in the Streets*. One of the first sheroes of paramedicine, Dr. Caroline cofounded Pittsburgh's Freedom House, an ambulance service that assisted underserved populations in the sixties and seventies. She became the first medical director of Israel's Red Cross and was often called that country's Mother Teresa.

Carrie then held up a fat textbook called *Emergency Care and Transportation of the Sick and Injured*, sometimes called the Orange Book, because it was orange. She passed it around.

This book, required for class, was over fifteen hundred pages long with an online curriculum. I flipped through the pages. It covered everything from bleeding control to emergency childbirth in the field. Just reading the words frightened me, and don't get me started on the pictures. People lay sick and dying between paragraphs, displaying infected fistulas and open fractures, cerebral aneurysms and third-degree burns.

Good God, was I really going to do this? At NYU I'd been highlighting gorgeous passages of Nabokov's *Pnin* and rereading Amy Hempel and James Baldwin.

Just then a tattooed guy with tribal cornucopias shoved through his earlobes, which were stretched wider than a perineum during birth, marched into the room and declared he was late because he'd taken a nap and his alarm didn't go off.

Nate yawned. "Lucky you got me as an instructor who gives no shit."

The late guy made a point to say he was not new. He was already working as an EMT and was taking the course as a refresher. EMT certifications expired every three years, so he was here to quickly recertify. He worked at Elderly Care.

"Elderly Scare," Nate said. "How many people have you killed?"

"I don't know, man," Cornucopia Ears said. "I honestly don't know."

After an hour or so of paperwork and chit-chat Nate and Carrie dismissed us early, telling us to buy the textbook and read the first several chapters, as we'd have a quiz the next class. Heading home on the train, I pondered how much I'd enjoyed meeting my classmates. But glancing at that textbook made me afraid of what I'd see on the street.

A few nights later, at my house, I told a detective I was sometimes dating—if you could even call it that—I was becoming an EMT.

Rafael was a Dominican immigrant who worked at a busy precinct in Brooklyn. He loved traveling, art, and wearing shirts with American flags on them in Paris, where I lived for four years before I dated the architect. Rafael was five foot eight, so in bed my legs looked like comparative chopsticks next to his. I wasn't a woman who discriminated against men based on height. I was taller than most people on earth, so I wasn't trying to limit my choices. And, as an Israeli Navy SEAL friend from the Vets Writing Workshop who was married to a taller-than-he-was woman once told me, "Height is a state of mind."

I asked Rafael if he thought I could handle being on the ambulance. He was a street guy, so I valued his opinion.

"I don't know why you'd *want* to do it," he said. "But sure. I think you can do it."

He said the worst things I was going to see on the street by way of trauma were train jobs and jumpers.

"I had this one dude who jumped off a bridge and missed the water. His bones came out of his body. Mostly his legs out of his buttocks. I'd never seen anything like it."

Just the kind of pillow talk I cherished.

Next class I aced my first quiz. Class after that, same deal. Month by month I winced my way through the bloody pages of the Orange Book. The material was dense, scientific, and not what I would describe as beach reading. I memorized a gazillion medical terms and facts I never wanted to know.

Who developed EMS standards? Department of Transportation. What were the flow rates for a nasal cannula? One to six liters of oxygen per minute. Define *distal*, *histamine*, *shock*. Farther away from the torso, the chemical in mast cells that triggers dilation and increased permeability in capillaries, shock, aka hypoperfusion, the inability of the body to adequately circulate blood to the cells in order to supply them with oxygen and nutrients—life-threatening.

The reading was torture, but I loved class. It was the people. Over time study groups assembled. We reviewed chapters together. Shared flashcards. Practiced splinting each other's pretend broken bones. Laughed our heads off at stories Nate told. I looked forward to nights I had class more than any other nights of the week and started to wonder if I'd been depressed.

Probably.

Being with my new EMT friends buoyed my spirits and gave me a likeminded community of emergency-drawn souls. The woman in class with scars on her wrists lived in my neighborhood. We took the train home from school together most nights and sometimes studied at my house, going over our lessons. Over time we got to know each other. She was like me, bookish and bespectacled and educated. We were the outliers in class. One night at my apartment we discovered we were both from equally shitty places. When I told her I was from Bakersfield she gasped, so I knew she was acquainted with my hometown.

This woman was from Fresno. It was like Bakersfield, only bigger, so she understood my Central California pain. Neither of us had any desire to return west.

One evening while we were studying I asked about her scars. She told me she'd been in a house fire as a girl, which had killed one of her siblings and injured her and her other family members. She and her family, those who survived, had been rescued by firefighters. She said she'd never forget them, the firefighters who pulled her out of the burning wreckage. They were her heroes. She sensed the tragedy had something to do with why she wanted to become an EMT.

I sensed the same was true for me.

I rolled up my sleeve and showed her the knotted vertical scar that graced my upper right arm. I told her I'd had cancer in my twenties. That I was diagnosed in July 1999, a year after I'd moved to New York City and a month after I got sober. There were countless ways to get sober. Hospitalization, inpatient, outpatient, detox, rehab, halfway house, AA. I did one of those. And in doing so, I met a firefighter named Patrick Brown. He heard my story and looked out for me like a big brother.

Pat was a fiery, fast-talking Irish guy in his forties who stood a few inches shorter than me but seemed larger than life. He worked at Ladder 3, on Thirteenth Street, where I used to live. We practiced yoga together before yoga was cool. Pat wasn't your typical firefighter. He was sober, for one, and he loved going to Broadway shows. He meditated, and prayed, and grunted when he contorted himself into yoga postures that brought him pain.

After I got cancer, Pat saw me all bandaged up and assured me I was going to be OK. "I'm not worried about you," he said. "You're going to make it."

And I guessed that because he was sober, and he was a person who spoke no bullshit and told no lies, and I guessed that because he was a firefighter, he must know a thing or two about sickness and death. So I believed him. I borrowed his belief and lived on it when I had none of my own. For years.

Getting sober was one of the hardest, scariest things I ever did, and the people who were in the room those first days and weeks when I staggered into recovery, hopeless and broken and doubtful I would ever get better, will always hold a special place in my heart. Pat was one of those people. He was solid and generous and reassuring. I thought he was a saint. I thought of him as my own personal rescuer. He was there at the critical hour, when I desperately needed help, and every time I saw him my shoulders dropped, and the world was safe. I'd never experienced such kindness before I got sober and met people like Pat. I was confounded by the love I received in early sobriety. I couldn't believe people like him were spending their free time helping me. That they wanted to hear my painful stories and share theirs. And that no story I told was too much for them, too shameful or ugly. No matter what, they stood beside me. Pat was there.

In September 2001 I lived in downtown Manhattan. In Little Italy, a block above Canal Street. My bedroom window looked out on the towers. That Tuesday morning when the planes hit and Pat went missing—

I was shattered.

Over the years I kept him alive by staying close to his old sober crew in New York and by going to his firehouse every year on the anniversary of 9/11. I was especially close with a woman named Ylfa, an Icelandic actress he was in love with before he died. Pat was my hero. And I suspected I was now replacing him by trying to be like him, signing up to become an EMT.

Also, by dating firemen.

* * *

Each class Carrie clicked through endless PowerPoint slides. I had a narcoleptic response to PowerPoint. Most nights, my eyelids fluttered and closed. Nate punctuated our boredom with stories from the street. I lived for these stories. We all did.

"Patient charts," he said one night. "You must document everything you do for the patient. Patient Care Reports are legal documents. If something goes wrong, you go to court. If you gave oxygen to a patient and you failed to write that in your chart, it never happened. It never happened unless you wrote it down. Let me say that again: PCRs are legal documents. They have to be accurate. Whatever happened, you must write it down."

"Tourniquets," he said another night. "Like many practices in the field, this one comes to us from the military. Tourniquets used to be discouraged in EMS, but the military found blown-up soldiers had limbs survive after tourniquets were applied, so now they're back in circulation. Only apply tourniquets to extremities. Do not apply a tourniquet to the head or neck. You'll kill your patient. It's called murder."

"Never be a motivational speaker," I said.

Nate said, "I happen to be a very good motivational speaker."

We memorized the Glasgow Coma Scale, used to assess stroke patients and measure their level of consciousness. The lowest score a person could get was a three out of fifteen: one point for failing to open their eyes, another point for having no verbal response, and a final point for having no motor response.

"Even dead, you're a three," Nate said. "You're never a zero, which is good."

One night Nate gave us a lecture about our scope of practice as EMTs in New York. While laypeople didn't differentiate between first responders, thinking we were all the same, Nate said there were important distinctions between us in terms of medical competence and training, which we had to respect on the street.

There was a hierarchy. Starting at the bottom, the most basic rescuers on the street were Certified First Responders and CFR-Ds. The D stood for defibrillation certificate. CFRs and CFR-Ds did the basics. They were trained to stop bleeding, perform CPR, and use an automated external defibrillator, or AED, the device used on people in cardiac arrest. In the city, cops were trained in Narcan (for opioid overdoses), CPR, trauma (tourniquets), and basic first aid. Firefighters were CFR-Ds.

Next tier of first responder was us, the EMT-B. Emergency Medical Technician—Basic. As EMTs, we had to pass this six-month class, then pass practical and written state exams that tested our knowledge of protocols and skills used in the field.

I blew out a breath. Just hearing about the state exams stressed me out. I could write my way out of a ditch, but I was a horrible test taker. That haunting answer option "all of the above" made me diaphoretic. I'd gotten into grad school not because of but despite my standardized test scores. Plus, I'd studied creative writing, I hadn't been dissecting frogs.

"Murphy," Nate said. "You look worried."

"I'm scared of the state exams."

"You'll be fine."

I was still worried. "Don't you have to be pretty smart to become an EMT?"

"No, that's paramedic. Any moron can become an EMT."

Indeed.

Paramedics, Nate explained, were the highest-trained medical first responders on the street. Like nurses, medics received between eighteen months and two years of training. They could do everything we could do as EMTs, in addition to administering medications and performing invasive procedures. On the street, medics gave people narcotics for pain management. Started IVs. Intubated. Interpreted electrocardiograms, or EKGs.

Nate let it be known that we had to stay within our scope of practice and not perform rescues outside our medical qualification. We had to stay in our lane. What did that mean?

"That means if you're treating someone as an EMT, you can't leave them with a Certified First Responder, meaning a firefighter or a cop, because they're medically beneath you," he said. "Keep in mind a lot of cops and firefighters started off as EMTs and some of them used to be paramedics."

"Like me," Carrie said. "I was an EMT way before I became a cop."

"Like her. But on the street, unless they're on an ambulance, if it's a *medical* emergency—you're in charge. You're going to have police and fire with you if it's a serious job. Cops are going to be directing traffic and doing crowd control. Firefighters are going to be doing what we call the Fireman's

Death Watch, meaning standing around staring at the dying patient waiting for you to show up and tell them they can go home."

Seriously? I couldn't believe what I was hearing. I couldn't wait to get out on the street and start bossing around some firefighters and cops. I'm in charge! Go home! What a dream.

Also, what a waste of resources, it seemed, to organize EMS this way. Firefighters arrived on medical jobs just for us to come on scene and tell them to go home? What was the point? If they had to be on scene, why not just train them as EMTs or paramedics?

Nate said many other major cities did it that way. Firefighters were cross-trained as paramedics in Chicago, Dallas, and Los Angeles, to name a few. The problem in New York City was historical.

Here, I later learned, EMS used to be its own agency. An organization called NYC EMS operated municipal ambulances under the New York City Health and Hospitals Corporation, which dispatched its own trucks and hospital units. But as medical emergencies increased, NYC EMS was unable to handle the 911 call volume. Sometimes people waited up to an hour or longer for an ambulance to arrive. In emergencies, response times mean everything. Speed equals life. If you're having a heart attack or choking on a steak and it takes an ambulance an hour to get to your house, you would almost certainly no longer be gracing the earth with your presence.

Flash forward to 1996, NYC EMS merged with the Fire Department. Where EMS was too busy, the FDNY was too slow. There were fewer and fewer fires, and it needed revenue to avoid closing firehouses. If the Fire Department hadn't taken on EMS, it likely would have bankrupted. Medical emergencies were increasing and generated revenue when a fire engine was sent to a job, and when a patient was transported to the hospital in an FDNY ambulance. The patient's health insurance reimbursed for the trip if it was determined to be medically necessary.

Contrary to public perception, fighting fires has not been the primary job of a New York City firefighter—of any firefighter in the country—for decades. Here, the reduction of arson-for-profit schemes, fireproof building construction, and a decline in cigarette smoking—a common cause of fires—has made fires a dying business. Mayor Bloomberg throughout his tenure proposed closing numerous firehouses for being grossly inefficient in order to balance the city budget. But firefighters are universally beloved, and their unions are powerful. In New York City they were rightly gilded as heroes after their sacrifices on September 11. Closing firehouses sparked political backlash, protests, and emotional outpourings of support from New Yorkers.

Firehouses in New York City were holy ground. To close a firehouse was to close a church and put sainted rescuers out of work. Like the police, firefighters were a protected class. Politicians cowered before their unions. As a rule, first responders operating in these hermetically sealed worlds felt roundly misunderstood by the civilian public, politicians, and the media. Cops were racist devils who stood around all day killing innocent Black people, and firefighters were godlike saints whose primary purpose in life was rescuing civilians from flames. No such thing as a good cop, no such thing as a bad firefighter. That was the binary, the master narrative. In increasingly divided America, to question or pressurize this narrative was to step on a grenade.

So, what did New York City firefighters do all day? This was one of my life's favorite questions. They were busy, just not with fires. In recent years, more than four out of every five jobs firefighters responded to were medical emergencies, around 83 percent of their workload. Fires comprised one out of forty calls, 2.6 percent of their workload.

That being said, when they worked a fire, it was often a bad one. They frequently got injured on the job and got killed in the line of duty performing dangerous rescues. The department trained some of its staff to respond to mass-casualty incidents like active-shooter events, chemical attacks, and terrorism of all stripes. Firefighters also responded to public-safety incidents and non-fire emergencies that didn't involve crime. Stuck elevators. Car accidents. Carbon monoxide detectors chirping. Smoking manholes. Gas leaks. Scaffolding snafus. Forcing doors (and breaking shit). Kitty cats stuck in trees. Cops stuck in trees. And they cooked! Always something simmering in a firehouse kitchen.

This was why my former cop colleagues constantly cracked jokes about firefighters not working as hard as they did.

"Be honest with yourself," one of them said to me. "When was the last time you saw a fire in New York City? Buildings have sprinklers now. All they do is sit around in logoed gym clothes and eat. Lemme tell you something. I have never worn an NYPD article of clothing off duty in my entire life. If they took away a firefighter's department-issued shit they would literally be naked. FDNY shirts, FDNY hats, FDNY underwear, tattoos. Jesus Christ. Get a fucking life. Climb out of your bunk bed and go buy some normal clothes. Slide down your pole."

When I told this to a Bronx-based firefighter I was chatting up online, he swung back. "Yeah, of course he said that, he's a cop. How fat is he? He can't wear any NYPD clothes because everyone hates cops. Why doesn't he go give someone a traffic ticket? Why doesn't he go make some 'collars'? How come they can't stop shooting the wrong people?"

In New York the rivalry between cops and firefighters was real. I cherished it. Many years I enjoyed attending the annual FDNY versus NYPD charity hockey match and watching the gentlemen beat each other up on and off the ice.

Back to our history lecture. Post-merger, FDNY EMS now controlled ambulances through 911, accounting for around 70 percent of units on the street. Voluntary hospital-based ambulances made up the remaining 30 percent of 911-dispatched units. In class Nate said the problem here was that when the two agencies merged in 1996, the functions of EMS and Fire were never truly integrated. The Fire Department treated EMS like its redheaded stepchild.

Come again? This redheaded student asked for clarification about the stepchild situation.

Nate hit us with some numbers. FDNY EMTs started at $35,254 a year, less than any other first responder made, rising to $50,604 after five years—half a firefighter's salary after the same period of service. FDNY EMTs got twelve sick days. Firefighters got unlimited. If an FDNY EMS worker died on the job, their beneficiaries received three years of their pay. Beneficiaries of firefighters with line-of-duty deaths received the fallen rescuer's full salary and health benefits in perpetuity.

Union representatives for the Fire Department's 4,000 EMTs and paramedics argued that gender and racial discrimination kept their wages low, relegating them to the status of third-class citizens on the street. In New York City, EMS was the most diverse uniformed workforce. Roughly 55 percent of FDNY EMS workers were Black, Hispanic, or Asian, and 30 percent were women, whereas firefighting was 78 percent white and 99 percent male.

For years, officials rationalized the enormous pay disparity by categorically devaluing EMS work, claiming it was "different" than other first responder jobs. Different meaning less dangerous than firefighting, police-work, and—drumroll—sanitation. It was hard to imagine, but in New York City saving lives was less valuable than collecting trash.

Nate finished class with a moral fable from the nineties to drive home his point about why it was important for us to stay within our medical scope of practice on the street. "Time for another true story," he said. Then he hit us with this zinger:

Two paramedics arrived on the scene of an emergency in New Jersey. They found a late-stage pregnant woman in cardiac arrest. In other words, she was dead. The paramedics worked up the woman and failed to revive her. She stayed dead. They followed protocols and called the medical director—the doctor available by phone to EMTs and paramedics on scene, responsible for overseeing challenging medical decisions in the field. They told the doctor about the baby trapped in the dead woman. The baby would die within minutes if it didn't receive oxygen. The medical director said the paramedics could attempt to save the unborn child.

They performed an emergency C-section in the field. The baby survived for a week. But later the paramedics lost their licenses since they'd gone beyond their scope of practice. They'd followed protocols by calling the medical director, who'd given them the green light, but state health regulations forbid paramedics from performing surgeries. They got punished because paramedics were paramedics; they weren't surgeons.

"But what do you think?" Nate asked us. "I want all of you to think about that when you go home tonight. Were the paramedics heroes or criminals? What would you have done? Leave the baby to die inside the dead mother? Or open her up to try and save the baby, and lose your license?"

One evening in March we went over mass-casualty incidents. MCIs in medical parlance range from responding to radioactive spills to collapsed buildings, mass shootings to terrorist attacks.

"Remember, terrorist attacks usually have at least two explosions," Nate said. "The first bomb is for civilians, to take as many human lives as possible. The secondary device is to wipe out first responders. That explosion is for you."

Meep.

My two biggest fears as a future EMT were another terrorist attack in New York City and a mass shooting. Those disasters seemed inevitable. Every New Yorker had to live with that fact. It was only a matter of time.

"Cycle of life," Nate said during a lecture on PTSD and first responders. "The old are supposed to die before the young. Mess with the cycle of life and see people die out of order, that's going to stay with you. That's going to stick. If you're an EMT who loses Grandma on the ambulance and you're crying every day for a month, you need to talk to someone, because that's a natural death. Find someone and talk about it. If, however, you see a child die on one of your tours and you *don't* cry every day for a month, also talk to someone, because something is fucking wrong with you. A note about that. EMTs have a high rate of what?"

"Alcoholism," I said. Educated guess.

Nate said, "Very good. What else?"

Cornucopia Ears said, "Divorce, man. My woman stepped out on me last year."

"Maybe it's because of those horns going through your ears. What else?" After a moment he said, "Suicide. EMTs commit suicide at ten times the rate of civilians, got that?"

The room fell silent.

Nate said, "If you notice yourself changing after being on the street, pay attention. If you're a person who always cries reading Hallmark cards, then after a while on the ambulance you find you no longer cry reading Hallmark cards, take note of it. Ask for help."

Ask for help. I took Nate's advice to heart. All these years later, Heather's murder still haunted me. I just couldn't wrap my head around that case. After Nate said that thing about being upset after seeing people die out of order, I understood why the event had stuck with me all these years.

One night at my house, I decided to talk to Raphael about it. He was a detective after all. I felt ashamed and weird about asking him for help. But the detectives who'd worked Heather's case were long gone by now. And also, what would I say if I could speak with them? I wasn't a cop or homicide detective. I wasn't a family member. I had no rights. And as an investigator, trying to obtain criminal records of military personnel was nearly impossible. That was a black box. I'd talked to my sheriff uncle about it, and he had some theories, but they were about the same as mine. I wanted Rafael's opinion, too. I coughed up the story.

"So when I was a girl, my friend and her entire family were murdered. Her father did it. My father had a bad temper, so it turned my world upside down."

Rafael sat up and leaned on his elbows.

"For real?"

"Yeah. Would you do me a favor and read the article about it and tell me what you think?"

"Of course."

I showed him the news story. He read it. VIOLENT END SHATTERS IMAGE OF AN ALL-AMERICAN FAMILY was the headline. Then he lay on his back and flopped his muscular leg over mine.

"Why would a man do that?" I asked him. "Shoot his own children in the head? And why did he stab his oldest daughter to death and not his wife? Stabbing is personal. It's up close. And her wound pattern indicated she'd fought him. The wife's the one I'd think would get stabbed."

Rafael took my hand and squeezed it. "This isn't the kind of thing you're supposed to figure out, love. This is not a murder mystery. It goes into the unknowable pile."

I found it ironic he said "This is not a murder mystery" about an actual murder mystery.

"Do you think it had to do with him being Air Force?"

I felt bad for being stuck on the military detail again.

"No," he said. "I don't think it had anything to do with that. The article said they were separated. His wife left him and took the kids. Then she came back. Killing them all was probably his fucked-up way of keeping his family together."

"Do you think there's something wrong with me because I want to see the dead and work on an ambulance?"

"Not at all. It's a calling. And it's normal to want to see the bodies after someone dies. I think you'll be great."

"You really think I'll be able to do it?"

"Why not? You're not going to see anything on the street that's worse than a murdered family, and you've already survived that. You'll be fine. You're fine now."

"But I didn't actually see the dead family. And I wouldn't say I'm *fine*."

* * *

The last month of EMT school in April included practical skills and handling equipment. There was only so much we could learn from a book and secondhand stories from the street. Knowing how to read the letters and numbers stamped on the collar of an oxygen tank was one thing. Cracking the cylinder with an oxygen wrench, fitting a regulator onto the valve stem so the pinholes lined up, and attaching connective tubing to the flowmeter from a bag valve mask was another. As was securing the combustible green tank so it didn't become a missile en route to the hospital.

By now I was comfortable acing weekly quizzes, hopeful in my ability to pass the upcoming state written exam, much less confident in my capacity to get through the half-dozen skills stations included in the practical.

Four testing stations were mandatory to pass: 1) patient assessment management for trauma; 2) patient assessment management for medical; 3) cardiac arrest management and AED application; and 4) securing a bag valve mask to an apneic patient. The final two skills were random; we went in blind to whatever scenario lurked behind the test partition. It could be upper airway adjuncts and suctioning or long-bone injury immobilization.

All of it terrified me. Over the years I'd become an impractical woman. I often wondered if my book smarts had bled the tank on the more hands-on aspects of life. Adulting required an awful lot of pragmatic action, which I was bad at.

As a crisis manager I could easily guide a tearful room through the ballistic aftermath of a mass shooting. I could travel to France and speak bad French. Later that month, I was heading off to Italy for a writer's conference. But the thought of going to the DMV to update the address on my driver's license short-circuited my brain. I lived in New York City for twenty years before I changed my California driver's license. The handle on my dresser had been broken for seven years, and I had no idea how to fix it. Every morning I looked at it and thought, "Well, that's still broken."

In class we practiced skills on dummies. The mannequins were scummed with fingerprints and stank of sour laundry. Most of them lacked extremities. It was hard not to laugh when instructors threw a plastic torso on the floor and told us to get on our knees and start compressions. Many nights we got reprimanded for doing inappropriate things to the mannequins. I can neither confirm nor deny my involvement in these pranks.

When we did skills drills, we practiced with other EMT classes as one big rowdy group. One girl had a huge scar slashed across her forehead from going through the window of a car when she was in a traffic accident.

We got to know other instructors, too. One of my favorite teachers was a fast-talking paramedic named Eyal. He spoke like a human textbook and took me under his medic wing, making sure I knew what I was doing. Three years later, when COVID-19 hit and New York City became a hot zone, Eyal lost his brother to the virus and worked the pandemic while he was emotionally destroyed.

One spectacular night a skills instructor who worked as an FDNY EMT made the mistake of telling us he had no gag reflex. Now there was a detail you didn't want going public. My eyes flashed with excitement.

Oropharyngeal airways, or OPAs, were devices used on unresponsive patients at risk of developing airway obstructions from their tongues. Protocols required that patients have no gag reflex for an OPA to be inserted. It was nearly impossible to practice jamming the airways into the inelastic mouths of dummies. But now a real-life mannequin stood before me.

"Can I put an OPA in you?" I asked the EMT. He hesitated, then agreed. He sat on a table and opened his mouth. I was ecstatic. The entire class gathered and watched with awe and horror while I asked my patient to open wide and slid the plastic OPA into his mouth, all the way down his throat. Stunningly, he tolerated it. My classmates gasped.

I threw my arms up in victory. "I did it!" I said. "Wow, you're much easier than the dummy."

The EMT choked and pulled the airway out of his throat.

Before taking the state exams we had to complete clinical rotations. Ride on an ambulance or work in an emergency room. I signed up for a tour with a private ambulance company.

Before I did my ride-along I needed to get medical forms signed by my doctor showing I'd been vaccinated against every disease and virus under the sun. Well. Every virus known to mankind prior to 2020.

I went to the doctor. I loved my GP. He was a funny, straight-shooting guy.

"What's this for again?" he asked in the exam room when I handed him my vaccination form. I was crinkling around on the paper-laced table.

"I'm becoming an EMT," I said brightly. "Can you believe it? I have to get this form signed before I can do my first ride-along on an ambulance."

He looked at me with raised eyebrows. "EMT? I thought you were a writer."

"I am a writer. And a private investigator. And crisis manager. I'm also a Plant Lady. Also love to bake."

"You're going to see heads roll. You know that, right?"

"Stop it. But wait—do you really think that's true?"

"As an EMT in New York City? Definitely."

"You're scaring me."

"I couldn't do it," he said, toggling back and forth between the form and his computer.

I was flabbergasted. "What do you mean you couldn't do it? You're a doctor. You went to med school and played with cadavers. I know who you are. I could never do what *you* do."

He grinned. "In med school, they kept body parts in garbage cans. One time our instructor rolled this garbage can into the classroom with a bunch of legs sticking out of it. He told us to get a leg to work on, so I went up to the garbage can and grabbed a leg. Another garbage can was full of arms. We did all sorts of crazy things, playing with the cadavers."

"Exactly. Doctors are sick. That's revolting. But back to me, do you really think I can handle it? Being an EMT? I'm afraid I'm going to see things I can't handle."

"Yeah, you can do it," he said. "You get desensitized."

"How long does that take?"

"It's almost immediate. You'll get to a point where none of it bothers you. I can sit in my office and eat soup while a patient is throwing up in the room right next to me."

After this inspirational story, he handed me the signed medical form.

"Good to see you," he said. "Good luck."

Evening of my first ride-along my doctor's voice haunted me. *You're going to see heads roll.* It was all I could think about on the train to Far Rockaway, where the ambulance base was located. I wasn't ready for this. That's how I felt.

The EMTs I rode with that night were two petite young women who lived in Brooklyn. They hadn't been told they had an observer, and their displeasure at having me in the back of the truck did not go unfelt. Mostly they ignored me, listened to rap, and talked about how this guy friend of theirs deserved to have his tires slashed for cheating on his girl.

Jobless hours passed. I was bored.

At some point my phone chimed. The firefighter I'd been chatting up texted. I liked Rafael, we had a lot in common, but we weren't heading toward love and we were on polar opposite sides of the political spectrum. It was tough for me to envision a future together. Same for him, I felt.

"Talk to me," the firefighter said.

I loved talking! I dove into my phone. His name was Tommy, and I was crazy about him. He was thirty-seven, an Army vet who worked at a busy firehouse in the Bronx. He had chestnut-colored hair ruffled around an open face with eyes that seemed to gaze at me from the deepest part of the forest. He was smart and quick and hilarious, an excellent sexter (sorry, Mom) and texter. He was so good at texting that some nights I stayed up late in bed, rereading things he'd said.

Also, Tommy was hot. Many nights I rowed my thumbs down the streamlet of his photographs. Look at him chauffeuring that rig. Look at him standing with his shoulders square to the camera, his biceps ripped and bulging beneath his dress shirt. There he was in a boat, sunglassed and hatted. Standing on a cliff overlooking the mountains. Now at the gym, lifting significant weight. Damn, I hoped he could cook.

"Not all firefighters can cook!" a firefighter friend scolded me. "That's a myth! I can, I love to cook, but some of the guys at my old house? They made the same stuff over and over. I used to be like, 'Come on, buddies. Mix it up. Try something new! Step out of your comfort zone, why dontcha?'"

Tommy and I had matched on a dating app six or seven months back. It had taken me all of ten seconds to bring up losing a firefighter friend in 9/11. Tommy didn't know Pat personally, but he'd heard of him for sure. "Legit hero," he said.

I'd tried to meet Tommy in person several times, but he always stood me up. Reasons he couldn't see me over the months: sore foot, bad cold, buddy's house burned down, working a double, back pain, outta town, hungover, sick mother.

Hero with a thousand excuses.

Tonight when I asked why he didn't want to meet me in real life he sent me the shrugging-man emoji. I'd put up with these nonresponses for months.

My girlfriends found this insane.

"If this were movie," Felice said one night on the phone, "if this were a rom-com and the couple hadn't met by now? After how many months? The audience would walk out."

But I waited. I could wait longer than anyone I knew. Once, I asked my EMDR therapist to define my core issue in life in one sentence. She nodded then said, "Chronically drawn to the waiting room."

Ouch. That hurt. But the good woman was right.

By now I'd pretty much given up on Tommy making a real-life appearance and settled for a text-based relationship situation. A situationship. It was a bit like having an imaginary friend. Some people talked to Jesus, I talked to a fireman.

Tonight on the ambulance Tommy and I texted for an hour or two. Then finally, at last, an hour before our tour ended, we got sent on a job.

Dispatch wanted us to transport an elderly man from his house to a dialysis center. We drove to the patient's home without lights or sirens since he wasn't having a medical emergency, he just needed a ride in an ambulance since he couldn't walk. We might as well have been in a U-Haul.

When we pulled up to the house some guy standing outside on a shaggy lawn, who I guessed was the patient's son, made some crack about how all of us EMTs were women. Astute observation, but he probably wouldn't win a Genius Grant. Then he said something about how he doubted we "girls" were strong enough to carry the patient.

"We can do it, sir," one of my partners said politely.

I gathered she'd received this note before.

Inside, a bed was shoved against a wall of a dark musty living room. A tiny elderly man lay curled in the sheets, his body contracted like a bleached snail, his skin so thin it looked like it would tear if a feather brushed against it. He couldn't have weighed more than eighty pounds. His sheets wreaked of warm death. It shocked and saddened me to look at him. Just being near him took something out of me.

"Do you want to grab his blood pressure?" one of the EMTs asked me.

No, merci. I stepped back. I was afraid to hurt him with my giant man hands.

One of my partners took vitals while the other one secured a nasal cannula to the man's face, then gave him a bit of oxygen. Easily the women moved him onto a stair chair, burritoed him in a sheet, strapped him in, and wheeled him outside. In the street they transferred him out of the chair, onto the stretcher, and into the ambulance while I watched. I was a watcher.

We drove slowly toward the dialysis center. That, too, was a crushing blow.

The dialysis room was a cold, fluorescent hell realm, an open floor walled with sea-green recliners stuffed with amputated patients in late-stage renal failure. Most of the patients were blanketed, since dialysis patients got cold.

The nurses looked miserable. They seemed annoyed we'd brought in a patient. "Weigh him then stick him in that chair in the corner," one of them said, as if we were delivering a lamp.

After that job I was impressed by my partners. They warmed up to me as the night went on, once they discovered my winning personality. I liked that they were tough and smart and pretty, the kind of women who talked shit about slashing some guy's tires when they were alone on the truck, then went inside a dying man's home and kindly helped him.

They gave me high marks on my observer sheet, despite the fact that I hadn't done anything all night. That was my clinical rotation. My patient care experience. Pretty heroic stuff.

"How was it?" Nate asked me the next class.

"We did one job. I was bored and scared and incompetent."

"Welcome to EMS."

A month later, in May, I took the state EMT exams and passed. We all passed, except one of the dark-haired sisters who failed by a few points. She sobbed. We patted her back and told her she'd pass next time. I believe she did. Now I was officially an EMT.

I knew almost nothing.

Carrie and Nate and Eyal took us out for pizza afterward.

"Congratulations, Murphy," Nate said, hugging me.

After dinner Nate stood up and gave a toast. "I'm proud of each and every one of you," he said. "You're going to deliver babies and see people take their last breath, and you're going to have a front-row seat to the greatest show on earth. EMS is a thankless, dangerous, rewarding job, and all of you are heroes now. You can call me any time. I'll always have your back. Welcome to the family."

As soon as it said it—*family*—I fought back tears.

Many of my classmates never went on to become EMTs for a variety of reasons. No time. Waning interest. Fear. Their first responder careers started and stopped in the classroom. To Nate's surprise, I was one of the first and only students from his class to put on a uniform and work as an EMT.

Tell me I'm part of a family, I'm in. All those months of school I'd been so happy. I always knew I would work on an ambulance. The only question was: Where?

3

DRIVING GRANDMA

Finding a place to ride as a new EMT in New York City felt daunting. I didn't know where to start aside from researching my options and talking to veteran first responders.

Here's what I learned:

Like the heart, New York City EMS had four separate yet interconnected chambers: volunteer ambulance companies, commercial ambulances run by private businesses, voluntary hospital-based units, and municipal ambulances operated by the Fire Department. I wanted to work serious emergencies, which, ideally, meant riding with an agency on the 911 system. Two of these four EMS agencies were on the 911 system: hospital-based ambulances (and a few commercial companies working in partnership with hospitals) and FDNY.

Trouble was, hospital companies required EMTs have 911 experience before being hired even part-time or per diem. Therein arose my dilemma: How was I supposed to get 911 experience as a new EMT when 911 companies only hired seasoned technicians?

Nate told me the Fire Department hired people straight out of EMT school. "They'll hire anyone with a pulse," he said.

Some aching, reverential part of me that missed Pat longed to join the department in his honor. He would love it, I thought. He would love it if I wound up in riding on an FDNY truck. He would think it was funny. Pat's friend Robert "Bobby" Burke, the actor known for his role as Tucker on *Law & Order: Special Victims Unit*, told me that Pat thought it was great when the Fire Department started sending fire engines on EMS jobs. "We can help more people," Pat said. To him, that was the whole point. Helping people.

But joining FDNY was a serious commitment. They only hired full-time EMTs. And the salary was pitiful. I couldn't live on $35,000 a year. Not at this age. And sure as hell not in this city.

Outside the 911 system, private companies and volunteer ambulance companies also hired new EMTs. Privates got paid and vollies worked for free. Both types of agencies bolstered citywide EMS when disasters struck and 911 call volumes spiked, as happened during heatwaves, hurricanes, coronavirus.

"Don't work for free," Carrie said when I told her I was thinking of volunteering. "If you're going to do this, get paid."

Since EMTs were some of the lowest wage-earning civil servants in the nation, the phrase "get paid" didn't hold much weight with me. I looked into volunteering somewhere.

Narrowing my new first-responder home search down to vollie squads didn't simplify matters. Around twenty-six active volunteer ambulance companies operated in New York City. Many vollie squads dated back to the 1970s and were formed out of communities' need to improve slow emergency response times.

In Brooklyn, Bay Ridge Ambulance Volunteer Organization responded to its first call in 1974, when city ambulance response times in the area were often over an hour. In Manhattan, Central Park Medical Unit established itself in 1975, when injured parkgoers frequently waited between forty-five to ninety minutes for a city unit to arrive. Due to its unique geography, rescuers who weren't familiar with the park's terrain often got lost. Community members in the area decided Central Park warranted its own rescue squad. They started off with twenty volunteers who used personal bicycles and a retrofitted Ford van.

Historically underserved communities were no strangers to the perils of slow emergency response times. A volunteer ambulance crew in Bed-Stuy was born of this pain. In 1988, it took an ambulance over thirty minutes to get to Bed-Stuy after a seven-year-old Black girl was hit by a car. The child's uncle, the late James "Rocky" Robinson Jr., was an EMT who worked for New York City EMS at the time.

Rocky climbed on the ambulance with his critically injured niece, who died en route to the hospital. The tragedy inspired him to form a volunteer corps in Bed-Stuy with a twofold mission. One, get ambulance response times down to a few minutes in the neighborhood. And two, train at-risk youth to become EMTs in an effort to get them off gun- and gang-ridden streets, with the operational belief that it was better to save a life than take a life.

Since I lived relatively close to the Bed-Stuy Vollies, it made sense that I would try to ride with them. I filled out the necessary paperwork and visited their base a few times, but nothing ever came of my application. It stalled for reasons unknown to me, which was probably a good thing. It was a Black-led, Black-community-based organization that met the mostly Black neighborhood's needs. While I knew one white guy who rode as an EMT with the Bed-Stuy Vollies, I didn't want to fall into that white-savior trap of installing myself as some well-meaning white lady in a Black organization that was doing just fine without me. Or worse, take up space that could have gone to one of the organization's at-risk youth.

People had great things to say about Park Slope Volunteer Ambulance Corps. I looked them up. They seemed legit. And not terribly far from my house. I filled out an application and got a reply saying the next step was an in-person interview. If I passed, I had to wait for orientation to begin. When was that? Winter, they hoped. December or January. That was too long to wait. It was summer. I surrendered to riding at a private company like the one I'd done my ride-along with in EMT school.

In June 2017 a private company with a base in Coney Island hired me. They paid EMTs minimum wage, which at the time was $13.50. Base was far from my house, a commute that took over an hour and a half one way. I knew from my observation tour that private-transport jobs were dullsville. Some first responders said riding with "the privates," as these companies were called, was not really EMS, since the bulk of calls were transports and nonemergencies. "Driving Grandma," they called it. But I didn't have a lot of other choices as a newbie. Nevertheless, when I finally geared up, I knew my grandma would be proud.

I loved my grandma. Fern Alberta Duggan was an ornery, stout, mouthy woman who made crazy quilts, demolished boxes of See's candy, read westerns, and adored going out to lunch, preferably for enchiladas. She taught me how to sew and make piecrust from scratch, and she drove her plum-colored Cadillac while sitting atop the fat yellow pages of a phone book so she could see over the steering wheel.

My grandma's love for me was perfect and absolute. They say that's all it takes in a child's life for them to survive—one person who loves them unconditionally. My grandmother was that person. She also taught me to believe in ghosts one day in 2003.

Two years before that, in August 2001, just before 9/11, I'd been laid off from my job writing for a dot-com in New York. I was more than fine with it, because I planned to go back to school and get an MFA in fiction writing at Brooklyn College. The novelist Michael Cunningham was teaching there at the time, and one day he called and told me I'd been accepted into the creative writing program. I remember exactly where I was standing when he rang, in my apartment in Little Italy, with vined plants hanging above a bathtub in the kitchen. And I remember thinking, I'm on the phone with Michael Cunningham right now. Michael Cunningham called me.

But then terrorism struck. The towers collapsed, Pat went missing, the economy crashed, I couldn't find work, I had no health insurance and cancer, I went into debt, and eventually lost my apartment. One of my doctors at Memorial Sloan-Kettering felt sorry for me and got me into a research study for free. For years I couldn't find adequate work, not enough to cover my expenses. Then two years later, in 2003, I gave up on New York and took a yearlong contract job as a writer for a dot-com in California.

I was bitter about my exodus from New York at the time, as I didn't want to leave the city and I hated dot-com life. But since the job was in California, it gave me an opportunity to spend time with my grandma for a year.

Weekends I drove from Laguna Beach to Bakersfield to visit her in the nursing home where she lived. My grandfather had died years before. He was a quiet, gentle man who worked for the Southern Pacific railroad, played harmonica, and washed his hair with bar soap long after the advent of shampoo. They'd been married for sixty-five years, so I figured my grandma must have longed for him something awful.

"Do you miss him?" I asked her one day in the nursing home.

"Not really," she said.

I was stunned. "You don't miss Grandpa?"

"No," she said, smiling. "I don't have to miss him, because he visits me every night."

"What do you do?"

"Oh, he just sits on my bed, and we talk."

The way she said it, the confidence in her voice, made me believe her. She was as sure of his nightly presence as she was of the crazy quilts she sewed.

For her, he was alive.

My first weekend tours working transport were a blur. It was so much to take in, this medical world and its incredible weirdos, present company included. I didn't know how to do anything practical. Reattach the metal feet to a wheelchair. Raise and lower a hospital bed. Use a Toughbook, the indestructible magnesium-alloy-cased laptop used to fill out Patient Care Reports, PCRs. Charts, as they were sometimes called. It was all new to me.

And then there was lifting. Since all of our patients were nonambulatory, we lifted like hell every tour. As EMTs we had to be able to lift 250 pounds between two partners, so a buck twenty-five each.

At training, when I'd tried to lift a stretcher weighted with sandbags in that amount, something humiliating had happened. I couldn't hold the weight in my hands, my forearms felt like they were about to burst, and the stretcher dropped and took me down with it. Boom! In one bedeviling swoop I fell to the ground like a spatchcocked chicken.

I worked out enough, I thought. Three or four times a week I hit the gym in my building and did a high-intensity interval training regime called BBG, short for Bikini Body Guides.

My Navy SEAL friend said, "I do Bikini Body. That program is hard, Jenger." Everyone called me Jennifer or Ginger, so he combined them. "Burpees, commandos, squats. That's some Navy SEAL shit."

He would know. But BBG was nothing compared to lifting the dead weight of paralyzed patients.

My first two partners were men. Ji was a warm, funny guy with a dark sense of humor and two kids and a wife at home, from whom he hid the fact that he smoked cigarettes, the trickster. Patients adored him. I adored him.

Our other partner, Ron, was Ji's opposite in many ways. A dark-haired manchild, he swore a lot and was fearless as an EMT, but irrationally terrified of girls. He teased Ji incessantly about everything under the Brooklyn sun and jovially made fun of patients, who ripped him apart right back. Ron was barely over the legal drinking age, but he'd worked in EMS since he was a teenager, which gave him the sad, crushed aura of a man approaching retirement.

I loved these guys. They taught me everything I knew. Which, admittedly, was not a lot.

For a while we rode three EMTs on a truck, rather than the usual two, since as a newbie I was fearful and experientially impaired. We laughed constantly and once got dinner at Target. I knew Target had everything before I became an EMT, but never in my life had I gotten a takeout meal from one.

Ji and Ron had nerves of steel and saintlike patience with me. They never made me feel stupid or called me out if I floundered. They were always with me. They had my back, literally. Feeling their flattened palms pressed against my spine to guide and support me when I rolled a stretchered patient backward down a ramp made me feel safe and reassured.

In EMS I was never alone.

Many of our transport patients were regulars. Over the months, I got to know them almost as intimately as my partners. We transported the same handful of people in late-stage kidney failure to and from their twice- or thrice-weekly dialysis appointments.

A notable majority of our chronically sick patients were brown or Black. Many were paralyzed or amputees as consequences to renal failure, which caused peripheral artery disease. I never got used to taking patients to dialysis centers. A whip of despair lashed my face every time I brought them inside. Hemodialysis treatment usually lasted around four hours, so sometimes we'd see the same patients twice in one tour.

One of them, Garrison, was a rascally Black Vietnam veteran and bilateral below-the-knee amputee with a feisty demeanor. I can't remember if he had insurance. A disproportionate number of Black veterans from various wars were discharged with bad papers, which made it impossible for them to get healthcare from the VA. Bad papers were oftentimes for minor "offenses." Lateness. Alcohol issues. Supposed insubordination.

The problem was rampant.

Black airmen were 71 percent more likely to face court-martial or non-judicial punishment than white airmen in an average year, according to one research study conducted between 2006 and 2015. In the Army, they were 61 percent more likely. Navy, 40 percent. And Black Marines were 32 percent more likely than white servicemen to get slapped with bad papers. Unlike "bad conduct" and "dishonorable" discharges, which went through legal justice reviews, bad papers were thrown at people privately, with no equivalent due process.

The federal government roundly abandoned and punished bad-paper vets who came home with life-threatening emotional, spiritual, and physical wounds from war, as the VA denied them access to much-needed benefits and healthcare services. Bad papers also made it harder for them to find work. The same thing happened with women servicemembers who were reprimanded with bad papers for reporting sexual assaults. Gay servicemembers, too.

I felt—still feel—the way we treat servicepeople in this country is a monstrous disgrace.

Garrison spoke mainly in curse words and had a fatherly, combative relationship with Ron. The two of them teased each other mercilessly, which Ji and I enjoyed. It was like watching macho-man tennis.

"Just throw me, dumbass!" Garrison yelled at Ron one night when we were in his bedroom, moving him from the stair chair onto his bed. "Just lift me up and throw me on the bed, I can do the rest. Just throw me, motherfucker!"

We surrounded Garrison's chair and lifted him up, then tossed him gently onto his bed. He got himself situated and, once he was settled, lit a cigarette.

"You get her phone number yet?" he asked Ron.

Ron had a massive crush on a nurse who worked at one of the hospitals we frequented, but he was too scared to ask for her phone number. "Not yet."

"He won't do it," Ji said. "He's too scared."

Garrison scoffed. "You're a pussy, man. Don't be a pussy. Locate your balls and ask the woman for her number. What's wrong with you?"

Ron shook his head and said to the floor, "I know, I know."

"No, you don't know!" Garrison snapped. "Next time you come here you better tell me you got her phone number. Don't come to my house and pick me up until you got it."

"I'll do it," Ron said. But it took another three months for that to be true.

Ji predicted that down the line Garrison would lose his arms in addition to his legs. He was right. "Garrison just has his torso now," he told me some years later.

Another weekend tour Ron told me and Ji he'd finally asked the nurse for her number. "She said she has a boyfriend. But she gave me her number and said we could chat."

"I'm so proud of you!" I said. "Congratulations! This is a victory for all of mankind."

Ji couldn't resist teasing him. "She probably lied," he said of the nurse's boyfriend. "She probably made that up."

"Stop it," I said, slugging him.

I told them about Tommy. How we texted all the time but he never showed up to meet me in real life.

"How long has this been going on?" Ji asked.

I squinted. "Eight or nine months?"

"Eight or nine *months*?" Ron said. "What the fuck, man. Who is this guy?"

"Delete his number and block him," Ji said. "The end."

"Agree," Ron said. "You deserve better. Fuck this dude."

It was good brotherly advice. I ignored it.

Until, one day, I couldn't.

That summer I bottomed out on Tommy not manifesting in real life. I knew he was busy. He worked a lot. He played hockey. Many times when he texted, he sent photographs of himself in dress blues on his way to a service funeral for yet another 9/11 firefighter who'd died of cancer.

"They're dropping like flies," Tommy said.

So he had his hands full with life—and death. But still. The guys were right; fuck this dude. First, however, I had to solve the mystery of Tommy's absence. I was a detective, after all. Tiger couldn't change its stripes. Neither could the Lioness.

One day I decided to ask Tommy about it directly.

"Just give it to me straight. Is the reason you're refusing to show up because you're married? I know you're a firefighter, so that would come as no surprise."

"No, I'm not married."

"Then what? Enough with the lies. Speak the truth."

Tommy confessed he had a girlfriend. They'd been together unhappily for many years. They'd been broken up when we matched online. But now they were trying and failing to work things out. He didn't know what to do. But the on-again, off-again girlfriend wasn't his solitary excuse for his absence. The underlying reason was misery.

Tommy was desperately unhappy. He felt stuck. The brain-drain atmosphere of the FDNY blighted his spirit.

"The other day I walked into the firehouse kitchen and said, 'Hey guys, read any good books lately?' And they were like, 'You're gay.'"

Tommy missed the structure and rigorous training of the military. He felt that comparatively, the Fire Department didn't measure up. "We're not ready," he said about the inevitable coming of another terrorist attack or mass-casualty incident in New York City.

Wait until we get to 2020 and see how right he was.

The job blunted Tommy's creativity. He used to write when he was at war—one year he kept a journal where he drew only skulls—and he wanted to start writing again, but he couldn't get himself to do it. He felt like he was living in a hole, and the hole was filling with water, too much for him to climb out of but not enough to drown.

Oh, boy. When he told me this my romantic dreams collapsed like a cooling cake and the crisis manager inside me flew out of my mouth and said, "That's no way to live. You're living in what other people would consider code red."

"Do you really think that? Do you think I'm that bad off? That makes me a little scared for myself."

"I think it's time to get help, petal."

Tommy agreed. But he didn't know where to begin. He'd never gone to therapy and worried about the cost. About his coworkers finding out. Firehouses were gossip mills. He didn't want all the guys to know his business.

"Are you a post-9/11 vet?"

"Pre and post."

"Double winner. Congratulations, today's your lucky day."

I sent Tommy a link to an organization called Headstrong. I knew about the nonprofit from military pals. Headstrong gave free, no paperwork required, confidential mental health services to post-9/11 military vets and their families, and they offered therapies like EMDR. I told Tommy I did EMDR, and that it was changing and rewiring my nervous system, essentially saving my ass. I suspected he would benefit from it, too.

He thanked me and said he'd look into it. I encouraged him to call right away. He said he would. But I had doubts.

In my experience, people who desperately needed help often dragged their feet asking for it, myself included. I could tolerate ungodly amounts of despair before I raised my hand and said, Help me. By the time I did that, I was in catastrophic pain. If there was one thing I learned as a crisis manager, it was this:

When people tell you they're in pain, believe them.

As for Tommy, tough guys who worked in civil service where therapy remained stigmatized, and where denying and compartmentalizing your misery and cheating on your wife while silently drinking yourself to death was championed as the correct way to be a man, asking for help was a stunning act of courage.

My college boyfriend once told me that when his parents sent him to rehab, his counselor made him wear a sign around his neck that said I'M DYING BECAUSE I REFUSE TO ASK FOR HELP.

I thought of that phrase often. I thought of military veterans like Tommy who were dying at chilling rates—up to twenty-two of them committing suicide each day, one every sixty-five minutes. I thought you could sew those words on the uniforms of most first responders and it would apply.

After our conversation I sent a prayer up to Pat, hoping that maybe some afterlife magic would get in there and nudge Tommy's boots-on-the-ground action.

It worked. Tommy texted a few days later and said he contacted Headstrong and got an intake appointment. I was shocked and proud and so relieved I hung my head and wept.

I couldn't believe it. This was some Irish ghost shit.

My favorite dialysis patient was a middle-aged churchgoing woman named Rita. She was medically obese and paralyzed from the waist down. She lived with her husband, two young kids, and a tabby cat in a cramped apartment on the second floor of a walk-up in Crown Heights.

We often saw cockroaches in Rita's building, which, in New York City, was nothing new. I ran into a lot of amazing bugs on the job. Cockroaches and houseflies and lice that looked like traveling sesame seeds.

I preferred my insects taxidermied, but they didn't bother me all that much. Some EMTs tucked their pants into their boots to keep pests from dashing up their legs or making babies in their socks. Also because it looked cool. If my uniform pants were long enough, that's how I would have worn them. A woman could dream.

Rita had just about every health problem available to womankind, and we took her to dialysis appointments to get her kidneys flushed twice a week. We often arrived at her house over an hour before her scheduled appointment because it took us so long to get her downstairs. Most days, we needed a second unit with four additional pairs of hands to help us lift. Bikini Body was helpful, but EMS got me stronger faster than any gym routine.

Sometimes when we arrived, Rita was on the toilet doing her business, unable to get up without our assistance. "Ji!" she'd shout when we walked inside, "Get in here and help me!" She always wanted Ji to help and not me or Ron. As I said, patients loved the guy.

I often wondered what Rita did on the days we didn't come to her house. Her husband was much smaller than she was and usually around, standing in the kitchen stirring a pot of something that smelled of curry with a slotted spoon, their kids running around the living room and the cat swatting our bootlaces. We helped Rita into her wheelchair then rolled her to the apartment door, where the real work started.

The stairs were steep and wooden. A stair lift that barely held Rita's weight was fitted along the wall. But first we had to get her out of the wheelchair and onto that lift, which took four EMTs and several sets of sheets we wrapped around her waist to steady her once we got her to her feet. The dead weight of paralyzed patients astonished me. Rita and the rest of us sweated crazily while we worked. Ji often took off his uniform shirt and wore only a T-shirt, which he drenched.

Once, a woman EMT from another unit came to give us a hand at Rita's house. She was muscular, had long dark hair flowing down her back, and wore tactical pants that fit her perfectly.

She flew off the bus with a set of sheets and straps, stormed past us, and immediately took charge of the scene. She greeted Rita and her family then got her out of the wheelchair and onto the stair lift faster than anyone I'd ever worked with. She was beautiful and capable and aggressive, and I wanted to be like her. It was powerful to see a woman show up and dominate.

I remembered how, in high school, my coach made me watch videos of professional volleyball players and study how those players excelled. He had me visualize being in the game, playing at their level. Then one day he brought two volleyball players to the gym. They were fiercely athletic girls. He asked us to sit down and watch them.

For twenty minutes he had the setter send them balls, and they stood in a hitting line and hammered the balls straight to the floor every time they swung. I'd never seen girls hit the ball so hard or fast, crushing it in front of the three-foot line.

Watching them, I understood in a new way what I needed to play like, how hard I needed to exert myself to get to their level. It was critical for me as a female athlete, and EMT, to see other women do things I couldn't yet do. Women who were more advanced than I was, so I could visualize myself in their position.

Most days at Rita's house, Ji and Ron and I took long breaks in the stairwell as we moved her along the back wall to the corner, where the automated stair lift did its magic and eased her down toward the exterior door, at which point we had to reassemble, unbuckle the chair belt, and lift her onto the stretcher.

Many spiritual conversations were had in that stairwell, which I enjoyed. We talked about God, family, illness, Brooklyn. After some months Rita came to know me and called me by name. One night in the stairwell when we took a breather, Ji asked Rita how she thought I was coming along as an EMT.

"Jennifer?" she said, speaking as if I weren't there. "Oh, I think she's doing good." Then she looked mournfully at her unmoving legs and back up at me. "But she sure picked a hard job. I don't know why she'd want to be here doing this kind of work. This isn't very pleasant. She could be doing something much easier."

"You're comparing my outsides to your insides," I said. "You don't know anything about my life, or why I do this."

"Mmm," Rita said. "That's true. That's deep." She looked at Ji and said, "She's deep."

"She is deep," Ji said.

"It's true I could be doing something easier, but I'm not a stranger to health problems. I've had my share. I had cancer when I was younger."

"You had cancer?" Ji said.

Then Ron. "Wait, what? You had cancer?"

"And I know it's hard work, but like being here with you," I told Rita. "It makes me happy."

"That's what matters. Doing something that makes you happy, right?"

"Right," Ji said.

Like Garrison, Rita's health eventually deteriorated. Years later, Ji told me she'd died. He didn't know how. None of us did. That was one of the trickier aspects of being an EMT. We didn't always get to hear the story of what happened to our patients. We met them, we helped, then we let go. Short-term care.

The news of Rita's death crushed me, even though I knew all of our transport patients were at the end of the yellow-brick road. Still. I'd gotten close to Rita. I loved her in some way. I still think of her sometimes, and our conversations in that stairwell.

I saw my first dead body working transport. Early one August morning in Coney Island, when I was riding with a woman EMT whose name evades me, we stopped at a deli to grab coffee and egg-and-cheese sandwiches at the start of our tour. We were waiting for our food when a frantic man dashed into the deli pulling his hair. He told the man behind the counter to call 911.

"I need help! Call 911! My buddy—oh, God. He's not moving! I don't know what to do!"

My partner and I looked at each other. We were in uniform. Our uniforms said EMT. We seemed to be the right people to help this guy out.

My partner went up to the man. "Sir, where's your friend?"

"He's out there!" the guy said, pointing outside. "Can you help him? He's in my van."

We trotted outside. I tried not to spill my coffee. For some reason it was still in my hand. My pulse raced and my breath thinned.

The man led us across the street, through a chain-link fence, into a parking lot where a solitary van was parked. I set my coffee on the ground and hid behind my partner as she approached the vehicle. She looked in the van then opened the passenger door and reached across to touch the body in the driver's seat. I looked over her head and glanced at a man who broke the tape in the marathon of death.

He presented with obvious signs of death as defined by EMT protocols. These included patients exhibiting decomposition, rigor mortis, dependent lividity, and my personal favorite, the rather philosophical, "injury not compatible with life," i.e., decapitation, patients burned beyond recognition, massive open or penetrating trauma to the head or chest with obvious signs of organ destruction. When we saw these things—nothing we could do.

"Can you help him? He's my buddy," the man said, pacing in circles.

My partner turned to the bereaved. "I'm sorry, sir. He's gone."

"Oh, God!" the man cried.

I glued my eyeballs to the dead gentleman in the driver's seat displaying rigor mortis, his body so still there was no way to mistake him for the living, no way at all. He was grayer than one of the sculptures gracing Tuileries Garden in Paris. His head was tipped back and his mouth frozen open. He had an expression of ecstasy on his face. He was shirted but naked from the waist down, his pants unbuckled and puddled around his thighs, where his penis had found its final resting place. His testicles were swollen. One was the size of a grapefruit.

The sirening sound of a fire engine filled the air. Heroes were here.

"This is my van," the man said. "I don't know what the fuck happened to him. He's homeless. I let him sleep in my van sometimes. I just talked to him yesterday. He was fine."

Well, he sure wasn't fine now. It seemed clear he'd been self-pleasuring at the moment his number was called, but that was just a guess. An educated guess. From a private investigator. And EMT.

"Did your friend have any medical problems?" my partner asked him.

The man said, "He kept saying his stomach hurt. He had pain in his stomach. I told him to go to the hospital, but he didn't have insurance. Isn't there anything you can do?"

"I'm afraid not sir," my partner said. She told him to wait for the cops. That they would be there soon. By law, cops had to stay with the body until the medical examiner arrived. It usually took the ME two or three hours to get on scene, so cops spent a lot of quality time with the dead.

The fire rig parked. A handful of tired-looking firefighters spilled into the parking lot and slogged toward the van. Soon they would be having a dead-on-arrival for breakfast as well.

An FDNY lieutenant came up to us while his men fell back. We shook our heads and tastefully made a slicing gesture across our necks, the universal sign for dead, finito, kaput. The lieutenant nodded. Then he peeked inside the van, turned around, and made the same neck-slicing gesture to his men. All of us loped out of the parking lot together. I picked up my coffee on the way out.

We went back to the deli, grabbed our cold egg-and-cheese sandwiches, and ate them on the ambulance. I was famished. Famished and pleasantly surprised by my ability to eat so soon after seeing my first DOA. I guessed my doctor was right.

You get desensitized.

After a few months of working transport I grew tired of being trained to work serious emergencies and responding to none. The gold standard for any first responder was performing a rescue that saved a human life. Ji and Ron had a few victorious rescues during their time at the private company. But I'd experienced no such saves. So far, I'd applied one non-rebreather mask to a single patient who had difficulty breathing. That was my "emergency."

I'd used none of the practical skills I'd trained for in EMT school. I was forgetting all the cool medical stuff I'd learned. What was the normal pulse range for pediatric patients again? How did you calculate the Rule of Nines to measure the percentage of body surface area burned for burn victims? Where were you supposed to cut the umbilical cord during an emergency childbirth in the field? Use it or lose it, and I was losing it.

Slow nights my tours felt longer than a war in Afghanistan. My back hurt from being squashed in the ambulance. I got dehydrated because if I drank water I had to pee, and I didn't love using filthy EMS-only bathrooms in hospitals or senior facilities, with toilet seats splashed with urine. I got headaches from being dehydrated. The trains never ran on time weekend nights, so I didn't get home until two or three o'clock in the morning. My paychecks were a joke.

One night I walked down my block in uniform while some of my neighbors were sitting outside, listening to music, hanging out. They saw me and screamed and clapped. "Woo-hoo! EMT in the house! Yes, girl! EMTs are badass!"

I waved and felt like a massive fraud. *You don't understand*, I wanted to say. *I'm not a real first responder. I'm with Grandma.*

Every year on the anniversary of September 11, firehouses in New York City opened to the public. They observed the six moments of silence and had a little Mass. That year, firefighters were hopping off the rig parked outside Pat's firehouse when I rounded the corner around eight o'clock that fateful morning. My eyes followed the weary steps of the dismounting men.

Faced with the presence of that bright, hopeful fire truck gleaming in the sun, I half expected to see Pat. There was always something in the air on this day that made me feel he was present. I remembered the torrents of wind that swept through the annihilated streets in the days and weeks following the attacks. Even the newscasters said it:

Ghosts.

Inside, firemen stood in dress-blued clusters around a little makeshift church. An arc of wooden chairs faced an altar where a candle burned in a bell jar. I stepped inside and immediately my eyes went to the ceiling, where Pat's smiling face hung on a banner draped beside the faces of his fallen brothers. Pat's house, Ladder 3, colloquially referred to as 3 Truck, had been one of the hardest hit on September 11. They lost eleven members and one chief, leaving eight widows and eighteen children without fathers.

From the back I saw sunlight catch the luminous, long, blonde hair of Ylfa, Pat's last love. She came up and hugged me, and I glued myself to her side. Firehouses were intimidating. The racks of turnout gear and stepped-out-of boots. The truck. The energy was so dense and electric I always felt like I was inhaling a rich, musky homebrew of vintage masculinity.

Ylfa was a refuge. I thought of her as someone from a different time. Born in Iceland and named in honor of her uncle Wolfgang, her grandparents fled Nazi Germany in 1938 and ended up in Iceland because her grandfather was a cellist, and he received a position with the then first Icelandic symphony orchestra. Ylfa played more instruments than I could count, and animals were drawn to her. When I thought of her, I thought of music. Mandolin. Violin. Flute. Every time we went for a walk in Central

Park, birds and turtles and squirrels and you name it approached her. She was a faery for sure. Her name meant female wolf, and rare was the person who pronounced it correctly: Ilva.

We wandered outside and stood on the sidewalk.

Then something extraordinary happened.

I looked up the block and saw Pat walking down the street. My skin goosebumped and the hair on my arms stood at attention. It was his brother Mike, who looked eerily like him. Same face, same disheveled mess of brown hair, same warm, smiling eyes. He was mustached, wearing a backpack that made him look like a little kid heading off to school. I couldn't believe what I was seeing. He hadn't been at the firehouse the year before, the first year I went, since I was living in California or Paris the years before.

"He looks just like Pat, right?" Ylfa said.

"I thought it *was* Pat."

"I know, it's crazy. Same DNA. They're Irish twins."

Ylfa introduced us. Mike was a firefighter turned ER doctor based in Las Vegas. He shook my hand and Ylfa told him I was a writer.

"Hey I write, too," he said. "I write terrible books no one reads. I'll give you one."

He opened his backpack and pulled out a book he'd written about Pat called *What Brothers Do.* Then he signed a copy for me.

Soon, everyone gathered on the sidewalk for the moments of silence. The weather was sickening, fair and bright. To this day I deplore clear-blue autumn skies. The firefighters lined up in formation. An officer stood in front of the parked rig and sounded out the times and events that ended so many lives. Bystanders paused. Cars slowed. I stood next to Ylfa and bowed my head. Tears splashed onto my skirt.

Between one of the moments, Mike came to me and put his arm around my shoulders. "Why are you sad?" he asked me.

I was taken aback by the question. Was there another way to feel on this day? Mike wasn't crying at all. He smelled faintly of beer and said he was still a little drunk from the night before. I remembered that feeling well from my drinking days. God bless, I thought. If drinking still worked for me, I'd also smell of beer on this painful day. I went home later that afternoon and slept. It seemed the hardest part of the year was behind me.

Or so I thought.

* * *

In October a mass shooter opened fire on a crowd at a music festival in Las Vegas, killing 60 people and wounding 412 in what swiftly became the deadliest mass shooting in modern US history.

I awoke the next morning to a flurry of e-mails from colleagues alerting me that my name had gone out to work the crisis. That happened almost every mass shooting nowadays, my name went out as part of a crisis team. Sad, but that was the math. Sad math.

As my name went out Mike Brown's name came into my mind. An arrow went through me. Right away I called Ylfa.

"Mike's alive," she said. *Oh thank God.* She said he was OK, but that one of his cousins had been shot at the concert along with one of his cousin's friends, a firefighter. The firefighter had been shot in the chest while doing CPR on a shooting victim.

America.

When Ylfa and I hung up I put my forehead on my desk and closed my eyes. I stayed like this for a long time.

Next day, a news story broke with Mike's name in it. The article detailed his cousin's injury was not life-threatening. Her sister had called Mike, who'd told her to call 911. Then he drove to the perimeter of the music festival and picked up three of his cousin's friends, including the firefighter who'd been shot in the chest. Mike helped the guy out.

I texted him later that day. "So relieved you're safe and that your family and friends are OK. Sending you so much love from New York. Nothing can ever happen to you. Good job with your cousin and the firefighter who got shot. You're a hero."

"I was blessed to be there and be able to help," Mike said.

Just then Tommy texted. "I just heard Pat Brown's brother got killed in Vegas! He got shot while he was doing CPR."

Firefighters.

"Mike is not dead," I told him. "I was just texting with him."

"Oh, shit. Sorry. Some guys at the firehouse just read a news story that said he got shot while he was doing CPR."

"That is NOT what the news story said." I sent the article to Tommy. "I'm going to teach a class for the FDNY called 'Teaching Firefighters How to Read.'"

"I'll take it," Tommy said. "Is it free? If it's free, it's for me."

I didn't wind up getting pulled into that shooting. But I did get pulled into Park Slope Volunteer Ambulance Corps. At last I'd been accepted for an interview. Orientation began soon. I was eager to move forward.

One of my last tours with Ji, we went to the hospital to fetch a ninety-something-year-old woman with dementia. She'd been admitted to the hospital after taking a fall. Now she was ours to return home. Her long white hair was done in a beautiful, swirling braid and her senility gave her a childlike demeanor. She was sweet and frail with blue cataracted eyes.

"Who braided your hair?" I asked her as we gathered around her hospital bed and piled her belongings onto the stretcher. "You look so pretty."

"One of the nurses," she said. Then she asked if we'd seen her mother.

Ji and I looked at each other. "Your mother?"

"Yes," she said. Then she started to weep. "I love my mother. I miss her so much. I want to see her. Have you seen her?"

I was no mathematician, but I was pretty sure this lady's mother was no longer on earth.

"We haven't seen her," Ji said, taking a shot at the truth.

"Where is she?" our patient pleaded. We quietly focused on the job we'd been sent to do. Our patient was feather light. It took no strength for us to lift her. Her crying grew desperate as we transferred her onto the stretcher. "Where are you taking me? Are you taking me home?"

"That's right," Ji said.

We bundled her up in sheets and rolled her toward the exit. An ornate gold barrette fell out of her hair, and her trembling hand flew to her head. "My barrette!"

We parked. Ji bent down and picked the barrette off the floor. Then he carefully brushed the patient's hair out of her eyes and took his time, fixing her braid. Watching him do this, so tenderly and gently, nearly broke me. He was a saint.

On the back of the ambulance the patient held my hand the whole ride. Her fingers were long and spindly, and she had the grip of an Ironman competitor.

She told me she'd grown up in Ireland. That her mother was her favorite person in the world. She repeated how much she loved and missed her mother, and Ireland, her home. The roses that grew in her girlhood backyard.

When we got to the nursing home and rolled her into the lobby, our patient started crying in outrage. "This isn't where I live! I live in Ireland! This isn't my house. Where is my mother? I want to see her. Am I going home?"

"Yes," I said. "You're going home."

Ji shook his head to say, Don't go there. Home means death.

We rolled her into her room and tucked her in bed. She stopped weeping. Ji left the room to clean the stretcher. The woman looked at me with wide, desperate eyes. Then she took my hand and squeezed it as hard as any human could.

"Am I going to see my mother?" she asked me.

I thought of my grandma in her California nursing home. How sure she was of my grandfather's presence at night. How peaceful she seemed, believing he was still around. How I always felt Pat's aliveness at his firehouse. Perhaps that was why Mike wasn't sad there. I, too, believed in ghosts. That there was more to this life than what I could see and touch.

"Yes," I told her. "You're going to see your mother."

She nodded. "I'm going home."

"Yes. We're all going home."

4

WELCOME TO PARK SLOPE

In December 2017 I had my one-on-one interview to volunteer as an EMT with Park Slope. I was excited to get out on the street. Gimme some emergencies! I hoped this would be the right place for me as a first responder. Fingers crossed. Little while before I would know. Interview. Orientation. Training. Then riding as an observer for three tours before being cleared as a member. I prayed I had what it took to get through each of these steps.

The ambulance base was a two-train commute from my house, the office housed above a garage on a busy street clotted with traffic that gushed out the Prospect Expressway. Dead cockroaches lay on their upturned backs outside the front door. I pressed the buzzer. It clicked open. Up I went a flight of stairs, fluorescent lights aflicker.

Inside, I waited alone in a conference room. After a while a tall, white, easygoing captain named Robert appeared and shook my hand. He was relaxed and around my age and asked all the questions I'd expected. Who was I? Had I worked in EMS before? Why'd I want to volunteer? Could I commit to riding once a week for two years? I was Jennifer. I'd worked transport. I wanted to volunteer for x and y reasons. Sure, I could commit.

Robert leaned back in his chair, crossed his legs at the knee, and told me about the all-volunteer agency, which provided EMS services in Brooklyn regardless of patients' ability to pay. Established in 1992, Park Slope had worked all the big citywide disasters. September 11. New York City snowstorm in 2011. Hurricanes Irene and Sandy. Three and a half years from this winter evening, COVID-19. But who saw that viral freight train coming? Reportedly, a lot of people in power. But we were not in power.

Robert plugged the organization. He said what made it special was its great people: a diverse group of first responders who were medically talented and generous with their time. EMTs who volunteered at Park Slope worked full-time as EMTs, paramedics, nurses, lawyers, and business executives, and many who cut their teeth here went on to become doctors and physician assistants.

I had no interest whatsoever in pursuing a career in medicine, which I didn't mention.

"A lot of people meet their significant other here," he said, wiggling his foot. "We've had several members get married."

"That's why I'm here," I joked. "To fall in love."

A moment later, Robert walked me into an office and presented me to Chief Suzy, a nurse with chin-length hair streaked with gray seated at a desk behind towering stacks of paperwork. I couldn't help but note her ethnicity, probably since we so rarely get to see badass Asian women in alpha roles when it comes to popular culture.

Suzy ran me through a few imaginary scenarios and asked me questions to test my knowledge of state protocols. I answered correctly, more or less. Days later I received a congratulations e-mail announcing my acceptance.

Then it was Christmas. I spent it alone.

A few days later I accompanied Nick to his annual World Trade Center health screening at Mount Sinai, where they monitored and treated sick 9/11 first responders. We sat in the waiting room, made small talk, and squabbled. About what, I cannot recall. Ronald Reagan, probably. We fought about him a lot.

"Yeah, he did a bang-up job," I often said of his hero. "Except for botching the AIDS crisis. And his racialized war on drugs that criminalized crack over cocaine and filled the prisons with Black people. And that little civil war he caused in Nicaragua, when he funded the Contras. But other than that, great job."

Even Rafael joked about cops' affection for Reagan. He called him "The Great White."

Nick and Rafael and I, as with most if not all of the cops in my life, we maintained mutual respect, trust, and love for each other as friends and colleagues and human beings. Same thing with my firefighter friends, many of whom I charged with being anti-Muslim, strung out on Fox News gushing out of firehouse TVs, just as they charged me with being a bleeding-heart communist. Periodically, all of us got into screaming matches that devolved into unkind words, slammed doors, and, at times, long, silent time-outs in our friendships.

Enraged as I sometimes got, I hated the systems they were part of, not them, if only because they were human, and because I understood, thanks to the intimate and painful stories they often shared with me, that beneath their politics was untethered rage, and beneath their rage, shattering personal heartbreak.

The same was true for me. Having lost Heather suddenly and violently as a teenager, and then Pat suddenly and violently on 9/11, one of my life's greatest agonies was being robbed of the opportunity to say goodbye to people I loved, to have last words. So I knew in my bones, from excruciating experience, that life was sacred and very short, it could go at any minute, and I couldn't bear the thought that if, God forbid, something happened to someone I loved, the last thing I might have said to them was "Fuck you and your fucking politics."

I guessed it was some sort of sacred pact I'd made with my soul, to never retaliate, never let myself bomb their village when they pissed me off. I fought with them to their faces rather than behind their backs. "True friends stab you in the front," as Oscar Wilde said. And I wouldn't allow myself to stay angry at them for long. Even after huge, tearful blowouts I never forgot their safety was provisional, as was mine, as was everyone's, and I always closed our tussles with "Have a safe night. I love you."

In the hospital, a mousy woman walked into the waiting room wearing a bomber jacket with the Twin Towers emblazoned on the back. Nick hated Never Forget paraphernalia. I told him I was going to get him a jacket like that and he shoved me.

We were there two or three hours. He saw a bunch of doctors. I perused some water-stained magazines. When he finished, we got omelets at a nearby diner. Even after his heart attack he still ate like shit. Typical cop. I asked what he'd scored on the depression questionnaire.

"Seven," he said, munching on bacon.

"That seems a bit generous. I would put you more around a nine or a ten."

"I lied to them. And you're a bitch. But seriously, Lioness, thank you for coming with me. I hate going to these appointments. I appreciate it."

I never minded. Felice had gone with me to my cancer checkups many times over the years, so I understood how comforting it was not to have to face these things alone.

Orientation at Park Slope started in January 2018 and was much more involved than what I'd completed for my transport job. I appreciated that. You can never be overtrained. As Creasy, played by Denzel Washington, says in *Man on Fire*, "There's no such thing as tough. There's trained, and untrained."

Class never bored me, as my fellow probationary EMTs were smart and hilarious. There was Chad, an Army vet who worked in some sort of systems management capacity at a hospital. He could talk to a rock and was dating half of Tinderized New York City. William, a muscular guy who wanted to become a doctor and had served as a combat medic in the National Guard. Aaron, a professional martial artist who aspired to work for the Fire Department. Raz, a shy EMT whose hands sweated profusely when he got nervous. MJ, a globetrotting woman who worked in marketing and played after-work soccer that resulted in impressive calves.

MJ and Chad and I were the only white people in the room. I was twenty years older than everyone in class, an EMS grandmother. It didn't matter. These were my brothers and sisters now. We bonded over our strange attraction to EMS and amused each other during hours of lectures.

For a week different chiefs and duty officers at Park Slope oriented us. I'd worked alongside paramilitary organizations my entire career. But I had a hard time wrapping my head around what power officers could wield in the context of volunteerism. What could the chiefs do if we did something wrong? Fire us? We worked for free. You're a volunteer lieutenant? Congratulations. What does that even mean? Was it like an Instagram model? You just decided that's who you were and crowned yourself a leader? It was difficult for me to understand.

Admittedly, I had problems with authority. I was a mouthy, defiant, know-it-all woman. Not all the time, but that was my shadow for sure. Tall woman, tall shadow. Most of my crisis clients were big shots. I was educated up to the eyeballs. That put me in a tricky position in terms of self-regard.

It also confused people in my life that "someone like me" would choose to work in EMS. Once, when I told a high-powered client I was an EMT in

Brooklyn, he chuckled and said, "They have no idea who you are, do they." I said, "No." But retrospectively, I didn't understand what he'd meant. Was I somebody?

As for authority, I longed to be told what to do. But I also deplored it. My general attitude toward paramilitary bosses was, Don't come to me with your white shirt and degree from John Jay College of Criminal Justice and start bossing me around like some knee-socked schoolgirl, I'm grown. So that attitude made me really fun to manage. Or as Nick said, "Impossible to manage."

I sent a prayer up for all the leadership officers at Park Slope who'd inevitably have to deal with the shadier side of my personality at some point. Possibly, many points. You'll see.

Park Slope was led by several chiefs. A young, educated woman and full-time EMT who everyone called by her last name, Hartford, did the bulk of operational heavy lifting. Smart and meticulously organized, Hartford had a commander-like personality scattered with islands of sincerity. I was scared of her. Her counterpart, Chief Beck, was a knowledgeable career EMT who seemed much older than his thirty-something years. He was married to an ER nurse.

One training session Hartford covered radio ten-codes, which we had to memorize. She told us the ominous 10-13 was the worst code we would hear come over the air, an SOS that meant a member of service's life was in immediate danger. When we heard this code, every first responder on the street would fly to the scene to help the endangered servicemembers.

"Do not use this code unless you're about to die," she said.

Hartford warned us that responding to emergencies where an MOS had been hurt or killed were especially distressing. She gave examples.

When a schizophrenic man hijacked an FDNY ambulance in 2017 and ran over EMT Yadira Arroyo in the Bronx, crushing her to death and dragging her through the street while her partner screamed in horror, that was a 10-13.

When two police officers were shot dead at point-blank range while sitting in their patrol vehicle in Bed-Stuy in 2014, killed by a man who wanted to avenge the deaths of Eric Garner and Michael Brown, two unarmed Black men killed by cops, that was a 10-13.

Rafael, the detective I used to date—he was in the wind—had been on the job that night. Those were his guys. Not long after the incident he wound up in the hospital with chest pain that turned out to be stress related.

Welcome to the world of feelings.

Another orientation day we learned the boundaries of our coverage area, which extended beyond Park Slope into other neighborhoods. We covered Bedford Avenue to the east and the Columbia Waterfront to the west, Sixtieth Street to the south and Atlantic Avenue to the north. Beck went over the locations of projects and homeless shelters, precincts and firehouses, Prospect Park and Barclays Center, hospitals and prisons.

Next, we learned which hospitals had trauma centers and which psychiatric ERs were locked; which handled strokes and where the nearest burn center was located. I really didn't want to see anyone who'd been badly burned. Those photos were some of the worst in the EMT textbook.

Onto history. Beck explained that most vollies in the city had been operating for ages, many of them since the late 1960s. Park Slope and the Bed-Stuy Vollies were the new kids on the volunteer block. Historically, before the 911 system existed, emergencies were handled by separate agencies. If civilians had an emergency, they called 0 for operator, or the police department's main phone line. If there was a fire, they called the Fire Department. If it was EMS related, the job went to one of the community-based volunteer ambulance companies, which sent EMTs and medics.

Fast forward to the creation of 911 in 1968. The Federal Communications Commission and AT&T identified an easy-to-remember, three-digit public-safety number as the emergency code for the country. It took years for the 911 system to cover all of America. In 1987, 911 was only available to about 50 percent of the country, according to the National Emergency Number Association. Today, around 240 million 911 calls are made each year, more than 80 percent of them from mobile devices.

Dispatchers now triaged the emergency at the call level. Based on what the caller said, dispatchers determined which first responders to send to a given job. Medical emergencies in New York City fell into segmented categories. For serious life threats where patient survival hinged on a fast response time, a multiplicity of first responders arrived on scene.

For Category Ones—cardiac arrest, choking, burn majors, confirmed shots fired—units from the NYPD, FDNY, and FDNY EMS got dispatched. Similar responses from various agencies arrived for callers reporting difficulty breathing, unconscious people, cardiac conditions, and major injuries. That's why a circus of emergency vehicles often arrived on scene: fire rigs, ambulances, and RMPs, radio motor patrol vehicles, as police cars were called. If you were about to be dead, the whole family showed up.

While responses from different agencies varied from city to state, for serious life threats, it was always quite a festival. In New York City, a Basic Life Support (BLS) unit with two EMTs or an Advanced Life Support (ALS) ambulance with two paramedics responded to all medical incidents and provided patient care and transport. Fire engines also responded to many serious medical emergencies in addition to an ambulance, as engines typically arrived faster, a minute or so before EMS. The fire engine was staffed with firefighters, of course, who in New York City provided a touch of medical care, having received training as Certified First Responders with defibrillation certificates, CFR-Ds. Tell a California firefighter that in New York City firefighters aren't paramedics and watch their eyes bulge out of their heads. Many states and cities that integrated fire and medical had required firefighters be trained as paramedics for a decade or more.

In New York City there were many long-running debates on how to improve EMS and provide better patient care. Some emergency management experts believed EMS should break away from the Fire Department. They argued that using fire engines and FDNY ambulances on medical runs was costly and ineffective, the Fire Department's unionized pretext for keeping staff that was no longer necessary due to the not-too-many-fires-anymore situation. As the adage about the fire services goes, "150 years of tradition unimpeded by progress."

From that vantage point, the question from a taxpayer perspective that every New Yorker should ask was this: Why did the city pay the Fire Department millions of dollars every year to provide EMS when hospital ambulances and commercial companies put themselves on the 911 system at no cost to the city? The operating cost of an FDNY ambulance was known to be significantly higher than that of hospital and commercial units. And hospital and private crews did just as good of a job as Fire Department EMTs and medics, if not better. In other cities that organized EMS separate from Fire, ambulances didn't cost taxpayers millions. Why did ours?

Others held that if EMS continued to fall under the Fire Department's management, FDNY should compensate and respect its EMTs and paramedics as it did its firefighters, and/or train all firefighters as EMTs and paramedics so they could treat more people on scene. Other suggestions for improving EMS in the city included staffing ambulances with one paramedic and one EMT, as was done elsewhere in New York state, since paramedics were in short supply.

Lastly, some argued progress could be made by putting the city's volunteer ambulance crews on the 911 system, since many of these agencies covered underserved communities. The Fire Department regularly pulled vollie crews onto 911 in times of citywide crisis, when call volumes surged and the FDNY needed help, so clearly vollies were needed, and up for the task.

Like all volunteer agencies, Park Slope got dispatched to emergencies from a separate entity. At times, volunteer crews co-responded to jobs with 911-dispatched units to improve ambulance response times, take pressure off the city's strained EMS system, and help the city's overworked, underpaid EMTs and paramedics. Initially, Park Slope dispatched ambulances in-house, from its base. But EMTs had different reactions to working as emergency operators. Some loved dispatching while others preferred to be on the ambulance. Eventually, the agency moved to using an EMS communications center that handled emergency and nonemergency comms for EMS.

Park Slope also had a direct emergency line—a hotline or "red-phone job"—wherein people called us directly rather than calling 911. Other volunteer ambulance companies had emergency phone lines as well. Hatzalah, a vollie squad that served the Orthodox Jewish community, dispatched all of its units from direct calls. The benefit to patients of having a volunteer crew was that we could transport people to their hospital of choice without having to ask a medical director for permission, within reason.

Reason meant if your stomach hurt because you had cancer, and you lived in Brooklyn but wanted to see your doctor at Cornell in Manhattan, we could transport you to that ER. If, however, you had a stroke and wanted to go from Brooklyn to see your doctor in Manhattan, a thirty-minute journey, at least, we could not grant your wish because of the nature of your illness.

Strokes were time-sensitive emergencies. Medical treatments needed to be administered within a certain window of time. The longer someone suffered a stroke, the higher their chance of disability or death. Every minute for a patient with a stroke equated to 1.9 million lost brain cells.

Last days of orientation at Park Slope, Chief Suzy went over how to write patient charts. Then Hartford brought us into the garage and had us practice lifting, working equipment, and responding to real-life scenarios we would see on the street.

It was amazing, how bad we all were. Before he cleared us to start riding as observers, Chief Beck gave us a talk about what we were getting ourselves into as volunteers at Park Slope.

"EMS is a dangerous job," he said. "Some of you will go on from here to work for the Fire Department, some of you will become doctors and PAs, and some of you will do this as a hobby. And I'm telling you right now—this is not like other hobbies. My neighbor rescues dogs as a hobby, and that is very nice of her. EMS is not rescuing dogs. You're going to have patients with hep-C spit on you. You're going to take combative patients to the hospital who try to punch and kick you. You're going to respond to suicides and rapes and DOAs, and get bottles thrown at you, and see little kids get hit by cars. Any of you want to quit?"

No one said a word.

After a pause he said, "Wonderful. We want you to have fun out there, but above all else we care about your safety. Next you'll start your observation tours. One of the duty officers will send you a scheduling e-mail to fill out. Welcome to Park Slope."

My first evening as an observer, waves of nausea crashed on the shore of my gut. My armpits filled with nervous sweat that made me reek like a cornered skunk on the way to base. I'd waited what felt like forever to start responding to serious jobs, but I was simultaneously terrified of it.

In addition to stinking, I looked dumb. My uniform wasn't a uniform yet. We'd been told to wear dark blue tactical shirts and EMS pants, but we wouldn't get patched until we passed our three observation tours to the satisfaction of our field training officers.

As newbies we didn't get to ride every week. We had to wait for a crew to become available to train us. Heading to work this February evening in my blank getup I looked like I could be any civil servant. Mail carrier.

Bus driver. On the subway platform a lost lady asked me if the Q train was running, mistaking me for a transit worker, I guessed.

Wasps of fear attacked me as I got off the train and walked to base. I was afraid of freezing on scene. Dropping a patient. Killing a patient. I called and shared my anxiety with Nick. Why I tried to squeeze emotional support out of a retired cop was beyond me.

"I never froze on the street," he said. "But it happens all the time. So does dropping people. Oh wow. Hang on, Ginger. I'm sending you something. OK. Check your phone."

I put him on speaker. And there on my screen a present from Nick. A photo of a dead rat.

"Tell me what I'm looking at," I said after I glanced at it.

"That rat, it was pancaked by something."

"Did you just interrupt our fucking conversation to send me a photo of a smashed rat?

"I thought you'd appreciate it. No?"

Cops.

"In terms of killing patients," Nick said, "you have to think of it like this: if you hadn't shown up, they would have died anyway."

Thanks a lot.

I arrived at base first, before my trainers. One of them texted me and told me to pick a truck and do the 800—provide a detailed inventory of the equipment on the bus as required by the State EMS Code Part 800 for ambulance vehicles, to ensure the truck was compliant with Department of Health regulations. I went upstairs and grabbed keys and a fresh run sheet with an 800-inventory checklist on the back. Then I went down to the garage and climbed on the truck.

I was so new this simple task, which seasoned EMTs could do in ten minutes, took me over an hour. When I finished, I sat in the cold fluorescent bus staring morbidly at the sheeted stretcher and holding my breath, having overwhelmed myself by the range of medical equipment I might need to use on critically sick and injured patients. Transporting grandmas had been one thing. But this, responding to serious emergencies, was a different world entirely.

For the life of me I couldn't remember why I'd chosen to ride on an ambulance. I was so far out of my comfort zone I could barely move. I heard

Felice's voice in my head, asking the question she'd posed miles back, when I'd decided to become a first responder: "Who becomes an EMT as a hobby? Most people learn a new language or take up cooking. But not my sister. She rides on an ambulance for fun."

At base I found Hartford and told her I was nervous. She assured me it was normal, that everyone was terrible in the beginning. She'd felt the exact same way when she was new. "EMS is a self-motivated field. You can study all you want. But everything you learn you're going to learn on the street."

That seemed like a rather high-stakes classroom.

Around seven o'clock my partners appeared. A fit Polish girl in her twenties named Lexi, short for Alexis, came to volunteer for the Tour 3 seven-to-midnight shift, after working all day as an EMT with a hospital ambulance crew. Lexi had a voluminous Instagram following and she laughed hard and easily at every joke I cracked, which was one of my favorite qualities in a person. Her partner, Vincent, was a hipster-looking dude with a technology job who looked like he lived in Williamsburg and played in a band.

For hours I sat quietly in the back of the truck and tried not to irritate them. It was a quiet night. Very few jobs came over the radio. But there was still a lot to learn.

Dispatchers spoke fast and in ten-codes. Lexi had me practice the codes and listen to the radio. Her head was made of ears. She could be talking with me and listening to the radio at the same time, then stop mid-sentence to respond to a run, whereas it was impossible for me to make any sense of the gobbledygook coming over the frequencies. I loved the radios. Ever since I was a girl, I cherished anything having to do with walkie-talkies, and the secret language of ten-codes made me feel like I had a key to a secret world.

For dinner we got steamed shrimp dumplings from Dumplings & Things. We got drinks at 7-Eleven. Peed in filthy EMS-personnel-only hospital bathrooms. At one point that night, when Vincent stepped aside, I asked Lexi if there was any chemistry between them, since they were both young and attractive and single.

She said, "Nah. I like alphas. I'm more alpha than he is, and I can't be more alpha than the guy I'm dating. I prefer guys in uniform."

Finally, another woman like me. A unicorn who came out and said it, articulated my weakness for men in turnout gear bearing Halligan mauls.

I liked being around Lexi, who later became my regular Wednesday night partner. And with whom, a year or so down the line, I worked one of my all-time worst emergencies, "An oasis of horror in a desert of boredom," to borrow the French poet Charles Baudelaire's words.

This night we went on a few runs that wound up being 90s, ten-code for no patient found. That concluded my first observation tour.

My second observation a few weeks later was with a young EMT named Gabriel and his partner Stephanie, a brunette in glasses who'd recently been accepted to medical school. They were street husband and wife, married to their core, though in real life, whatever that was, Gabriel was gay. I loved them.

Gabriel rapidly became one of my favorite first responders. Everyone at Park Slope agreed he was one of the best rescuers. He was medically talented, wonderful with patients, and fun to work with on the truck. He was applying to paramedic school and, like me, was an empath. Many medical professionals fell into this archetype. The street was their church, helping people in healthcare crises their ministry. There was a sainted quality to them when they treated patients. They were angels, basically.

There also existed in the field a sort of psychopathic first responder who hated people, enjoyed screaming for sport, and had the emotional life of an empty refrigerator. Scores of doctors fell into this category as well. These rescuers enjoyed medical trauma and didn't seem to mind seeing people fall apart. Whenever I encountered these buried-alive medical professionals on the job, I tried to manage their dead-inside qualities when they were near patients and family members, since they were incapable of providing solace.

As far being a newbie went, scientists thought the sloth was the slowest-moving land mammal until they saw me try to get off an ambulance in an emergency. Unlike transport, at Park Slope I had to fly off the truck fast, because patients were badly hurt or sick or dying. During my observation tour with Stephanie and Gabriel, by the time I'd figured out which doors to open first, which handles turned up instead of down, and how to wrestle the bulging tech bag out of the cabinet, my trainers were already down the street treating the patient.

"So," Gabriel said between runs. "I've noticed you're a little slow to get off the ambulance."

I crumpled with laughter. I told him it was a technical issue. He understood.

"Practice doing it now," he suggested.

And so that night I practiced the idiot task of getting off the ambulance until I could do it with acceptable velocity. I was almost done with my observation tours, but I still hadn't responded to a proper emergency. I was getting frustrated. What would it take?

My Brooklyn block was a historic award-winner for being one of the greenest in Brooklyn. When the weather permitted, my neighbors were outside puttering, potting flowers, rewilding their gardens and tinkering with their brownstones.

Everyone looked out for one another around here, looked out for me, too, and I never got any frowny faces for my tall white presence. That being said, gentrification was a problem, and I was part of that system. Being a white woman in a mostly Black neighborhood suffering the rent-spiking consequences of gentrification was a charged position. As was denying the fact that Bed-Stuy continued to have problems with guns, gangs, and drugs on the streets.

My area was considered, to use a phrase from the street, "a busy neighborhood." Most first responders who worked in busy neighborhoods took great pride in their locations, since the best rescuers often got routed to the busiest spots in town. Bed-Stuy Volunteer EMTs treated more gunshot wounds in one week than a Park Slope EMT would see in their entire career.

My approach to inhabiting postures of conflict was mostly to ask people impacted by my position how they felt about it, when appropriate. I didn't canvas the neighborhood or anything.

One afternoon at lunch with my neighbors, the ones who'd called me a badass back when I transported grandmas, I asked the question. "How do you feel about my people being here?"

"Your people were here first," my neighbor said.

I never knew that. I was historically ignorant. I came here in peace. Also, in ignorance.

He told me German, Jewish, Italian, Chinese, Greek, and Irish immigrants lived in Bed-Stuy prior to World War II, when it became mostly Black. Across the street from my building there lived a slender, elderly Black veteran. He often sat outside in the morning, reading the paper, wearing a Korean War cap. We always waved to each other and said hello.

But certainly not everyone felt cozy about my presence. One afternoon, walking down Patchen Avenue, a Black man saw me on the street and screamed, "What are you looking at, fucking white girl? Fucking cracker! Get the fuck out of Bed-Stuy!"

A month later, in March, it happened at last: I finally got an emergency.

My third and final night with Lexi and Vincent we got a run for an EDP, street-speak in New York City for emotionally distressed person, meaning someone having a psychiatric emergency. It used to be emotionally disturbed person, but the people who named things were trying to PC the language. I wasn't sure they'd gotten there yet, by switching out disturbed for distressed. Or, in 2019, when Mayor de Blasio tried and failed to get cops to stop saying EDP and use "mental health call" instead. As Nathan Englander used to say of unready student stories in grad school, "This one's still cooking."

Tonight, before I knew what was happening, Vincent radioed dispatch that we were 63, heading to the EDP. Lexi in the driver's seat blew down the street, taking the red lights like stop signs and occasionally blasting the air horn. I almost had a heart attack sitting in the back, my body shot with a blast of adrenaline so hard and fast I understood how mothers of imperiled children were able to lift cars in emergencies in order to save their baby's life, and why paramedics injected adrenaline into cardiac-arrested patients to try to jumpstart their stalled hearts.

I'd drunk my share of vodka and taken some bedazzling hallucinogenics in my youth, but never in my life had I felt, had I even come close to feeling, the tachycardia-producing, adrenal-gland-pumping, blood-pressure-spiking, deeply euphoric, roller-coaster ride, three-headed hormone high of epinephrine, norepinephrine, and cortisol slamming into my primal nervous system at once.

By the time we arrived on scene and I stumbled off the truck I felt like I'd been dropped off a cliff. Meanwhile, Lexi and Vincent waltzed up to a stoop where the emergency was unfolding as if they were picking up their dry cleaning.

"What's up?" Lexi asked one of the cops, a bulky, light-haired fellow who looked like he lived in on Long Island, in one of those bar towns colonized by cops and firefighters. He seemed overjoyed to see her.

"I'll tell you what's going on," the patient said. She was a Black, six-foot-three trans woman wearing the highest of high heels and a sparkly dress that reflected the moonlight. She stood on the stoop smoking a Newport with a cute little box purse looped over her shoulder, and she had an awful lot to say about the cops at her door, which went a little something like this:

"These two fucking idiot police officers here just came inside my house because my bitch-ass landlord called 911 on me because we was having a fight because she's a dumb fucking bitch who calls 911 on me all the goddamn time because she don't like the fact that I live here and I wasn't doing nothing wrong, OK? I was just playing my music and singing Rihanna because that's my girl, that's my queen, and that is my name, Rihanna, I am motherfucking Rihanna, which I explained to these officers, I tried to explain the situation but these dumb fucking racist midget-ass cops believe my landlord and don't believe me. And I *told* them not to come in my house. I *told* them I just cleaned my floors. I said, 'Officers don't you *dare* come in my house with those big dirty boots and ruin my clean floors,' and do you know what they did? You know they came in my house and left their muddy-ass footprints all up and down my floors which now I have to clean again. That's what happened. And I don't want nothing to do with them and I'm not going nowhere with any of you especially not to no hospital and FUCK THE POLICE!"

We were all of us silent. I was so impressed I almost clapped. Suddenly the trees and nighttime air pulsed with aliveness. I felt fearless and at home. I wanted to hear more from Rihanna. I could have listened to her all night.

And just like that I fell in love with EDPs and made a decision to prioritize responding to mental health emergencies above all other jobs for the rest of my time at Park Slope, transporting distressed patients to hospitals so often that some cops hugged me on scene whenever they saw me show up, and psych doctors shook my hand.

Tonight the doting blond cop looked at Lexi, then at the patient, and said we needed to take her to a locked ER. I was impressed he got the patient's pronoun right.

Lexi shut down his suggestion since we were only a few blocks away from the nearest hospital, the locked psych wards were fifteen minutes out, and the patient wasn't violent, she was simply animated. Made sense to me at the moment, but wow did this decision boomerang back to us later. We couldn't leave the patient on scene, which was what she most wanted.

* * *

Every city responds to mental health crises differently, and how these calls are handled is an issue of intense debate.

In New York City at this time, EMTs co-responded to 911 mental health emergencies with police officers. EDPs were medical calls, so we led on scene and interacted with patients. Cops made sure the scene was safe for us to operate and then generally stood back unless we needed them, or the patient was actively violent. As a rule, cops did not enjoy these jobs, and emotionally distressed people did not find it relaxing to see police at their door. But once dispatchers classified the call as an EDP or EDP-C, meaning critical—patient was emotionally distressed *and* actively violent, suicidal, homicidal, or barricaded with or without a hostage—cops could not under public health law leave these patients on scene unless they downgraded the call to something else, like "domestic incident."

As EMTs we could have patients sign an RMA—Refuse Medical Assistance form, which allowed them to refuse treatment and/or transport—if they qualified for our protocols. But the police had a must-act obligation to take people first responders reasonably believed were in a psychiatric emergency to the hospital and make sure they were in a safe environment.

The historical background for this patrol obligation came from a series of emergencies in the late 1990s that involved people with untreated mental illness becoming violent toward themselves and others, resulting in what was known in New York as Kendra's Law. The state law was named after Kendra Webdale, a young woman pushed to her death into the path of a subway train by a schizophrenic man who wasn't taking his medication. Originally proposed by the National Alliance on Mental Illness, the law granted judges the authority to issue orders for people who met certain criteria to receive regular psychiatric treatment. Failure to comply could result in commitment for up to seventy-two hours.

The results of this law were considered by many mental health experts to be exemplary in terms of giving people with serious mental illness a better chance at long-term treatment and community integration while simultaneously ensuring public safety. Around forty-seven states had adopted some version of the law, known in mental health circles as "Assisted Outpatient Treatment." Kendra's Law was reportedly proven to reduce a patient's risk of hospitalization, suicide, and violence, and was especially helpful in plugging systemic cracks in the healthcare system the seriously mentally ill often fell through.

In Ms. Webdale's case, the man who pushed her had been hospitalized over a dozen times before killing her. In the case of slain EMT Yadira Arroyo, the man who ran her over with her hijacked ambulance was schizophrenic, likely on drugs, homeless, and repeatedly hospitalized, and had a history of violent assaults. Advocates of the law noted that when it worked, it worked well, but it continued to be underfunded and underutilized. Many family members of mentally ill people still didn't know the law existed.

But like all solutions, Kendra's Law came with a subset of broader systemic problems. The American Civil Liberties Union argued that it caused incarceration of the seriously mentally ill and that the state should not have the authority to compel people with psychiatric disabilities to undergo treatment. Advocacy group New York Lawyers for the Public Interest found that Black people were nearly five times more likely than whites to be the subject of court orders stemming from the law. Some experts attributed the racial disparity to the fact that three-quarters of court orders were issued in New York City, which had a large Black population. Others stated that Black and Latinx people with mental illness might not have access to preventative, early-measure healthcare, making them more likely to suffer from severe crises that result in court-ordered intervention.

The primary duty of all first responders is to preserve human life. Is the street a safe environment for someone who says they want to push someone in front of train, or who reports being noncompliant with medications to treat their mental illness, resulting in them hallucinating and hearing voices others don't hear? No. Many of the problems that plagued us on the street commenced at the call level, making it difficult for us to act outside protocols based on the 911 call type. No matter how much we wanted to, we couldn't easily unring that bell.

Now it was time to convince Rihanna she had to get on the ambulance. Quite a feat, since she didn't want to go.

How to gracefully convince someone to get on an ambulance often comes down to training. Crisis communications. De-escalation. EMTs in New York City receive almost no training in responding to EDPs and volatile patients, which comprise a considerable percentage of the 911 call volume. In EMT school and continuing education courses we get between two and four hours of education on psychiatric emergencies. Paramedics get a little more. A few days. In 2015, the city said it would train cops in de-escalation strategies and crisis techniques to respond to emergencies involving the mentally ill. But it only trained a third of officers.

First Lexi tried and failed to coax Rihanna into the back. Then Vincent. Then the cops, who were the least successful and received more heated words from my queen. I felt Lexi's hand on my back. She shoved me forward. Apparently, it was my turn.

I don't remember what I said that after a long conversation convinced Rihanna to get on the ambulance with us. I made my voice as soft as a lullaby—"Angel Voice," Lexi nicknamed me—and asked if she felt like hurting herself or anyone else. Negative.

For psychiatric patients that's what we had to find out fast: Were they homicidal or suicidal? If they were suicidal, did they have a plan? If they had a plan, did they have means to carry it out? If they had means, had they picked the date they were going to do it? Answer all four questions, or even two, and you were pretty far along on your suicide journey, a metaphoric "jumper up," a call type used to describe someone on a ledge, staring hellward.

Rihanna wasn't suicidal, so I asked if she had a diagnosis. Bipolar. Was she compliant with her medication? Nope, she couldn't remember the last time she took her meds. We then had a long circular chat about her landlord's unfairness that repeatedly resulted in cops at her door. She stepped off the ambulance and smoked a few relaxing cigarettes.

We'd been with her almost an hour by now. There was genuinely no place I would have rather been. People feel that. Not just psychiatric patients. All people can feel it when someone has time to truly listen to them. Finally, she agreed to let us take her to the hospital. A little miracle.

On the back of the truck I belted Rihanna to the bench and complimented her dress, which was truly joy-inducing. She wasn't having the blond cop who'd messed up her floors sit beside her, so he sat on the stretcher. A cop almost always rode on the truck with us with EDPs since it was a volatile and sometimes violent call type. People frequently awoke from psychotic stupors en route to the ER, realized they were on an ambulance, and attacked us. Cops rode along to make sure we remained safe.

I sat next to Rihanna, and Vincent sat in the captain's chair at the stretcher's head. Rihanna stuck a cigarette in her mouth and reached for her lighter. I told her she couldn't smoke on the ambulance because it was full of oxygen so we would burst into flames. That made sense to her. She put the cigarette away.

Crisis communications. It's not rocket science.

En route to the hospital the cop apologized to Rihanna for dirtying her clean floors. Some understanding was reached. They tolerated each other. Vincent opened the Toughbook to fill out Rihanna's information.

With trans patients what mattered on the medical chart was the name and gender marked on their driver's license. If they identified as female but their driver's license said male, we had to put what their ID said, which often created psychic pain for the patient. Vincent must have expected this when he reviewed Rihanna's license, because when she handed over her ID he shrieked with delight.

The cop and I looked at each other, confused. Vincent handed me the license. I looked at her legal name.

Rihanna.

"I told you," she said, shaking her head. "I don't lie."

At the hospital we walked Rihanna into the triage line and gave the nurse the lowdown. Then we got signatures and said goodbye. We cleared the hospital and returned to the street. Less than forty-five minutes later a run came over the radio for an EDP at the exact same address.

"It's Rihanna!" Lexi said, slapping the steering wheel.

Now I understood why the cop had suggested we transport our patient to a locked ER. That was the logic of the street. First, we faced and survived the emergency. Understanding came later. Sometimes the same night, if we were lucky. Sometimes months or years later. Sometimes it never arrived at all. In terms of the cop's previous suggestion, finally it all made sense to me.

Here's why:

Many ERs had a psychiatric section. But most of them were unlocked and structurally blended with the main floor, where patients lay in beds crammed together, separated by a thin curtain. People experiencing a mental health crisis often got rowdy and loud, which was hard on sick and dying people. Imagine being laid up in the hospital in pain from metastasized tumors, and suddenly your roommate is an untreated schizophrenic belting out the lyrics to "New York, New York" because they think they're Frank Sinatra.

General ERs had a tendency to check and release EDPs fast, to get rid of them, so these patients wound up right back on the street within hours, sometimes minutes, having received no lasting care. Then someone called 911 on them again, and a fleet of first responders returned to their door. States like California, Arizona, and Texas, all of which did a better job of responding to psychiatric emergencies, provided mentally ill patients with alternatives to hospitalization and jail. New York did not. In 2015, Mayor de Blasio promised the city would provide "diversion centers" for nonviolent people experiencing a mental health crisis by 2016. But it didn't open any centers until 2020. And even then, it only opened one center. In Harlem.

This was our healthcare system, New York City.

A few hospitals had locked psychiatric ERs that were separate from the general ER. Locked wards had the security, structure, and medical resources necessary to treat patients suffering a mental health crisis. They evaluated patients and kept them for up to seventy-two hours, releasing them only when they deemed patients were no longer a threat to themselves or others.

In Brooklyn, we typically only transported the street's most violent EDPs and combative patients to locked ERs, since they were fewer and farther away than our other options.

For the second time that night went back to the same block with the same cops and found our beloved patient, whose landlord had called 911 on her again. By now we were all friends. The only difference was that this time, Rihanna had to pee. I knew more than I needed to about that emergency. Lexi told her she could use the bathroom at the hospital and granted the cop's original wish to transport her to a locked ER.

Soon we were together again on the back of the ambulance, rolling happily and chit-chattily down the avenues. The facility we went to had gated entrances. First, we waltzed through sliding-glass doors and stood in a locked glass box, telling the registration lady why we were there. Then we entered a second locked glass box, where we waited for eons for nurses and doctors to free up and accept their next patient.

There was nothing for us to do but stand around and talk. The nurse behind the glass partition was reading her horoscope. Rihanna repeatedly reminded us she had to pee, and we repeatedly apologized and explained she could release her bladder once we got inside. It was taking an eternity.

"What's your sign?" the flirty cop asked Lexi.

She told him her star sign, and he hers. The nurse joined in. A conversation about star sign attributes ensued.

Rihanna stomped her heel. "Well, I'm a motherfucking Scorpio, and if you people don't let me use the goddamn bathroom, I'm gonna open my purse and pee in that!"

"Please don't do that," the cop said.

Eventually, the ER doors opened. It was time to go inside, and for Rihanna to say goodbye to the police. She and the cop shook hands, said it was nice to meet each other, and respectfully said goodnight. Peace reached. I almost keeled over with pleasure.

Inside a little windowless room, a gathering of psych nurses and doctors talked with Rihanna. We gave them the story of why we were there. Rihanna explained her medical history, untreated bipolar disorder. We got the nurse's signature so we could go.

Suddenly I was sad our work was done. I loved my patient. That's how I'd come to think of her these last few hours, not as "the patient," but as mine. She liked me, too. She said I looked like Julianne Moore.

"Thank you for everything you did for me, baby girl," she said when we hugged goodbye. "Don't forget who you are."

Then she opened her mouth and bellowed the lyrics to "Diamond," by Rihanna—her queen.

That completed my observation tours. All of my field training officers gave me rave reviews, which was kind of them. Park Slope accepted me as a member and sent my blank uniform away to get patched. At last, I was cleared to ride.

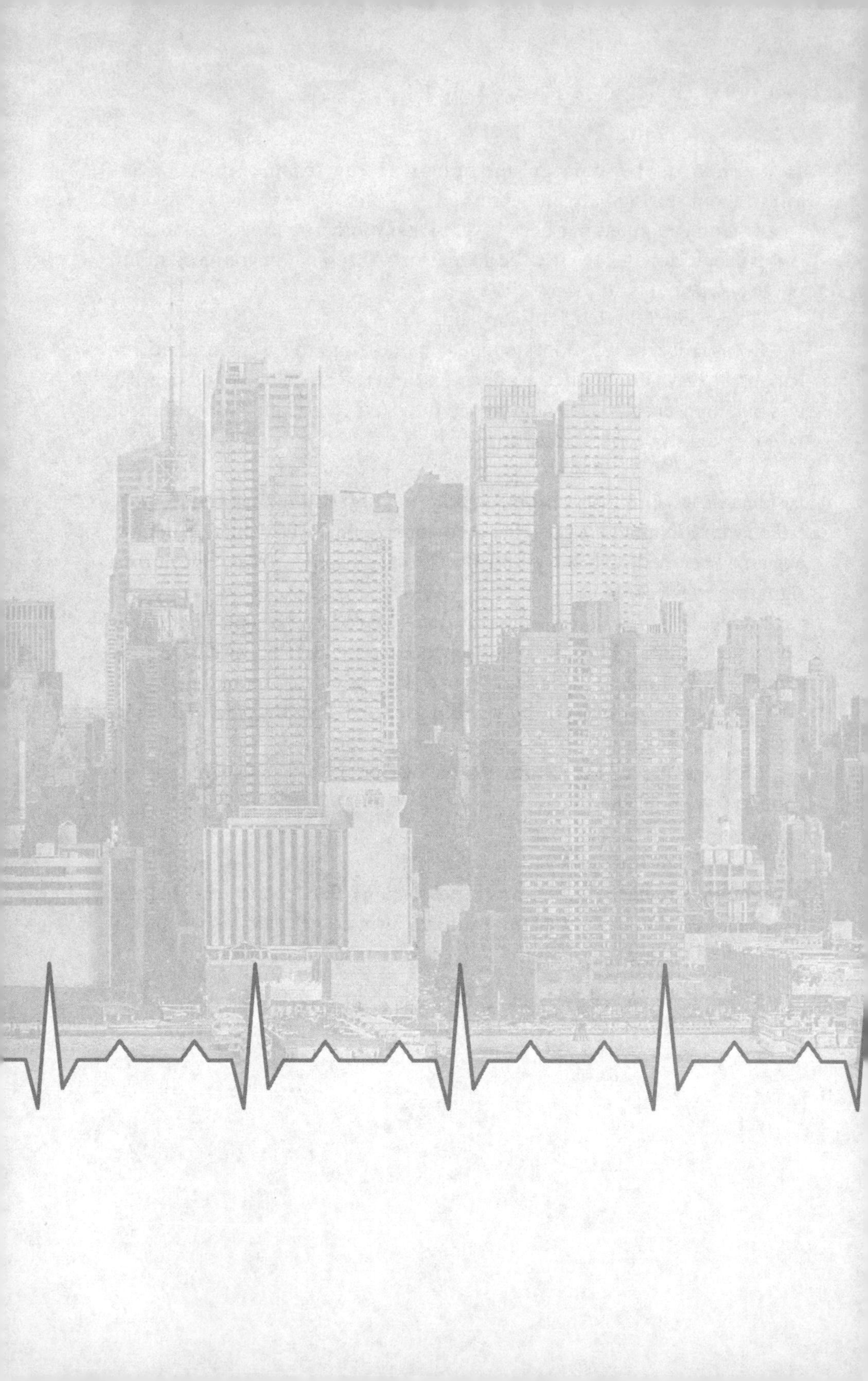

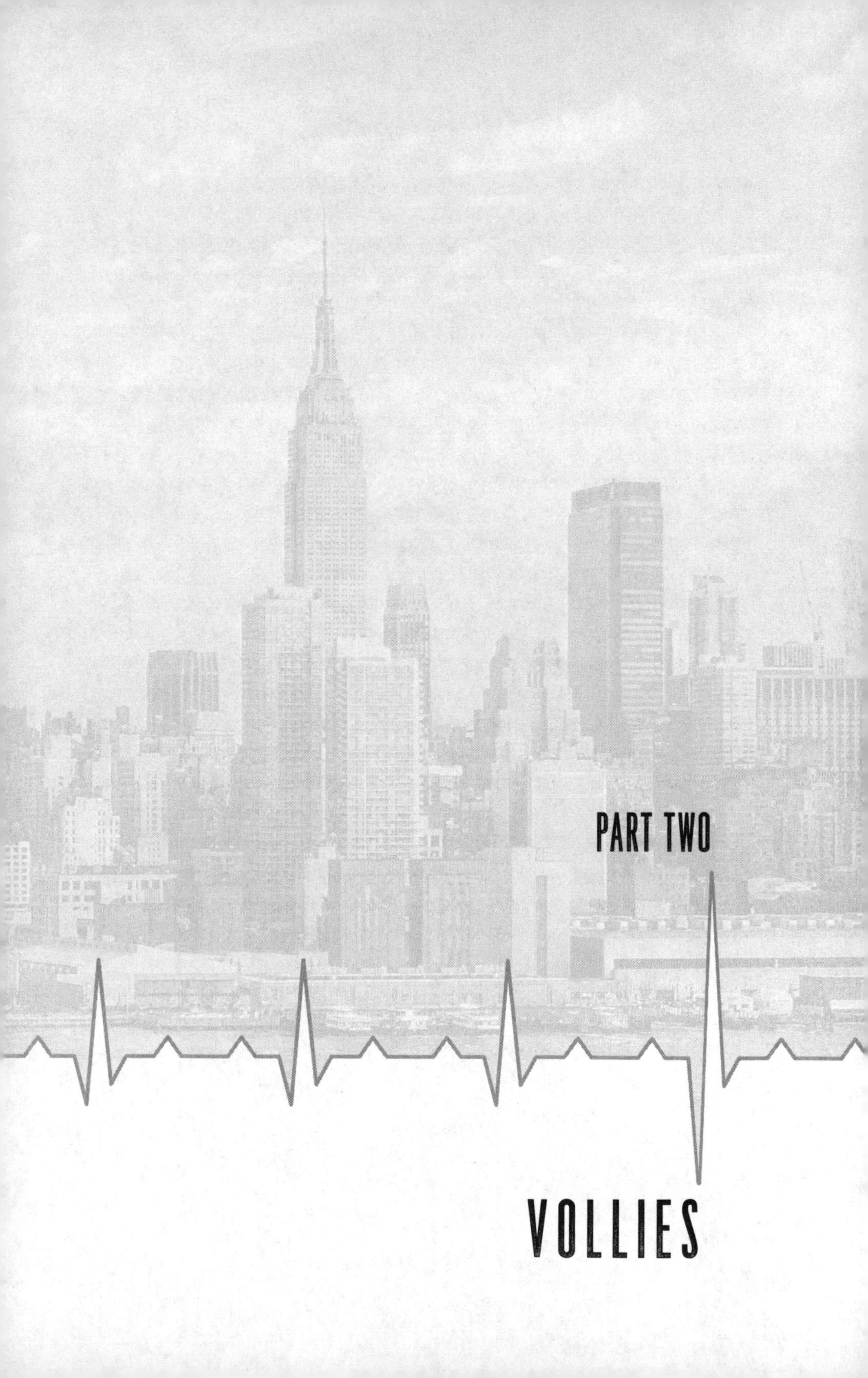

PART TWO

VOLLIES

5

STREET WIVES

Lexi and I spent nearly every Wednesday riding on the ambulance together from six in the evening to midnight that first year at Park Slope, and I came to feel she was my partner in the deepest sense of the word. I trusted her with my life.

You fall in love with your partners, is what it is. Shootings, heart attacks, seizures, car crashes, dead tours with no jobs but ripe with stories and hours of downtime to talk. On the street the stakes are so high, the consequences so violent and terrifying, the rules of the world so twisted, you come to trust your partners with every cell of your being. You can ride with a total stranger and fall in love with them after one emergency. As first responders, your relationships with one another advance fast. They outpace your oldest, deepest friendships. They change you.

When I was new at Park Slope a lot of talented EMTs offered to pick up tours with me, which was cool. I fell in love with my other regular partner, Nina, at the Red Hook Criterium, a fixed-gear bike race in Brooklyn that took place in April 2018. It was one of our organization's mainstay community events.

Unlike other volunteer ambulance companies, Park Slope received no large endowments or copious amounts of government funding. To survive, we relied on revenue generated from patient insurance billing as a result of transports, and community events. These ranged from concerts to marathons, bike races to food fairs. While event tours provided a great service to the community, offering a standby crew of first responders in case people got sick or hurt, as EMTs who enjoyed being out on the street, these tours weren't always a thrill ride.

Many events were unbearably eventless. Smorgasburg, the largest open-air food market in the country, involved sitting on an ambulance all day long in Prospect Park, waiting to rescue foodies who'd choked on a gourmet hot dog or passed out from heatstroke. Rarely did an eight-hour tour result in a single job. It was like going on a long road trip, only when you stepped off the truck in the evening, you were headachy and exactly where you'd started. Smorgas*bored*, we called it.

In contrast to Smorgasburg, everyone at Park Slope wanted to work the Red Hook Crit, as the bike race provided loads of medical trauma. One sixteen-hour day at the track offered more exposure to traumatic injuries than six months of community tours on the street. Racers on brakeless bikes crashing into one another, slamming into barriers, resulting in massive pileups of ten or twenty road-rashed athletes heaped and bleeding on the asphalt with concussions and broken clavicles.

We saw it all. That's why we became EMTs: to help people who were critically injured and sick. As rescuers we never wanted people to die or get hurt. But if they were going to die or get hurt, we wanted to be there.

The first time I worked the Crit I got stuck in the medical tent with other newish EMTs while veteran first responders got to work the better posts on the track.

Most of the bikers who limped over to the tent were lacerated from crashing but otherwise unharmed, whereas bikers who ate it on the course were usually critically maimed.

For hours I stood in the balmy spring heat beside Chad, the talkative young Army vet from my orientation class. We handed out ice packs and Band-Aids, bantered and made fun of each other. Mid-morning, Chad pointed at the sparkling river and said, "I think after a full day in the medical tent with you, I'll just drown myself in the water."

Repeatedly, like a typical dude, Chad intercepted my patient care and made me write the paper PCR. Never had I met an EMT who could talk more and obtain less relevant information than Chad—until later, when I met his partner, Nathan, who trained him. Twenty minutes with a patient and Chad knew the make and model of the athlete's bike, but he could not tell me the individual's name, where they lived, or where they were injured.

"You're treating me like your secretary," I bitched in the tent. "It's bullshit."

He chuckled. "You love it. You're a writer, that's why I make you do all the charts."

At one point an injured Italian biker stumbled up to the tent and sat down, complaining of pain to his elbow. As usual Chad shoved me out of the way and treated the athlete with an ice pack, assessing the guy's busted wing while I got going on the chart. When Chad finished, the patient looked up from his chair and said, "Thanks, but that's not why I'm here. I have a bigger problem."

Oh? Say more.

"I think I tore my ball sack."

With immeasurable joy I watched the blood drain out of Chad's face as he winced and tiptoed around in imaginary pain, suffering from too much empathy.

"Could one of you take a look?" the biker asked.

One of us sure could. I placed my hands on Chad's shoulders. "This is all you, buddy. Army strong. This is what you were designed for, one man to another. Time to be a hero."

Miserably, Chad walked the limping patient to a Porta Potty, where he examined what indeed turned out to be a ruptured sack of testicles. I heard tragically elaborate details about this injury after the patient hobbled away, having refused ambulance transport and mumbled that he'd take a taxi to a hospital later, for stitches.

Most of the Red Hook Crit racers were from Europe. Italy mainly. Scores of injured bikers chose to take Ubers to the hospital or walk-in health clinics like CityMD after the sun fell and the track cleared. These athletes enjoyed universal healthcare at home, and they knew a thing or two about the American healthcare system. Namely, not to step on an ambulance without medical insurance.

EMS in Italy fell under the provision of the Public Health Authorities by region and no distinction was made between volunteer and paid EMTs. Local hospitals, private companies, and, in many instances, volunteer organizations like the Italian Red Cross provided EMS services, and emergency transport was free.

Italians respected, even revered emergency services. It wasn't looked down on or considered beneath accomplished citizens. During COVID-19, when Italy got hit hard, former Ferrari boss Maurizio Arrivabene volunteered to drive ambulances, helping coronavirus patients get to the hospital. Formula 1 Pirelli "Tire King" Mario Isola also rushed to Italy's front line, working as a paramedic during the pandemic. Imagine that level of service and humanitarianism from the luxury class here.

If only.

In New York City, as was the case elsewhere in America, the cost of an ambulance ride to patients varied widely and depended on numerous factors: the medical training level of first responders dispatched to the call (paramedics or EMTs); the type of company that transported the patient and what that particular company billed for ambulance services; how many miles the ambulance traveled to the hospital; medical interventions delivered by first responders (oxygen, IV, et cetera); and how much of the cost the patient's insurance company covered. My ambulance transport after laparoscopic surgery was around $775. My insurance covered a few hundred bucks of that.

Later that afternoon at the race, a duty officer pointed across the track at Nina and told me to go stand next to her. She was alone on the inside of the course, where it curved. I was intimidated.

Nina was slender and Russian, in her early twenties, dark-haired and petite and drop-dead gorgeous, although she didn't think so. She hated her nose. And she maintained the stone-cold gaze of a statue, which gave people the false impression she was angry. I'd heard she was a really good EMT and that she talked very little, whereas I was a person who could rarely shut up. I wanted her to like me so I could ride with her sometime.

She already had a street wife—Austin—a young Asian EMT who worked seasonally during summers and holidays at Park Slope and often joked that all white people looked alike, which was why she so often got us confused. She was presently in graduate school in Boston. And besides, in EMS, street marriages were polyamorous. We enjoyed multiple husbands and wives.

I walked over and stood beside Nina and tried to make small talk. It was a little painful. Quickly I learned that, like me, Nina enjoyed responding to psychiatric emergencies, particularly those involving violence. Her dream job was an EDP with a knife. Suddenly, as if she'd beckoned disaster, a swarm of bikers flew around the bend and a racer hit something and sailed airborne over his handlebars, landing square on his face. A dozen onlookers gasped in unison. I'd never seen anything like it. The biker was completely still for a moment. Dazed. Then he sat up, cupped his palm, and spat up blood and teeth. Jesus!

I was sweating and panting. I couldn't believe I was an EMT, that I was supposed to help people who were critically injured. *Quelle horreur.* I lunged for the tech bag stuffed with bandages and trauma gauze, ready to sprint across the track to help the bleeding biker.

Nina didn't budge. She looked at me then made a barring gesture with her arm like a mother telling a child it wasn't time to cross the street. With her chin she pointed at the pair of EMTs standing in front of an ambulance on the outside of the track, one of whom was Chad.

"Let them take it," she said. "They're in the parking lot so they can exit faster."

Her face was blank as a firefighter's plate. I'd never seen anyone be so calm in an emergency in all my life. I wanted to be like her.

"I love you," I said. "I love that this doesn't affect you at all."

Nina smiled. "I've always liked you. I liked you right from the beginning."

Later, she asked if I wanted to do a tour with her sometime.

Woop woop!

Soon, we started riding every Thursday night, in addition to my Wednesday evening tours with Lexi. I was now on the ambulance twice weekly, giving double the amount of time that was asked of me. I could be like that sometimes. Martyr. Voracious overachiever. But in giving more I received more. Those evenings on the truck with Lexi and Nina were probably the happiest of my life.

That summer things were looking up for me. I was happy on the street. And Tommy was knee-deep in EMDR therapy at Headstrong, having finally ditched his ex and moved forward into a hopeful future. I thought maybe once he felt better, we would meet up. We still texted and talked often about our dreams. He really wanted to get back to writing. We chatted about books and authors, and he cheered me on as I worked on my novel—about him. And I had other things to look forward to in June.

Half a dozen of us EMTs from Park Slope decided to do the Tunnel to Towers stair climb for military and first responders, in memory of a firefighter named Stephen Siller who'd been assigned to Brooklyn's Squad 1. Park Slope EMTs usually participated every year.

On September 11, Stephen finished his tour and was headed to play golf with his brothers when he heard over his scanner that a plane hit the North Tower. He canceled his golf date and drove to the entrance of the Brooklyn Battery Tunnel, but found it closed. He strapped on his gear and ran on through the tunnel to the towers, where he perished.

A firefighter who worked as a personal trainer helped prepare me for the event. Running was one thing, climbing stairs another. I wasn't sure how to get in adequate shape for climbing 104 flights of stairs with a thousand first responders. I was afraid I'd be unable to finish. I was even more terrified I'd fall apart in the stairwell of the Freedom Tower, since Pat had died in the stairwell of the North Tower on 9/11, having received and refused the evacuation order and stayed, not wanting to leave burn victims flooding down the stairs to die alone.

No one dies alone—no one. Not if we can help it. On the street, that's one of our codes.

My trainer, Mateo, once worked at the Fitness Unit in the FDNY. He came to my building gym a few days a week and ran me ragged. Mountain climbers! Burpees! Sprints! It was exhausting and fun. Mateo gave me pep talks and assured me I could complete the climb. He had me run up and down the stairs of my building and, later, the FBI building in Manhattan. In case you've never been inside, don't go. It looks like a prison.

Up and down flights I ran. Mateo told me to take the stairs two at a time, which used the larger and more powerful glute muscles rather than relying on my hamstrings and quads.

"I'm scared I'm going to lose my shit and start crying in the stairwell," I told him one session, relaying the story of Pat.

He said he understood. Then he told me he believed I could do it. "Your friend would be proud of you. And you'll finish. You're ready, and you have more tenacity than most firefighters. Plus, everyone walks up the stairs. Not very many people run, and if they do, they tap out fast. Not even the firefighters run when we do the climb with gear on. Everyone walks."

I was delighted to hear this.

* * *

The morning of the climb, I happily discovered Mateo was right.

Chad and Aaron bolted up the stairs from the jump. But I took the steps two at a time at a steady walking clip and caught up with them on the hundredth floor. Aaron and I finished together, in twenty-five minutes. We made a video of each other, and he bragged in his lilting Jamaican accent about finishing the climb fast. Then I asked him to tell our imaginary audience my time, which was the same as his. We cracked up.

The Tunnel to Towers Foundation people looped ribboned metals around our necks on the observatory deck and took a group photo of us first responders, in which I made Chad pick me up in his arms. Tall girls never get picked up. Everyone go pick up a tall girl.

At one point during the event, a TV newscaster approached me and Aaron. The journalist ignored me and asked Aaron who he was climbing for. "Climbing for?" he said. He was in his twenties. He wasn't climbing for anyone in particular. Standing unseen beside him with Pat buried in the collapsed tower of my heart, I felt quietly destroyed.

I hadn't shed a tear during the climb. But the next morning the grief dam broke upon awakening. I felt so infested with despair I couldn't get out of bed for two days.

Not long after the Tunnel to Towers event, I flew to Mexico and took myself on a romantic vacation for one, to a beach getaway in Tulum. For a week I drank virgin piña coladas alone, and ate breakfast alone, and slept alone, and went to the beach and swam, you guessed it, alone.

Curiously, I started to feel lonely.

It was hurricane season in Mexico. After two days of sun, rainstorms ravaged the beach. There was nothing to do but watch the wet leaves of palm trees thwack against the windows and lie in bed and read. Reading was one of my greatest pleasures ever since I was a girl longing for escape, so I didn't mind the bad weather.

That week I read *The Twelve Lives of Samuel Hawley* by Hannah Tinti, who'd been one of my favorite professors at NYU. Hannah had given us tips for enduring the writing life, which was one of solitude and constant rejection. She suggested we find other writers and befriend them, then tie ourselves together with survival rope. That was what Felice and I did for twenty years. We were in a writers group together. Whenever our work got rejected, which was often, we called each other and said, "Congratulations, sis! You're in the game!"

In addition to befriending other writers, Hannah had said, "Don't forget to leave your house." This was something that only had to be said to writers. Tulum was a rain-soaked bust. But at least I'd left my house.

When I returned to New York, Tommy unexpectedly announced he'd met someone.

Um, what? Excuse me, I was here first.

Apparently, while I was in Mexico, some woman had cut me in line. This was bullshit. I lied and said I was happy for him. Then I addressed my loneliness and resumed swiping around online, looking for someone to stop the bleeding.

Rather speedily I matched with an Airborne paratrooper named Marko. He was in his late thirties. What a beautiful name, Marko. Ukrainian for Marcus, meaning warlike. How auspicious. The app geolocated him in New Jersey.

Frown. I wasn't trying to spend my life on the Jersey Turnpike.

I resented the Garden State for razing my social life in my thirties. Once my girlfriends got married and had their rent-spiking second kid, they invariably moved to Jersey towns with fecund names like Maplewood. They always promised nothing would change in our friendship when they relocated.

Lies.

Once they set foot in Jersey, they were never to be seen on Brooklyn soil again. So I wasn't a fan of that state. But I made an exception. For Marko, I made an exception.

The café I picked for our first date was in Hell's Kitchen. Cement overpasses arced over the trafficked avenues. Drivers honked their way forward. I covered my freckled ears as a fire engine blared by and cursed Manhattan for being so loud, crowded, and natureless. Why did I live here? A New Yorker wonders this every other week.

I turned down Tenth Avenue and there in the middle of the block was the little café. Inside it smelled deliciously of bread. Marko texted that he was stuck in the tunnel. He'd be here soon. I took a seat at the bar and talked to the restaurant manager for a while. Ten minutes. Fifteen.

"Hello," a deep male voice said from behind me.

I turned, and in front of me stood a man so strangely beautiful he looked like one of the Greek gods in Tuileries Garden, Theseus slaying the Minotaur, walking out of sculpted marble into the heart of Manhattan. I was so overloaded with feeling I couldn't speak. The blown fuses of his eyes were blue and his I've-seen-some-shit stare so wide, blank, and unfazed I knew straightaway he'd seen combat. He had dust-colored hair and broad shoulders and was almost my height but seemed skyscraper tall. I stood, and for reasons beyond my understanding threw my arms around his neck. I felt his hand on my hip bone. When we peeled apart, the bell of my body tolled with desire.

"You're beautiful," he said. "And I can tell you right now I already want to see you again."

The manager winked at me and seated us by the window. My pitter-pattering heart dumped a fresh bucket of sweat into the armholes of my dress. I hadn't felt this excited to meet someone in a long time. I ordered a sandwich. Something involving arugula. Marko passed on food. He'd eaten a late lunch and was driving back to Washington, DC, after our date.

Wait. "DC? I thought you lived in Jersey."

"No, I'm at Fort Belvoir. I'm teaching a course there in the fall. I'm from Jersey."

"But you currently live in DC."

"For now. I'm applying to PhD programs next year at Princeton and NYU, so hopefully I'll be living back east again soon."

Marko had just returned from his fourth tour overseas, one in Iraq and three in Afghanistan, and now he was on leave for a month. His ex-wife and son lived in New Jersey. He was here spending time with them. He was driving to DC for a training and would be back next week.

We talked for an hour or so. He'd been overseas for a while, so he had some questions about changes to the country that confused him. What was avocado toast? Title gave it away, an avocado mushed on toast. Why was there so much incest porn online now? *Game of Thrones* was my guess.

For the first time in his career Marko had no deployments on the calendar, so he'd be visiting his son once a month now that he was stateside. He had an amicable relationship with his ex-wife; they'd divorced four years ago. Their marriage fell apart after he was wounded during his first tour. She wanted him to leave the military. He wanted to stay in.

"Your turn," Marko said.

As the waiter delivered my sandwich, I told him I was a writer and said what I did for work, which, unlike the rest of the human race, he understood without me having to explain it for three hours. He liked that I had a serious career.

Politely, he excused himself to use the bathroom, saying, "My bladder's fucked up from the war."

My bladder was fucked up from that surgery! Twins.

While I waited for his return, I shoved a peppery sprig of arugula in my mouth and did math on the chalkboard of my head. Could I date someone based in DC who visited Jersey once a month? Um, yes. Absolutely. I loved solitude. No place I'd rather be than alone, reading and writing. Once a month seemed like the perfect amount of time with a man.

When Marko returned from the bathroom this, him, all of it suddenly seemed too good to be true. I had an inrush of fear that he was fake. The small child, the dashing Army officer job, the war, the wound, DC. Maybe it was unreal, and he was impersonating a soldier. The investigator in me awakened. Military romance scams were a huge problem. There were loads of bots online, and Felice never let me forget the time years back when I got bamboozled by one.

"Are you really a soldier?" I asked. "You're flagging for all the indicators of a military romance scam."

"Am I? That's funny."

Marko pulled out his phone and showed me a photograph of him shaking the killing hand of Secretary of Defense General James "It's-fun-to-shoot-some-people" Mattis, and another where he stood smiling beside Elizabeth Warren, who he referred to as his wife.

I felt a pinch of jealousy toward Senator Warren. I brushed it off. Brush brush brush. In another photograph Marko stood in dress blues while being awarded a ribboned medal.

"Where's your saber?"

"We can wear our blues anywhere, but we have to get permission to wear the sword."

"I'm not buying it. You're not real."

Marko took out his wallet and slapped his military ID on the table. "I'm real. See? And if you want to see my divorce papers, I have those on me too, because I need to hand them over at Fort Belvoir."

Newly confident he was legit, I asked Marko if he still loved her—his wife. Ex-wife. He said he respected and admired her. Without her, he would have killed himself after his first tour in Iraq. She'd stuck it out with him and given him a son after he'd been injured three weeks into his first deployment. He got blown up and suffered a traumatic brain injury and lost all his front teeth. He had shrapnel in his neck. When the medic arrived the first thing he asked the guy was if he had everything. Meaning his limbs, I intuited. "Yes sir," the medic said. "But your translator is dead."

Marko felt guilty about that for a long time, asking about himself before his translator. But he knew his translator was dead because the gentleman's severed torso was what blew him against the dashboard, at which point he sat up and started vomiting blood and hard little bits he later recognized as his teeth.

My eyes flashed with wonder. I could picture this exactly, having seen that biker crash at the Red Hook Crit. I felt grateful I could visualize some of what he'd experienced at war and impressed that he gave credit where credit was due, to his ex-wife who'd saved his ass after his first tour.

Marko asked if I felt like going for a walk along the water. Sure thing. I closed out and we stood up. I took his warm, handsome face in my hands.

"Smile, let me see."

He smiled and clicked his fingernails on his front teeth. "These are all fake."

"They look great. They look even better than real teeth."

Outside, we strolled down the bright, loud, romantic street, toward the river. New York seemed like the most impressive city in the world. Marko made sure I walked on the protected side of the sidewalk, away from the flow of traffic, so if a car hopped the curb and crashed into us, he would get hit first.

When we got to the river, he pulled out his phone and took a photo of us together, and he said, "This is going to be the picture I frame and put on my nightstand after we move in together."

Swoon.

For hours we walked along the river and talked. I clutched onto the trunk of his arm like an endangered orangutan. With ease, openness, and a sense of comfort that made me feel as if we'd known each other a thousand years and been parted by a thousand wars, we fed each other the wretched and lovely stories of our lives from antiquity to present, listened sympathetically when the other spoke, and laughed at the tragic bends in the road where laughter was the only salve.

Things I learned as we looked out on the Intrepid Sea, Air & Space Museum: Marko loved to read and hoped to own a bookstore one day. He also loved the mountains and wanted to build a cabin, maybe in Colorado or Maine. He learned I grew up in the Mojave Desert and summered in the Sequoia National Forest as a girl. And that I loved trees, and reading, and was an EMT.

He looked at me with lit-up eyes. "That's really admirable, that you do service. We have the same archangel. Saint Michael, patron saint of EMTs, medics, police, and military. I want to see you in uniform."

"Really?"

I'd never once considered men might like women in uniform. Was it possible they had the same weakness, the same reverence for service and bravery that plagued me? What kind of man desired a woman who thought of belts as tourniquets and carried a CPR pocket mask in her purse, as I was carrying now? The thought blew my mind.

"Of course I want to see you in uniform," Marko said. "It works both ways."

It worked both ways!

"Was your wife military?"

"Librarian. But after my divorce I dated this badass Air Force officer. Then I dated an Army psychologist. Then an FBI agent."

"Oh, God. We're the same person."

"I've dated a lot of women in uniform," Marko mused. "I blame Trooper Wendy. She came to my class in fifth grade and told everyone to Just Say No to drugs. I wanted to be a trooper because of her, but then I joined the National Guard. I ran into her the day after 9/11, actually, on the way to Ground Zero, when the New Jersey Guard got called in to help, before the New York National Guard kicked us out. I went up to her and said, 'Trooper Wendy, my name's Marko. I met you in fifth grade and you're the reason I said no to drugs.'"

I told Marko I lost a firefighter friend in 9/11.

Immediately his expression turned serious. "I'm so sorry. I worked the site for a few days after the attack, and what I saw in those forty-eight hours was worse than everything I saw in Afghanistan in all my tours. It never gets better, losing someone in the line of duty."

I turned my face away.

Later, as sun scattered across the river, we kissed. I felt like I could finally breathe. Like the universe gave me a pat on the back and said to me in the kindest voice, You're not alone. You thought you were, but you're not. Here's someone just like you, to love.

My highest hope was that Marko and I would fall for each other, and maybe he could come with me to Pat's firehouse this year, since he understood the profoundness of my grief. Now that he was stateside and without a deployment calendared, he planned to apply to doctorate programs to get a PhD in the weaponization of data. "Like what Russia's doing to us right now."

Looking back on this day many years later, playing it and replaying it in my head, I came to recognize the moment Marko uttered those amorous three words—weaponization of data—as the moment I fell in love.

One Saturday in July, I picked up a Smorgasburg tour with Luna, our dispatcher. She was a young, bespectacled, easy-to-laugh Ecuadorian woman who worked overnights and got less sleep than a giraffe, which topped out at 1.9 hours a night. Most Thursdays when Nina and I finished our tour and returned to base at midnight, we lingered and hung out with her.

Luna worked alone in the dispatch room, sitting at a desk crammed with phones, radios, two-screened computers, bags of candy, and enormous cups of coffee. We chatted about the street and emergencies and love. Often, Luna fell asleep and snored in the middle of a sentence. We gave her a few minutes then poked her awake. "Don't tell Beck I fell asleep" were always the first words out of her mouth.

Spending time with servicepeople who work overnights and twenty-fours—dispatchers, cops, soldiers, firefighters in busy battalions—I couldn't help but remember sleep deprivation was a tool of war, creating a plethora of harmful symptoms in its recipients. These ranged from hallucinations to aggressiveness, memory deficits to accelerated aging, performance degradation to derelict conduct, most commonly with excessive alcohol use and high-risk sexual behavior, not to mention shorter lifespans and double the risk of death from cardiovascular disease than well-rested human beings.

Symptomatically, as with people suffering from diabetic emergencies, lack of sleep mimicked alcohol intoxication. If you were working with a first responder who hadn't slept, you were essentially dealing with a cognitive drunk. Of all the great and idiotic suggestions made for improving the behavior and lives of first responders, I often wondered why "let them sleep" went undiscussed.

"Do you think it's the job?" Tommy asked me one night after he'd forgotten something I'd told him ten times and found himself wondering why he was sexually aroused after coming off a sleepless twenty-four at his Bronx firehouse.

"Yes," I said. "Next question."

This blue-skied Saturday in Brooklyn, Luna drove the ambulance to Prospect Park. She positioned the truck beneath the shade of a tree near an assembly of tented food stalls erected for Smorgasburg. We commenced our eight-hour event tour with our seats reclined as far back as they would go, our knees bent, and our unbloused boots on the dashboard.

Like me, Luna had quit online dating apps, where she had one of the best and simplest descriptions of her work life I'd ever read. "Unusual hours," her Tinder bio said.

First responders, like celebrities, tend to date one another. Cops date nurses, nurses date firefighters, and firefighters—firefighters date everyone. I suspected it had to do with the cruel and unusual nature of our jobs, which came with a fair share of toxic stories. The stories I acquired on the street had the potential to horrify civilians and made me feel lonely and sick if they went unshared. Not everyone on a first date wanted to hear about the baby who got hit by a car while they were sniffing aromatic wines. But first responders did. First responders would listen to anything.

Luna was in a new, choppy-watered relationship with a firefighter who kept breaking up with her then returning. It flummoxed her and made her tearful, as she loved him, though she wasn't ready to use that word yet—love.

I could relate.

That summer I started to feel Marko was my soul mate. Even Tommy, my therapized firefighter, was happy for me. He liked the line-cutter woman he was seeing, too. Win-win.

We thought we were winning.

Marko and I called and texted and videoed each other constantly. One day driving around Brooklyn together, a jaywalker crossed the street on a red light while looking at his phone.

"That guy's getting hit by a car tonight," I said. "Ped struck. He'll roll over the hood and be hospitalized with a concussion in an hour."

Marko burst into laughter and said, "My baby's an EMT!"

Baby was.

Often I read Marko funny e-mails my mother sent me from California that read like a police blotter. A weather report followed by a cooking update followed by the deaths of church ladies and neighbors she knew, e.g., "It's hot in Bakersfield. One hundred and three yesterday. Way too hot. I made Italian wedding soup for the church. Milburn died."

I didn't know Milburn.

Marko said he couldn't wait to meet my mother.

Whenever he was in town, we made love at my house until we had unsteady gaits. I cooked him the only dish I could make excellently, a cast-iron roasted chicken with leeks. He ate two plates to make me happy even though he'd already eaten dinner with his son. He gave me his soft-worn T-shirt to sleep in and before I put it on, I pressed it against my face and inhaled his musky scent. But there were some hiccups.

Burps?

One weekend we'd gone upstate for a romantic getaway. We booked an Airbnb on a glimmering lake in Kingston. There, I started to notice some things about Marko that worried me. One day he drank ten beers. That was a lot. Sometimes he texted me drunk, in a blackout, having forgotten what day it was.

I could put up with almost anything a man threw my way—my therapist would say too much—but not substance abuse issues. That's where I drew the line. I buried my worry and told myself to relax. Marko was just back from war. And he was a happy drunk. Whenever he got shitfaced, he wept about maps, "because maps created the world."

In Kingston one night he showed me a video of him as a paratrooper, jumping out of a C-17.

"Are you scared when you jump? I'm still scared on the ambulance."

"I'm terrified every single time."

"That makes me feel better."

Later that same night a storm rolled in. We fell asleep early as the rain tapped on the windows. In the dark I prayed Marko would ask me to be his girlfriend. We took a lot of pictures together in Kingston, and I hoped maybe he'd put one of them on Instagram and show the world we were in love. We said it to each other now, "I love you."

But the next afternoon when we drove home, in the car, Marko said to me, "What I love about you is that you're a modern woman. You don't need to get married or put some relationship title on what we have. There's no need. What we have is special. And we can keep dating other people when I go back to DC next month. You can keep your virtual firefighter," he said, referring to Tommy. "My baby loves her firefighters."

I stared out the window the rest of the drive home.

Luna and I discussed this and much more that jobless summer afternoon at Smorgasburg as the shade disappeared and we boiled inside the ambulance, the air-conditioner vents blowing out lukewarm air due to the idling engine.

I asked why she never rode on the truck. She told me she became a dispatcher because being an EMT gave her too much anxiety. No matter how many times she tried, she just never settled into the job, which perhaps more than most occupations, was certainly not for everyone. She made an exception to pick up this event tour with me because she knew we'd get no calls and we could sit on the ambulance all day and talk.

"I have to warn you," I said. "Last time I worked this event we got no jobs for eight hours straight. And then five minutes before our tour ended, we got a flagged for an injury."

Luna kicked the dashboard. "Don't say that! I can't believe you just said that! Now it will happen!"

First responders are superstitious. We work in the realm of life and death. In what the Irish call "thin places," where the dividing line between the real and eternal vanishes, creating an ephemeral atmosphere and, often, direct talk about the existence of otherworldly signs, symbols, and ghosts. Put plainly there's a lot of weird shit that goes down on the street and operating in this surreal realm comes with its own laws and purple sortilege about what you're allowed and not allowed to say.

One of the widely held beliefs in EMS was that if you said it was a quiet night, you'd soon be slathered in a rich buttery flying cake of jobs. Incantation equaled manifestation. If you said the last time you drove down that street a child got hit by a car, an hour later you'd respond to a child hit by a car on that very same block. So imagine Luna's anger at me when five minutes before our tour ended, we got flagged for an injury. Ha.

"That was your fault!" she screamed at me after we transported a lady with a dislocated shoulder to the hospital. "You said that happened last time, so it happened to us!"

She still brings it up to this day, my beloved Luna. Years have passed, and I continue to hear about this and repent for causing us to have a job five minutes before our tour ended.

As for Marko, we didn't survive September. None of my relationships ever did.

Labor Day weekend he was supposed to be in town. He said we could see each other late Monday night in Jersey, then he would wake up early Tuesday morning to take his son to his first day of school, then drive back to DC. It wasn't much time together. It was scraps. But at least it was something. I grew up in emotional deprivation. That was home. Ignore me, I'd be yours forever.

I wondered what Marko was getting up to that holiday weekend. I figured he was busy moving into his new place. It was hard for me to articulate how badly I needed to see him as the anniversary of September 11 approached, and I became a haunted woman.

Sunday morning, the day before we were supposed to meet, out of the blue, a bomb. Marko posted a photo on Instagram from a Jack Johnson concert in Colorado. I was sitting in a group meditation in Tribeca with Pat's girl, Ylfa, when I saw the photo. I had no idea my not-boyfriend was in Colorado. I liked music. How come he didn't invite me? He didn't even bother to tell me he was there. I thought he was in DC. I felt so unconsidered and stupid. Immediately my love for him fled. I bolted out of the meditation room.

Ylfa called me after she discovered my seat was empty. I told her what had happened, and she ran downtown to the little park across from City Hall and found me sitting on a bench with my splotchy face in my hands. I cried in her arms for I don't know how long.

When I got home, I called one of my friends in Paris, a writer named Josh. He knew me better than I knew myself. I trusted him to catch my tears but also give me the hard truth in regard to how I got myself into this despairing situation. I was a smart woman and yet in matters of the heart, so dumb.

"Read 'Bardon Bus,'" Josh told me. "By Alice Munro. It's about a successful woman writer who suffers horribly in her love life. She always falls for the wrong guy and has a huge bounce-back factor."

As soon as we hung up, I ran to my bookshelf and pulled out Alice Munro. Then I crawled in bed and filled my literature prescription. The medicine worked.

What a relief, reading this story, to learn I wasn't alone. Books really were, for me, a form of lifesaving first aid. When I came upon this passage, I highlighted it in green:

"There is a limit to the amount of misery and disarray you will put up with, for love, just as there is a limit to the amount of mess you can stand around a house. You can't know the limit beforehand, but you will know it when you've reached it."

I had reached it.

But knowing this didn't stop the pain. The next week I wept through my ambulance tour with Lexi. She was outraged Marko had hurt me.

"What'd you do to my partner!" she screamed as she drove. "She's always so happy and now she can't stop crying!" She sped lights-and-sirens to buy me ice cream, and I loved her for that.

Nina, too. Hearing the story the next night, she hated Marko from the bottom of her Russian heart.

These women. My street wives, sisters, partners. I didn't know how I would get through this life without them. Much has been written, perhaps a bit too much, if you ask me, on the importance of brotherhood. Of sisterhood we hear almost nothing. But time and again, my life has been saved by women.

This year on the anniversary of September 11, I was marinating on the idea of joining FDNY as an EMT, in remembrance of Pat. I often talked about this with Pat. I didn't speak to him out loud or anything. But sometimes in my prayers I consulted him and asked him for brotherly advice. I somehow felt like I wasn't a real EMT unless I worked for his beloved Fire Department.

Pat's brother, Mike, was unable to attend the ceremonies in New York this year. He was stuck in Vegas being an ER doctor, so at the firehouse I clung rather desperately to Ylfa. But of course, at times she chatted with other people.

At one point a tall, dark-haired firefighter about my height saw me standing alone, looking glumly around the firehouse. Before I knew it, he was planted in front of me. He introduced himself as Gonzo, short for Steve Gonzalez. He asked who I was there to see. I pointed to Pat's bannered face. Immediately his smile brightened with the same joy and sorrow washed across the faces of other men standing nearby. He swiveled on his foot and called other men over.

"Hey Mike, Johnny, Richie, guys, get over here. Come meet Jennifer, she's a friend of Pat Brown."

Retired firemen appeared and shook my hand as if I were someone special. I was so touched. I shook hands with them all, one after another, and we stood around and told stories about Pat that brought him back to life.

"We used to practice yoga together," I told a wiry white guy named Mike. Half the guys at the firehouse were named Mike. Ylfa later told me I'd been talking to Michael Daly, a writer and beautiful person, one of Pat's close friends.

"You look like you knew him from yoga," Michael Daly said. "You know what Pat used to say? He'd say, 'Hey Mike, there's a lotta hot chicks who practice yoga, you should try it. Lots of beautiful women, but they're all fucking nuts!'"

He shook with laughter, as did I.

Pat had been quite the ladies' man in his day, but I was more like his kid sister. He looked out for me, and everyone else he came into contact with, so it wasn't like we were especially close. Pat was an important person in my life, but I was just one resident in the city of people he helped. Anyway, I didn't want any of the guys to think we had that kind of thing going on. Whenever they introduced me as a friend of Pat's, I swiftly followed it up with, "Not that kind of friend. He was like a brother."

Constantly the veteran firefighters checked on me, asking if I wanted coffee, or tea, or anything to eat. They had a spread in the kitchen. I was starving and undercaffeinated but afraid to go deeper into the firehouse without Ylfa.

"How tall are you?" a retired firefighter named Johnny asked me. He made a visor out of his hands and ran it over my head.

"Six-one? Two?"

"Six-one."

"Six-one! Amazing."

"You play basketball?" Gonzo wanted to know.

"I played volleyball in college."

"What do you do, Jennifer?" Johnny asked. "Are you a nurse?"

Never in my life had I wanted to become a nurse.

I started to say I was an investigator but instead blurted out, "I'm a writer and an EMT. I think Pat would find it funny."

Johnny said, "Pat would love that! Why don't you become a firefighter?"

"I'm old. And I grew up in the desert. I don't like the heat."

"Got it. EMT then, like you're doing. I started out as an EMT. Boy do I got some stories for you. Remind me to tell you about the one with the eyeballs."

"Jennifer, don't listen to him," Gonzo said. "He's fucking crazy. He collects knives. He has all kinds of knives. One day when we were at the firehouse, I opened his locker and I seen all these knives. I said, 'Hey buddy, whatcha planning on doing with all these knives?'"

We roared laughing. It felt so good to laugh. A little break from the crushing grief, this year mixed with heartbreak over Marko, who took a meat cleaver to my heart with that dumb and unpredictable Instagram photo. I was someone who still suffered the aftershock consequences of terrorism from 9/11. The unpredictable was not a cozy experience for me.

The second Gonzo turned to speak to someone else, Johnny launched into his EMT story. Once someone knows you're an EMT, they hit you with their craziest stories.

"One time I saw this guy after an MVA," he said, describing a motor vehicle accident, "a drunk driver whose eyeballs came out of the sockets. They were dangling by threads. Then when the medical examiner showed up, he was fucking crazy, he snipped the threads right in front of me with these weird scissors on account of the driver was an organ donor. Then he stuck the eyeballs in a plastic bag with some clear liquid in it and he shook the bag in my face like the eyeballs were a couple of goldfish. I never drove drunk after that. Never. Not once in my life."

Just then Ylfa came up to us and handed me a mourning band. I ran my fingers over Pat's name and a little green shamrock. I felt like she'd handed me the most precious gold.

"It's so nice," I said, handing it back.

"Do you have one?"

"No."

"Take it," Ylfa said. "It's mine."

It seemed like too big a gift. Again I tried to give it back. "I can't take yours."

"Take it. Bobby's got a whole bag of them. I'll get another one."

Johnny said, "You can wear it on the street when you're out there doing your EMT thing. That way Pat will be on the ambulance with you."

I put it around my wrist and imagined Pat's hand clasping onto mine. It was magic, this band. It was Irish.

Gonzo said, "Jennifer, come into the kitchen. Eat something. You look like you need to eat."

He took my hand and we glided past silent rows of slack-armed young firemen who cleared the way as we walked by. "Hey, guys, this is Jennifer," Gonzo told them. "She was a good friend of Pat Brown." In the kitchen he poured me coffee and said, "You coming down to the memorial with us after the moments of silence?"

I said, "I don't know what I'm doing. I've never gone down there on 9/11."

I worried it would be too much. Today it was only open for family and service members.

"OK," Gonzo said, "what you're doing is, you're coming down there with us. We'll do the moments of silence here, then a few of us go down to the memorial with Pat's sister, Carolyn—you're coming—and then we come back here for the Mass."

"Are you sure it's OK for me to come?"

"Whaddya mean? Of course it's OK. You belong here. You're one of us."

An hour or so later, down at the memorial, Gonzo's demeanor changed. He became somber. The other veteran firefighters had stayed behind at the firehouse, saying forlornly they weren't up for going "down there." We walked up to Pat's name and stared into the dark twin wells. I wept standing next to Pat's sister. Gonzo dashed off and returned with a pack of tissues. He handed them to us.

"You're a gentleman," I said. "One of the last."

"I saw you crying, so then I went and grabbed 'em off that table over there."

"We're not crying," Carolyn said. "We have allergies."

Gonzo glanced around at the flocks of weeping mourners. "Everyone here has allergies."

We stood shoulder to shoulder in agonized silence. Gonzo bowed his head. When he raised it, his eyes were glassy and distant. After a long time, he spoke. He talked about being close with Pat. He told me stories. As I listened, I tried to memorize every word he said, carve his stories of Pat into my heart so I'd never forget them. These stories were all we had left.

"They were murdered," Gonzo said. His lip quivered, and his voice cracked with anger. "That's what they never say in the papers, but that's what happened. My friends, all of them, they were murdered. It was a massacre down there. I don't have guilt like some of the other guys who survived. I didn't get inside the towers on time, and everyone in the towers died. I turned one way and they turned another, and I lived, and they didn't. That's just what happened. That's how it is. Pat used to say, 'When your number's up, your number's up.' So I don't have guilt. But they were murdered, those guys. Each and every one of them was a great guy, and they didn't deserve it. It's a horrible way to die. I wouldn't wish that way of dying on anyone."

"I'm so sorry," I said. I knew Pat's firehouse had been one that suffered some of the most casualties. I knew it, but now I felt it. And I could feel Pat's presence, his spirit mixing with ours. He knew we were there. He knew we were together.

"That's why I hate coming down here," Gonzo said. "I hate putting on this uniform. I can't bear it. I haven't been down here in years and this is why. It's agony, being here. That's what it is. When I'm down here I get so angry. We lost eleven guys that day. Twelve, with a chief gone. It was a fluke that I lived. We had one guy who lost a brother. Then we had the widows, and little kids. Everyone at the firehouse asking for their husbands and fathers. The whole company was missing. It was a nightmare. And it went on and on. It wasn't just that day. We worked the pile. We dug. It took them a long time to find their bodies. To find even parts of their bodies. It took months. And some guys—there was nothing for the family to bury. How do you move on when there's nothing to bury?

"We were going to funerals every week, twice a week, every month for years. Then when you get a little break, a few years later, the cancer starts. Practically everyone who worked the cleanup got cancer. I got cancer. I don't know how I'm still alive. By now I've buried most of my friends. It's still going, the cancer. It makes me so angry. I know beneath the anger is sadness and fear and beneath that maybe there's something else."

He took a moment, then said, "I'm sorry I'm like this. It's just being down here all I can feel is anger."

"Pat used to be angry, too," I said. "Remember how angry he'd get sometimes?"

"Oh yeah."

"He was a great guy," I said.

"Yes, he was."

"He helped a lot of people."

"He helped everyone. Wasn't a person who knew him he didn't touch. Never left anyone behind. Just the type of person he was." Gonzo took a deep breath then said, "They're gone, but we don't forget 'em. They were great guys, each and every one of them. Oh well."

"Oh well," I said.

Oh well.

Back at the firehouse later that afternoon, Gonzo hugged me goodbye. I was so grateful to have spent time with him, with all the guys who knew Pat. There weren't that many of them left, fewer and fewer every year. After we hugged, Gonzo took me by the shoulders and said, "You keep going as an EMT. Stay safe, and next year I want to see you back here in uniform."

I wanted him to see me in uniform, too. There was nothing in my closet I loved more than my uniform. Each time I put it on I felt powerful. I wanted to make Pat proud, and every time I put my uniform on, I felt like I accomplished it. But what Gonzo said at the memorial, about hating putting on his uniform, that haunted me. I was so pleased working on the street as an EMT I couldn't imagine going from this sense of gratitude to feeling like my uniform was not a prayer or an offering, it was a sheet draped over a corpse. A garment of agony.

6

THE 99 PERCENT

Soon I was back on the ambulance, now with Pat's name wrapped around my wrist. Wearing the mourning band made me feel divinely protected. As I fell in love with my EMT nightlife, my daylight career grew less compelling to me.

Sure, my clients were in crises. But many of them were heading some of the world's most powerful companies. They were millionaires. They drove Audis and had second homes in the Hamptons.

It wasn't that they didn't suffer, the 1 percenters. They had disabled children who got bullied on the Internet. Family members on suicide watch in prison. They got wrongfully accused of hideous behavior and persecuted on Twitter based on social media pseudo-truths. But compared to the crushing healthcare disasters I was seeing on the street, the bare human need of patients requiring medical care, my clients began to feel somewhat luxurious and predictable.

So did desk life. Writing. Sitting inside alone all day, staring at a computer screen, working on a novel.

Occasionally, I toyed with the idea of becoming an EMT full-time, despite having no interest in riding for a private company or hospital crew, and no idea how I could live on the salary of an FDNY EMT. That seemed like career suicide.

Meanwhile, my job involved a lot of client meetings, flying around the country to have hushed business conversations in hotel bars and Michelin-starred restaurants. Now I was so at home in my uniform that whenever I slipped on a dress and heels—kitten heels—I felt like I was performing a strange version of myself.

When people saw me on the street in business attire, they often called me gazelle-like and graceful. One barista in my neighborhood told me he imagined after I got coffee, I flew off to the White House. More like the firehouse. Another time, I was in SoHo when an older man standing next to me on the street asked if I was a model. I told him I was not. He shook his head disappointedly. "That's too bad," he said. "You could have been someone." I could have been someone!

Wait, I thought. I am someone.

But I was an itchy someone. I became an EMT because I wanted to help people. I wanted to save lives. After being on the street for over a year I was astounded by how little lifesaving actually went on in the field. Bullshit nonemergency jobs swallowed most of our nights whole.

All these tours, and I still hadn't caught a single cardiac arrest. I felt like the other EMTs who'd joined Park Slope when I did were outpacing me. MJ and Chad rode with Nathan, a known black cloud. By winter 2018 they were charging headstrong into big crashing waves of medical trauma, working loads of arrests and femur fractures, leapfrogging me on the experience front. Even Raz, whose hands no longer shook on scene, had caught an arrest. I was itching to work more serious emergencies.

Be careful what you itch for.

While we worked Wednesday nights and she waited to get into nursing school, Lexi frequently repeated the idiom that EMS was 99 percent bullshit, one percent "Oh, shit."

In contrast to working transport, where patients were nonambulatory, many of the people who called 911 could walk; a pleasant surprise. I lifted half as many patients as an EMT at Park Slope than I had when I'd transported grandmas and bilateral amputees like Rita and Garrison.

Lexi underscored the importance of physical preservation and working smarter, not harder. "Assist before lift," she often said. "If a patient has a broken shoulder, walk them to the ambulance. Their legs aren't broken. Save your back."

Given that paramedics and EMTs were at greater risk for occupational injuries and assault than workers in any other profession, with eight to nine

EMTs and medics out of every hundred treated in the hospital for on-the-job injuries, compared to two workers out of every hundred in other jobs, I heeded her advice.

On the bullshit front, we responded to people who called 911 for an ambulance because of a toothache. Patients whose stomachs hurt after they ate ice cream. People with runny noses, blisters, scraped knees. Patients who thought they may have twisted their ankle while shopping at Target. Many things went wrong for people at Target. And nearly every job that came over for an injury at McDonald's was an intoxicated fast-food patron who'd fallen off their chair. Minor tragedies ensued that perfumed my hair with the fragrance of French fries.

Then there were people who milked the EMS system and used ambulances like Ubers, inspiring first responders to call their emergency vehicles Uberlances, resources misused to transport barely sick people to the hospital when a car service to a walk-in medical clinic would have sufficed.

Sadder jobs were the reverse. People our healthcare system pervasively failed. "Frequent fliers," we called them. Patients we saw once, twice, sometimes as often as eight times a month.

Regulars were often EDPs, intoxes, or a powerful concoction of both. Alcohol intoxication is tied to a stunning number of 911 calls and strains EMS systems nationwide. Excessive alcohol use results in over 2.7 million ER visits each year, an average of 2.3 million years of potential loss of life, costing the country around $249 billion dollars annually. Some states addressed the crush of 911 calls for intoxicated patients by dedicating special EMS resources just to meet the needs of chronic drug and alcohol abusers.

Almost all leaders in the field of emergency management agreed that unnecessary use of ambulance services and misuse of 911 for nonemergencies must somehow, in some way, stop. In Nevada, innovative programs had nurses answer 911 calls to determine whether or not the patient required emergency care and, if not, helped them find non-ER resources. In Houston, a telehealth program allowed arriving EMS staff to assess whether or not the call was a genuine emergency and offered video physician consultations. In a mobile healthcare pilot program in Dallas, fire-rescue crews made preventative community health visits to "frequent fliers" who constantly called for ambulances. This resulted in an 82 percent reduction in 911 calls.

In much of Western Europe, where I'd had the luck of living and working at times, doctors and/or nurses commonly rode on ambulances and assisted first responders. I'd fallen sick in Paris (where firefighters are also paramedics) on several occasions. There, you could call SOS Médecins, a 24/7 medical emergency service line that sent a doctor to your house instead of an ambulance. The doctor came to your door with a briefcase full of medical supplies, examined you, drew blood or took a urine specimen or whatever was needed, prescribed medicine, and left you at home—all for about seventy-five euros last time I checked, about eighty-eight bucks. Similar adoptions of this medical home-care model could be found in London, Rome, Geneva, Brussels, and other regions.

Universal healthcare. We are in the dark ages with this shit.

The streets of New York City provide no similar widespread offerings. Here, we treat and transport chronically intoxicated patients to the ER, where they sleep it off and then get released and sent home as soon as they're able to walk. They continue to drink, someone calls 911 on them again, and bloop—they're back on the ambulance, headed back to the same hospital to sleep it off. It's a vicious cycle. Or vicious circle. One of those.

Intoxicated patients are also frequently linked to traumatic injuries. Drunk people constantly fall down and crack their heads open. They get violent and assault people or try to kill themselves. They get behind the wheel and weaponize their cars. On the ambulance, they pee their pants, shit their pants, and often throw up on themselves, and on us.

There are EMTs on the street who've worked so many intoxes they have adverse, allergic reactions to these patients, and respond to them with a mixture of revulsion and disgust. If you didn't want to become one of these pathologically emotionless rescuers whose chest X-rays would show a dark empty void, you had to constantly produce new hearts.

As for me, doing the meditation, prayer, gym, sobriety, and healthy eating work required to stay fresh, stay sensitive, and stay kind on the street started to feel like a part-time job.

My favorite regular of the intox stripe was Kentaro, a flirty man in his fifties who got hammered in bars then passed out and had a siesta on the street. Inevitably, bystanders found him heaped on the sidewalk, and, believing he was dead, called 911. Kentaro usually came over the radio as an "unconscious" or "other," vague call types that were either nonsense or fatally serious.

Time after time we'd pull up with a blaring fire engine only to find our beloved, intoxicated Kentaro having a snooze. We'd tap his shoulder and rouse him—"Kentaro, wake up, my love. Time to go to the hospital." "Kentaro, honey, are you dead? These people called 911 because they think you're dead."—shocking bystanders who had no idea what the hell was going on. Most nights Kentaro looked up at me from the sidewalk and smiled. Then he closed his eyes, puckered his lips, and asked for a kiss.

Smooch. Love you, Kentaro.

He was in love with an FDNY EMT named Sally. He told me this one night as we headed to his favorite hospital, which he called his home, where ER nurses knew his date of birth and Social Security number by heart.

"Have you ever gone out drinking with him?" a nurse once asked another nurse when we brought him into the ER. "He's a lot of fun."

Fun, and dying of ethanol abuse, which was what we wrote in the chief complaint box of Kentaro's chart every time we picked him up: "ETOH abuse." Had things not turned around for me in my mid-twenties, and had I not had a model for how to live a sober, meaningful life like the one gifted to me from people like Pat, I could have been Kentaro. I thought this whenever I saw him. *There but for the grace of God go I.* I thought about my brother, who'd been drunk most of his adult life, and refused all sisterly help. I'd heard he was doing much better. I wouldn't know. We were warmly estranged.

Being a first responder was tough. But being a sober first responder was a thousand-layer cake of pain.

It wasn't just chronic alcoholics we transported often on the street. Quickly I discovered many people who called 911 were suffering from loneliness and its headless horseman cousins: sexual assault, opioid addiction, poverty, and hate crimes.

Going on runs with vague descriptions like "other," we frequently arrived on scene and got the story of what went south for the patient, and discovered things were much graver than we imagined. It was like waking up on Christmas morning to a room full of beautifully wrapped gifts with endless opportunities for astonishment, but when we yanked the red ribbon and opened the boxes, all the presents were sad.

Sad presents. That's what we opened most nights on scene.

The call that came over the radio for the "unconscious" turned out to be a white woman lying naked on the sidewalk with a military ID and a used condom at her side, drugged to the eyeballs and suspected of having been roofied, raped, and left for dead. The "assault" job turned out to be a transgender, female-identified patient jumped by a gang of boys, the victim of a hate crime. The "other" was a large Black man we found sitting on the subway stairs with Taser wires streaming out of his back like the copper hairs on the tail of a horse, handcuffed and surrounded by cops.

That job I cursed the police under my breath and felt sorry for my tased patient. Next morning I woke up and saw his face in the newspaper, and learned he was a repeat sex offender who liked to pull his magic hose out in front of children on the subway, a guy transit cops had been trying to arrest for years.

When I told this story to my dentist, a Black woman Felice introduced me to, she said, "They *should* tase that guy." So then I felt a little less sad? Sadder? Sadder in a different way?

All of these calls occurred on the affluent and supposedly safe white streets of Park Slope and Cobble Hill. And people gave me shit for living in mostly Black Stuyvesant Heights, casually referring to my neighborhood as a war zone.

Mmm-hmm.

"That was a sad job," Lexi often said after we cleared the hospital.

Yes. Merry Christmas. Here are some EMS presents. They're all sad.

One evening Lexi came to base in tears after seeing a homeless man on the street drinking bleach. When she asked what he was doing, he told her he didn't want to live anymore. She knocked the container out of his hands and called 911, reporting a suicide attempt.

That's what that was, by the way, before *and* after then President Trump suggested drinking bleach was a solution to COVID. Bleach was poison. Drinking it was a suicide attempt.

As a first responder your heart breaks each tour and a new heart grows in its place. Then that one breaks, too.

One quiet winter night when Nina and I rode together, we did some forgettable jobs, got fish tacos, and made several trips to 7-Eleven. Inside, we bought each other cheap joke presents. Globe roses floating in strange clear liquid. Matching "stone" bracelets that looked like plaqued broken teeth strung on elastic. No gift from 7-Eleven was too cheap or magical.

That cliché held. The cops were always at Dunkin' Donuts, we were always at 7-Eleven, and not a tour went by that we didn't see a fire engine pull up to the grocery store. "The heroes ran out of chicken again," we joked.

Nina and I both loved to bake and watched *90 Day Fiancé* and *Love After Lockup*, as did Felice and I, so there was a great deal to discuss during quiet nights on the truck.

This night I told Nina about a cop who always hugged me on scene, at EDP jobs. No one I told this story to could understand how or why this happened.

"He *hugged* you?" Rafael said one day on the phone. We weren't dating anymore, but we stayed in touch. "On scene? What do you mean he hugged you? That's not normal. Tell me what happened. Start from the beginning." After I told him he said, "I know exactly what's going on. You want me to tell you?"

"I would love nothing more."

Have you ever heard a detective read someone? It's fascinating. Reading people is a detective's job. I love readers.

"This cop's a really nice guy, OK?" Rafael said. "He's sweet and childlike. He's wanted to be a police officer his entire life. He loves the job. But he's not smart enough to pass the tests to get promoted. He lives at home with his mother. His mother is the most important person in his life. He's never been married. He's a virgin. If he dates, he brings the girl home to meet his mother, and they all sit down and eat soup. The mother goes on every date with him. He's rich, because he's never paid rent in his life. We've got a guy like that at our precinct. We call him The Broom. Really nice guy. Always sweeping the floors. Wouldn't hurt a fly. That's who hugged you. The Broom."

On the ambulance I told Nina the detective's theory about The Hugger. And about Tommy, my fire muse. He and I still texted, now more as friends. So much for love. What's that?

I was grateful Tommy was in therapy and feeling better as time passed, and I forced myself to keep telling him I was happy he'd found someone. But I didn't have anyone to love.

I still wanted to meet him, grab a coffee sometime, since we kept in touch and I loved chatting with him. But he still wouldn't show up. He said something about how he held me in such high regard he worried if we met, I wouldn't turn out to be what he expected, or he wouldn't be what I expected. Imagined disappointment would ensue, and he didn't want to experience that. He was over his threshold for how much disappointment he could bear in this lifetime.

I understood. Fantasy is sacred. The world is already much too real.

Tommy said he loved me now, and I said it back. He thanked me profusely for saving his life. I reminded him I didn't do anything, just pointed him in the right direction. He did the work.

"No," he said. "You saved my life."

Sigh. Being heroized was lonely.

Once you're the hero, no one helps you. By definition, heroes have their shit together. They have everything under control. It was a trap, and I had to get that animal's fangs out of my neck. People died in that narrative.

In exchange for my stories shared on the truck, Nina opened her life to me.

The only thing she ever wanted to be since she was a girl was a doctor. But she was getting Ds in organic chemistry so that dream was out. She had no Plan B vision for herself. She lived unhappily with her parents in East New York. She said casually and repeatedly that she was depressed. Tonight I asked if she was suicidal. She shrugged. What stopped her from being suicidal was that she was terrified of being dead.

After she said that, I wasn't terribly worried about her committing suicide. People who talked openly about being depressed were less likely to kill themselves than people who suffered quietly then took life-ending action. A psychiatric doctor from Bellevue had explained this to us at a Continuing Medical Education training session at Park Slope.

The psych doctor said that when patients experiencing a mental health crisis said they were suicidal they didn't mean they wanted to be dead. They meant they didn't want to go on living the way they were living.

Later that night, after we dropped a patient with a minor injury off at the hospital, I saw The Hugger standing outside the trauma room. It was that thin-place Irish magic. I'd told Nina about him so now he'd appeared. I manifested him, basically.

Nina cleaned off the stretcher and I strolled up to him. He was a medium build white guy of Jewish heritage, which I knew because he talked often about not working on Jewish holidays, and he gave very strong hugs. After Rafael told me he was The Broom, I saw him in a new way. Tonight he stared straight at me, but he didn't see me. His eyes were vacated buildings. Nobody home.

I waved my hand in front of his face and said, "Hey."

"Oh, hey," he said, snapping out of it. He hugged me, and I could feel Nina's eyes on my back.

"What's going on?" I asked.

"It's a bad night." He pointed at the trauma room, abuzz with nurses and doctors working up a patient, and said, "I brought in that job."

"What was it?"

"Jumper. Young girl. She tried to commit suicide."

"Oh no. Did she succeed?"

"I don't know. We did our best. We started CPR and they're working on her now, but she landed on her head, so half her face was gone. She didn't have half her face. It's a bad night."

"That's awful. I'm sorry you had to see that. Is this your first jumper?"

"Me? No. I've worked decapitations and seen dead kids and train jobs where people were cut in half. I've seen it all."

"Got it. Well, I'm still sorry."

"Thanks," he said. Then for the third time: "It's a bad night."

Our stretcher was clean. I degloved and said farewell to the shattered cop. Nina and I walked outside.

"That was The Hugger," I told her as we shoved the stretcher back on the truck. "Or The Broom."

"I saw him hug you. He likes you."

"No, he doesn't."

"Jennifer. He hugs you. Cops don't hug people."

True. Nina and I didn't know the cop's name, so we made one up. Larry, we named him. He looked like a Larry.

Over time, I came to know other first responders in our area by name and unit number. EMTs and paramedics who rode for the Fire Department, private companies, and hospital ambulances. I looked forward to seeing them on the street and co-responding to emergencies as one interconnected, unruly family.

Nationwide, the EMS workforce was largely male and white. New York City was anomalous in terms of the racial and gender diversity of its EMTs and paramedics. Most of the Fire Department EMTs we worked alongside were young dudes in their twenties of all races and nations. Many of them commuted to Brooklyn from Staten Island and lived with their parents, since they couldn't afford to live alone. The majority of male FDNY EMTs had aspirations of becoming firefighters, so they could make double the money and work less (sorry not sorry). Their words.

By contrast, women first responders riding on FDNY trucks were either EMTs who wanted to advance medically and become paramedics, or they were paramedics, lieutenants, and conditions bosses already. None of the women EMTs or paramedics I met on the street expressed any intention of becoming firefighters.

That came as no surprise.

Firefighting across the nation remains a career dominated by men. For decades, New York City broke the ribbon for having the lowest percentage of women firefighters out of all major departments in the country. In 1982, FDNY's first batch of women swore in thanks to a discrimination lawsuit filed against the department alleging harassment and hostility against women who wanted to become firefighters. Even with an increase in women in the department in recent years, as of 2018 a mere 3.1 percent of FDNY firefighters were women.

In EMS, by contrast, there were loads of women rescuers and there existed a palpable Ya-Ya Sisterhood on the street between us lady first responders.

One of my favorite sheroes in the field was an FDNY paramedic named Laverne whose pants fit her perfectly, which made me jealous. Laverne was phenomenally competent and went out of her way to be kind and instructive to us women EMTs, teaching us medical tidbits as she worked up patients and asking us how we were faring on the job.

Any time we went on a serious run and saw Laverne on scene, Nina and I thought, Whew, Laverne's here. Everything's going to be OK.

Once, Lexi and I went on a run with a hospital EMT crew that called for paramedics because the patient was AMS—altered mental status, a treacherous state for the brain to occupy and often indicative of graver medical problems. Our patient was a short, speechless man who'd started a fire in his kitchen and now smelled like a bonfire log. On the ambulance he couldn't answer any of the four questions we used to assess a patient's mental orientation.

Where are you? (oriented to place); What happened? (oriented to event); What day is it? (oriented to time); and my personal favorite, Who's the president? (oriented to person).

Responses to that last zinger during the Trump administration were highly entertaining. I heard patients who were mentally obliterated and hovering on the brink of death respond to that query with panache and style.

"Yes, I know who that fucking asshole is! Don't let me die while he's in office!" "Ah, fuck. Really? You're asking me this? Yes, I know who the goddamn president is. Piece of shit." "Yes, he wants to deport us. He's putting our children in cages. Is going to the hospital going to get me in trouble?"

No. Going to the hospital will not get you in trouble if you're undocumented. ERs don't ask for your immigration status and must help anyone who needs medical care regardless of health insurance. When they ask about health insurance, you don't have to mention your citizenship status. You can simply say, "I'm not eligible for health insurance and I don't want to apply."

That night, our patient stared out the back of the ambulance in a daze. One of the hospital EMTs suspected the poisonous smoke inhalation had made him AMS. Soon Laverne arrived on scene and climbed on our truck. She looked at the patient.

"I know him," she said. "Hey, Harvey, what's up? What'd you have to drink tonight?"

"Vodka," he said. He'd refused to answer a single question from any of us before.

"He's a regular," Laverne told us. "He's not AMS, he's intox. You guys don't need me for this, he'll talk to you. But watch out—he's handsy."

When Laverne turned her back to him and leaned over to get something out of her bag, Harvey's hand went straight to her ass. I grabbed his arm and put his hand back on his lap. Immediately he returned it to Laverne's butt, as if his arm were on a coiled spring.

"You *are* handsy," I said, removing his hand once again from Laverne's rear. "Listen, Smokey Bear, this isn't a strip club. Keep your hands to yourself."

* * *

As women, we had to put up with a certain amount of male incivility on the street that flew in our faces from every direction. The civil service world wasn't exactly marching in step with modern times.

Listen to this one. I knew a woman EMT whose male partner was a terrible weirdo. Between jobs he watched videos of women getting injured with the volume turned all the way up, so all she heard for eight hours straight was the sound of women screaming in pain. Repeatedly he asked her if she wanted to watch the videos. Repeatedly she said no.

"What's your favorite word?" he asked her one night.

"I don't know," she said. "I don't really have one. What's your favorite word?"

"Cunt," he told her. "I love that word. I love saying it. Cunt, cunt, cunt."

So that was her partner.

"I just disassociated," she said. "I tried to pretend it wasn't happening."

When that stopped working, she brought it up to her male boss. He stuck his flattened palm out and said, "Stop. If you tell me stuff like this, I have to report it and do something about it."

I cannot tell you how many times I got that exact response from male bosses over the years in my many jobs. What happened to her happened to #MeToo. It happened to the majority of us women in some way, at some point in our careers.

Why even bother reporting that kind of behavior when that was the reaction? And suing didn't exactly help. Quite the contrary. In my work life I'd seen women emerge victorious from sexual harassment lawsuits only to discover that no one wanted to hire them, because now they were branded as "the woman who might sue you if you looked at her funny."

The whole situation was disgusting. It was never the man grabbing your ass or the guy watching torture porn on the ambulance who was the problem. It was the women who told the story. The storyteller got persecuted. It was our fault. We were too "emotional." Too "sensitive." We were "crazy."

God forbid men change.

It wasn't just women who suffered in cruel, usual ways on the street. Luna told me it upset her how often people called dispatch to report vague nonemergency complaints against Black and brown people. "Black men gathering." "Female Hispanics looking suspicious." "Smell of marijuana."

We heard these calls come over the radios constantly, too. What was wrong with gathering? What made the Hispanic women look suspicious? Smoking weed was illegal in New York City, but come on. It wasn't exactly homicide. Half of my home state of California was high. Didn't callers have anything better to do with their time?

Luna felt callers didn't understand they were putting entire groups of people at risk when they called dispatchers with meaningless complaints.

Or, alternatively, they did. She said sometimes she could hear hatred and fear in their voices when they described alleged wrongdoers, and casually tossed around degrading identifiers like "ratchet" and "ghetto." She wished people would stop calling dispatchers with these complaints. She wished people gave better descriptions than "Black male" or "Hispanic women" that put a target on people's heads.

I agreed.

Countless of my Black male friends were relentlessly stopped by the police because they "fit the description," begging the question, Description for what? Dispatchers noted the race of the person cops were sent to find. But they weren't required to write down the race of callers.

I'd love to see that data. I have a terrible suspicion my people, white women, were placing an awful lot of garbage calls. The Amy Coopers of the world, white women calling 911 on Black men falsely stating they were being assaulted or threatened when a Black man was, for example, simply birdwatching in Central Park.

If only those callers knew real violence.

Violence against EMTs and paramedics was another huge unaddressed, unspoken-about problem on the street. The National Association of Emergency Medical Technicians found that four out of five medics have experienced some form of injury as a result of the job. The majority of these injuries—52 percent—were from being assaulted by patients. The rate of assaults against EMS workers is twenty-two times higher than all other occupations. Fatal assaults against EMTs and medics are three times higher than the national average. Injuries sustained by medical first responders inflicted by patients were severe and at times disabling, and many of them went unreported.

Known examples from an EMS conference I attended with Park Slope that year: First responder struck by patient on the head resulting in laceration above eye. First responder punched in the arm, jaw, shin, and breasts during a struggle with a patient. First responder punched in the face by an intoxicated patient. Tackled by a large patient resulting in contusions to chest. Struck by a patient resulting in knee injury. Punched in the eye while escorting a patient through hospital triage. Headbutted by a patient resulting in broken jaw.

This was why, as EMTs and paramedics, it gutted us when politicians suggested EMS was "different," less dangerous, than other types of first responder work. As one firefighter put it when I described a violent night to him, "People are scarier than fire."

Commonly, rather than talk to bosses about it, we reported assaults we received on the truck to each other.

"Jennifer, can we come see you?" Nina asked me frantically one gray November Saturday. "Ship and I just had the worst job and I need to cry."

"Of course," I said. "Come cry to me, my bride."

I was at a nail salon in Park Slope with my friend Dr. Anna, a redheaded, freckled clinical social worker, therapist, and trauma expert who looked like my twin, only shorter and with bangs.

"My EMT partner's going to swing by," I told her in the nail salon. "Something bad happened, she's upset."

"Oh no," Anna said. "I can't wait to meet her. Is this the one you work out with?"

"No, that's Lexi. We do Bikini Body workouts. This is Nina. The one in my Halloween picture on Instagram with the dog mask."

This November Saturday I'd baked a salty honey pie from *The Four & Twenty Blackbirds Pie Book*. I couldn't eat the whole thing by myself, so I'd planned on seeing Ship and Nina anyway, to give them something sweet to eat on the ambulance.

Minutes later they walked into the nail salon in uniform. All the women in the salon—Asian women doing the labor, white women reaping the gel and acrylic rewards—stopped what they were doing and stared at them. I stood up in my leopard-print dress and shuffled over to them in paper slippers. I handed Ship the pie.

"It's salty honey. What happened?"

"Craziness," Ship said. His eyes were flying saucers.

Nina relayed the story. I'd never seen her so shaken up.

Apparently, they'd picked up a job for an intox. When they got on scene it was nothing special, just a dude who walked with a cane and had some alcohol on him acting up on Atlantic Avenue. It was really a job for PD, but the cops didn't want to deal with it, so they asked Ship and Nina to take the guy to the hospital for intoxication so he could dry out.

Nina told the patient they were going to the nearest hospital and he was cool about it, so when PD asked if they wanted a police escort on the truck, they declined. But once they got inside the ambulance and Ship started driving to the hospital, things turned violent.

Things turn ugly fast once you're alone on the truck with the patient.

Midway through transport, the man said he wanted to go to a different ER. When Nina explained they couldn't do that and were almost at the hospital, the patient got enraged. He unbuckled the straps that secured him to the stretcher, stood up, and escalated from an intox to a full-blown violent psychiatric emergency. He cursed out Nina, weaponized his cane, and swung it around trying to hit her. She screamed for help.

Ship, in the driver's seat, hit the sirens and gunned it to the ER, radioing dispatch 10-85, 10-85, unit requesting police backup, a code that roughly translates into: Send cops, pronto, members of service have lost control of the situation and need help, things have turned violent. The radio codes 10-85 and 10-13—MOS in immediate danger of dying—cut the elevator cables of your heart and dropped it to the basement of your gut.

Ship got to the ER bay before the cops, and they ran inside to seek safety with the violent patient in tow.

The security guard at this hospital on this particular day was a thin, polite, elderly man. In situations like this you needed a burly guard or cops to restrain the patient long enough for medics and nurses to run a line and sedate. In the triage line the patient continued acting out while Nina tried to give the nurse a report about the situation.

That's when an ER doctor appeared out of nowhere and opened fire on my beloved.

"What the fuck are you doing bringing a violent patient to the hospital without police?" he screamed at Nina in front of the entire ER. "You don't know your protocols! You can't do your job! You're endangering the safety of everyone in here! What the fuck is wrong with you? I'm calling your chief!"

Nina got so enraged she yelled back, and the two of them faced off in the middle of the ER having a screaming match. Ship stood silently beside Nina and pulled her back by the shirt every time she stepped closer to the doctor.

Listening to this story, I loved Nina so much. She was tiny, with the body build of a wood sprite, so people misread her as timid. But she was ferocious. Screaming at an ER doctor after being attacked on the truck. That's my girl!

At last the requested police officers and a sergeant arrived and resolved the situation. Humiliated, Nina burst into tears and ran crying out of the ER. (That's also my girl.) The sergeant went outside and tried to console her, but she was too embarrassed to be near anyone and wanted only to get away from the hospital as quickly as possible.

In the nail salon I hugged Nina, who was not a hugger. Ship peeked inside the bag with the pie. "My poor baby," I said.

"Jennifer," Nina said, a little calmer now. "It was so embarrassing. Everyone saw him scream at me. I never want to go to that hospital again. I hate EMS. Why do we do this?"

"Because we also love it. We're in an abusive relationship with EMS."

Ship and Nina went back to work and I returned to Anna's side.

"Is your partner OK?" she asked me. "She looked so upset."

"She'll be alright. She got assaulted. It happens all the time."

On a lighter note, one winter night in 2019, Nina and I worked on the ambulance during a snowstorm. More like a blizzard. The twenty-minute drive from my house to base took us two hours.

Weather-related emergencies saturated the radio. Downed power lines. Downed trees. Crush jobs and injuries.

Wind lashed the ambulance and caused it to rock. Our uniforms were garbage when it came to hard weather. We froze in winters and sweated our eyeballs off in the summertime. How designers could make uniforms that were so impractical and ugly at once was beyond me. Park Slope gave us puffer jackets. That helped, but I'm mostly legs.

On the job front I had low expectations for this stormy night. Mainly I hoped a snow-weighted tree didn't fall on our truck, or on us. At some point a stray cat pawed its way across the street in front of our low beams, and Nina wailed with sorrow.

Nina was a person who valued animals over people. She could work an arrest and lose a patient without shedding a tear, but if she saw a stray cat cross the street, she broke in half. Whenever she ran late to pick me up for our tour, it was always because she was giving her dog a footbath.

"Oh no!" she cried this blizzardy night. "Jennifer look at that poor little kitty! He's all alone in the blizzard. What if he gets hit by a car? Who's going to help him? Where are his parents?"

I looked up from my phone. "It's a cat."

"I know it's a cat, but look at him, he looks so lonely. He must be freezing."

"He has fur. Why don't you become a veterinarian? You're crazy about animals."

Nina said she could never become a vet, because then she would have to see her furry friends get sick and die. Also, because veterinarians endured significant medical schooling, and Nina was coming to terms with the fact that school wasn't her thing.

Toward the end of our tour, we took a patient whose identifying details and medical complaint elude me to the hospital. I think the wind ripped scaffolding off a building and bopped our guy in the head? Cannot recall.

Whatever it was, in the ER triage line we ran into an FDNY conditions boss we loved, a fifty-something Black lieutenant in turnout gear with snow sparkling in her bunned hair. She had over twenty years on the job and a hyphenated surname, John-Nichols. She looked relieved to see us.

"You girls be careful out there tonight," she said. "There's a lot of trees coming down."

"No kidding," I said. "Did you hear the run that came over for the tree that fell on the dog?"

"No," John-Nichols said. "But I heard the run where the tree fell on the lady."

"Ugh. That's terrible."

Nina looked at the floor and said, "That poor dog."

That was our night. That was the majority of our nights. Intoxes. Sexual assaulters. Violent patients. The 99 percent.

More frustratingly, every time I banged out and Nina picked up a tour with someone else, for instance, Nathan—pow! A call for shots fired came over the radio in our area, where shots were rarely fired, and they ended up doing CPR on a traumatically arrested shooting victim, complete with their picture in the newspaper the next morning, looking like the heroes they were.

Well. Nina looked like a hero. In my favorite photograph of the two of them on scene, Nina could be seen doing chest compressions on the shooting victim inside an open-doored ambulance while Nathan stood on the street with his back to the bus and his hat flipped up, looking like he was on vacation in Hawaii. Nothing surprised Nathan. That guy was truly cooked.

As Chad was Nathan's regular partner, I immediately drew graffiti on the digital photograph from the news, typed a caption on it, and sent it to him. The caption had arrows that pointed at Nina and Nathan and said,

"My partner doing CPR while your partner chills."

Chad laughed. "Typical Nathan. I love him."

It wasn't just us women partners who enjoyed marriages. Chad and Nathan were massively codependent street husbands.

As for when I would get the serious jobs I craved, EMS was an occupation that gave you no choice whatsoever in terms of how experienced you'd be when the street threw you its scariest, wildest wild card. Some first responders worked years without having a challenging run. Others responded to 9/11 their first week.

I'd been on the truck some years by now and yet still hadn't worked a cardiac arrest or craziest-ever job. I compared and despaired. I started to feel worn down by the 99 percenters. I felt like a fraud, and often referred to myself as a fake first responder.

"I'm not a real EMT," I told Larry one night in the ER.

I knew The Hugger's name now, Sebastian, but I still called him Larry. He allowed it. I'd also discovered, because he told me, he was miserably married ("It's cheaper to keep her than leave her.") and he had a young son ("He's my life and my heart, the reason I live. The bane of my existence."). This drilled some holes in the detective's theory that he lived with his mother.

Larry and I texted de temps en temps. Once, when I was off the truck, he ran into Nina on the street and asked where I was. I was in Paris. She mentioned to him that I'd told her he was the cop who hugged people, and she saw him hug me herself.

"I do *not* hug people," he said. "I only hug Jennifer. She's impossible not to like."

Impossible not to like! And yet many have succeeded at this impossible task.

After explaining about 300,000 times I wasn't going to sleep with him, Larry accepted it, and we fell into a bantering textual comradery.

"What do you mean you're not real?" he said tonight in the ER after I moaned about being a fraud. "If I get shot on the job you can do CPR on me, right?"

I shrugged. "Probably. I'm pretty sure I remember."

Everyone at Park Slope assured me I was a terrific EMT. But still. I was a white cloud. All my jobs up until now had been somewhat pedestrian, even the overdoses and strokes. And still no cardiac arrests.

Nina said, "I don't know what to tell you, Jennifer. Patients see you, and just they want to live."

"It will happen," Lexi and Austin promised. "You'll get an arrest."

Robert, a duty officer, said, "Arrests are easy, because the patient is already dead. The worst has already happened. You can't fuck it up. You can only make things better."

Maybe I had bad luck. Everyone told me to have patience, that it would happen. They were right. White as a cloud I was until one day—thunder.

7

OH, SHIT

The first time I drove the ambulance with a critical patient and two paramedics in the back I almost shit my pants.

As an EMT at Park Slope I'd started driving the truck a while ago, around six months in. New EMTs started off teching—being the one in the passenger seat, responsible for patient care on scene, patient care during transport, and, most of the time, typing up patient charts. After being a tech I got trained to drive. In EMS the driver was, in many instances, the more experienced first responder on the bus. Both rescuers were either EMTs or paramedics, so while people often called us "ambulance drivers," no such thing existed. It was considered an insult.

As for driving the ambulance, people thought we were Mario Andretti out there sharking down the trafficked streets. But driver training was brief and chilling.

First, we took a short class called CEVO, Coaching the Emergency Vehicle Operator, for driving an ambulance. It lasted a few hours and included learning extremely not-fun facts.

For starters, emergency vehicle crashes were a nationwide problem. Vehicle fatality rates for drivers of fire trucks, ambulances, and police cars were estimated to be almost five times higher than the national average. And because first responders drove at higher speeds in emergency situations, these accidents often resulted in severe injury or death.

Ambulance crashes were an especially harrowing type of motor vehicle collision, since the back of the vehicle contained one or more rescuer and a patient who was already not having a great day. A nationwide study found 84 percent of EMS workers in the patient compartment rode unrestrained. I'd worn my seatbelt when I was riding transport, but that was because I was rarely (never) providing patient care on the way to the hospital.

In emergencies, I never rode belted in the back. None of us did. We worked, securing non-rebreathers on patients, splinting limbs, washing wounds, handing patients urinals and emesis bags, hovering above the stretcher, often swinging from the oh-shit handles on the ceiling when the driver hit a speed bump, jamming the steel toe of our boot beneath the stretcher to try to keep from falling down. And while patients were belted to the stretcher with three or more straps, in 44 percent of ambulance collisions, patients were ejected from cots. Imagine being sick or injured on the stretcher, and then your rescuers crash, and you're spit out the back of the ambulance. Double espresso of misfortune.

CEVO training included a driving video with examples that were true to life. We learned how to drive defensively, giving enough spatial padding between the ambulance and cars around us, how to examine traffic patterns under stress, and analyzing driver reactions to sirens while maintaining vehicle regulations.

In New York City, the sound of sirens was so common that people rarely, if ever, responded effectively to them. Many drivers stopped at red lights with an ambulance blaring behind them, not knowing what they should do: ease carefully through the red light and pull to the side, OUT OF OUR FUCKING WAY! (Sorry, rage). Other drivers ignored sirens completely. Still others drove close to the truck to chase its elevated speed. Hence the term "ambulance chaser."

Transport had offered the same online course, so I got all the answers correct on the CEVO test. But Park Slope supplemented driver training by playing an educational horror video related to driving ambulances.

Someone cut the lights. In the darkness an EMT emerged on screen and spoke in excruciating detail about the day that ended his career. I covered my eyes while a sorrowful man told the story of how, while he and his partner were on the way to a job, he went through an intersection and hit a car, killing the woman driving.

The first responder—*former* first responder—was initially charged with manslaughter. Later, a medical board cleared him. But his gavel-wielding conscience found him eternally guilty. "It's a mental block," he said in the video, tears glassing his eyes. "I have nightmares where I see the woman's face right before I hit her. We're meant to do no harm, and I took a human life."

After the classroom portion of CEVO, I did the practical, on-the-road test with Hartford and Lexi as my guides. A bunch of us EMTs went outside base and drove around an obstacle course. We drove zigzag through traffic cones while Hartford timed us. We had to pretend each cone was a person, so if we hit it, we killed someone.

Very lighthearted thing to visualize.

Hartford and Lexi taped the backup camera on the truck, and we had to back the ambulance into the garage using our partner as a spotter and our side mirrors. We learned how to work the sirens. Left hand went on the wheel, right worked the sirens and air horn. It took about ten minutes to do the obstacle course. That was the extent of our driver training. I passed the CEVO road test. It was the only exam I'd ever taken I wished that I'd failed.

Lexi had been in a bad car accident as a girl, so she got nervous every time I drove. She liked to be in control. Nina was the opposite. She hated driving. She hit things constantly. "No one at Park Slope has hit more things than I have," she said.

True.

I started out driving to jobs only—not transporting patients. That's how we learned. In the beginning, Lexi worked the sirens for me, since it took me a while to get the hang of steering the truck with one hand and working the sirens at the same time while weaving through heavy, uncooperative traffic.

Our ambulances didn't have built-in GPS. We used our phones and mapped the location of jobs on Google Maps or Waze. Some EMTs at Park Slope knew the coverage area so well they could get to an emergency and the hospital without looking at a map. But I hadn't memorized all the necessary locations yet, so a lot of the time I relied on my phone.

Nick, when I talked to him about my fear of getting lost while driving the ambulance, told me to memorize all the streets in my battalion. He did that, back when he was a cop. He knew his area so well that his coworkers thought he was a snitch from internal affairs. Most career first responders knew their coverage areas by heart. Give them a sheet of paper, they could draw without a map every street, hospital, prison, homeless shelter, project, and chronically frequented building. "Sensitive address" was how those locations came over the radio, describing places where people who chronically called 911 lived: commonly people like EDPs or domestic violence complainants.

Many first responders in their areas had close ties with community members, patients, and families who called 911 a lot, which helped everyone involved in the emergency by way of reducing potential violence and misreading of scenes. People on the street may or may not read books, but their job was always reading people. And reading mattered. The best first responders were good readers.

As part of my training, Lexi and Nina had me drive to all the hospitals in our area and park in the different ER bays. Some bays I had to double park, others I parked on the street, still others I had to back into, and others, squeeze into tight spaces next to other trucks. Two of our ambulances didn't fit under a moldy, collapsing awning at one of our most frequented hospitals. After a few weeks Park Slope cleared me to drive.

I dreaded this.

My wifeys said I was a good driver. But every time I got behind the wheel my mouth went dry, my hands gushed sweat, and I felt pure, unfiltered terror. Double-parked cars were the bane of my existence. I developed looming fears of getting lost on the way to the hospital with a critical patient in the back. I'd heard stories like that. Paramedics doing CPR on an arrested patient while the lost driver circled the blocks with a human life on the line. The thought of that happening when I was at the helm tormented me. As did the fear of crashing into something. As did hitting someone. As did flipping the truck with my partner and a patient in the back, killing everyone on board.

One night I ran into MJ on the street. She was riding with Nathan. MJ was driving now, too.

"I'm driving tonight," I complained.

"Me too!" she said. "I love driving the ambulance. It's so exciting!"

So exciting? Was she nuts? I couldn't believe she felt this way. How come I didn't feel that way? We were different stripes of alpha women, I supposed. MJ was naturally fearless. I was—I didn't know what I was. Definitely not innately brave. My driving terror wasn't a woman thing, either.

Whenever I saw a fire truck blaze down the street, taking the red lights and blasting unfettered through traffic as if the chauffer were on a wide highway in Nebraska, I presumed the driver was brave. But after talking with some firefighters, they informed me that wasn't the case.

Many firefighters were terrified to drive the rig. Some of them hesitated to step up when it was their turn to advance and get behind the wheel. They weeded those guys out of the firehouse. You couldn't operate in an emergency with your life in your colleagues' hands when they were locked in fear. And they hit things all the time.

"All the time," one guy told me.

Speaking of all the time, late one night at home, my across-the-hallway neighbor Jeremy called because he'd locked himself out of his apartment, again. No one locked themselves out of the building more than me and Jeremy. I buzzed him inside.

Jeremy was one of my favorite people on the planet. Like me, he was the green-thumbed parent of numerous houseplants. A high-powered media executive in his thirties, he had a five-year-old son named Bill, whose favorite superhero was Super Why, because Super Why had the power to read.

From time to time I watched Bill, who called me Miss Jennifer. When he heard police sirens, he said, "Lawyer." Early on, Jeremy had given Bill The Talk. Taught his son about police. To always act respectfully in their presence and ask for a lawyer. "Lawyer, lawyer," Bill said when police sirens flared in the neighborhood. He was a *five-year-old child.*

Some nights Jeremy and I stayed up late and watched TV together and talked. He was five-foot-seven, and we often discussed how much different—better—our lives would be if only he were taller, and I were shorter. We agreed that jokes about height were the last PC jokes comedians could safely make.

"Do you think poorly of me because I work with cops?" I asked him one night on his couch.

"Not at all," he said. "I respect what you do. I admire detectives. And you never try to pretend police brutality doesn't exist. You know it exists. You admit it."

Yes. Anyone who denies it hasn't spent enough time with cops or worked on the street.

One night with Lexi my worst fear materialized as a driver. We did a job with a pair of FDNY rescue paramedics we liked. One of the medics was an affable white guy named Chase with a wedding ring the size of a lug nut and a warm demeanor. His partner was a tall Black rescuer whose name I never knew but who I liked because he laughed at my wisecracks.

The highest-trained paramedics in New York City, FDNY rescue medics were the crème de la medic crop, trained in crush injuries, hazmat operations, confined-space emergencies, trench jobs, and high-angle rescues. They had a reputation for being arrogant and swaggering, but I never found the Tour 3 guys displaying anything more than friendliness toward us.

Most units on the street roundly expressed joy and relief to see Park Slope EMTs on scene. Perhaps more than most EMS organizations—including FDNY—we had a lot of very medically-advanced rescuers on the trucks. If I ever need an ambulance again, I'll be calling Park Slope. Two of my former partners at the agency were in medical school studying to become doctors, others were nurses, and still others, paramedics. I'm a crisis communicator, so cops were overjoyed to see me on EDP calls. I preferred psych emergencies to straight medical, but I loved helping out on rescue medic jobs, as their calls were often serious and provided opportunities to learn new skills.

Our patient that fateful night was a white lady in her seventies we found seated in the living room of her home in the company of her doting, slippered husband. She presented like a stroke patient when our quartet of first responders arrived on scene. I'd had to pee for half an hour, and we'd been en route to swing by base to use the bathroom, but then we got this job, so now I was in a bit of a urinary hurry.

The rescue medics assessed the patient. She was a mess. She couldn't raise her arms or keep them raised without one of them drifting (fail). Her grip was strong and equal (pass). Her smile, too. No facial drooping (pass). But she could barely speak. She mumbled (fail). She didn't totally blow the Cincinnati Stroke Scale. But she didn't pass it with flying colors, either. Accordingly, we couldn't rule out a possible stroke. She was a 'tweener.

We asked the husband for the story. Husband said she'd taken some CBD oil their son had mailed from California, to help with chronic pain. I asked to see it.

Cannabidiol oil was gaining momentum on the street in terms of 911 emergencies related to people taking it. Derived from cannabis, CBD was believed to have medicinal qualities that helped people with pain—many doctors recommended it—but it didn't get people high, which came from another cannabinoid known as THC.

In the kitchen the giddy husband showed me a half-eaten brownie.

"She ate this?" I said.

"We both did."

"Are you sure it's CBD and not an edible?"

Edibles were weed baked into food, an alternative to smoking. If you ate the brownie you got high.

The guy didn't know the difference. Neither of them had anything to do with weed since their rebellious years in the sixties. But the thing about marijuana from California was, that shit was strong. And CBD oil was unregulated. You never knew what you got. Let this woman's symptoms be a lesson to all the takers-of-things out there. The patient's reaction to this "CBD" brownie was so severe that while she might have simply been stoned off her rocker, we suspected a stroke.

The four of us loaded the patient into a stair chair and swaddled her in a sheet. The patient was dead weight, and wow, was she heavy.

Somehow, I wound up at the head of the stair chair with Chase at the foot when it came time to carry her up a few stairs. The Black medic stepped aside and grabbed my bag, letting me do the harder physical work of lifting. I teetered and almost fell over at the top of the steps but thankfully cleared the sidewalk. When I set the patient down, I was heaving and panting, and my back killed. I dragged my sleeve across my sweaty forehead and said to the medic, "Thanks a lot for letting me lift. Gallantry is dead."

"Gallantry is dead!" the patient's husband screamed laughing.

I believed he was high.

Chase looked at me instructively. "You're tall, so next time grab the foot of the stair chair and I'll grab the head. You should always be on the bottom."

I should always be on the bottom.

Outside, I realized with horror, Lexi and the rescue medics were loading the patient onto our ambulance, rather than theirs. The medics wanted to work up the patient in the back while Lexi drove their empty truck to the ambulance. *Oh, shit.* That meant I was driving two rescue medics, the possible stroke patient, and her husband. Realizing this, I almost shit my pants. I'd transported patients, sure, but none of them had been time-sensitive yet. And there hadn't been this many first responders and family members in the back, a festival of people.

I blew out a breath and climbed into the driver's seat, then radioed dispatch that we were 82, headed to the hospital with medics on the truck. The medics had already called a note to the ER, since stroke patients needed immediate brain scans and medications if they had any chance of surviving the event without lasting impairment. The stress was magnificent. I hadn't known anything like it until now.

Slowly, I pulled into the street and talked to myself. I pretended I was MJ. "I love driving an ambulance. It's so exciting."

Things went well, at first. Then I turned down a fatally narrow street with double-parked cars on both sides. Gadzeeks, as my mother would say. Driving the ambulance down this street was like trying to get an overweight person into a child's dress. It was impossible to squeeze the big box truck through with cars on both sides and before I knew it, "Pow! Crash! Bam!"

I hit something. Many things. I must have taken three mirrors off cars. I peed my pants a little. I was still driving. Chase stood up and poked his head into the front cabin.

"What'd we hit? Did we lose an oxygen tank?"

I was barely breathing. I wondered if I was dead. "No, we're cool," I said. "We're good. Everything's fine."

He went back to work. I inhaled and exhaled like I was in labor. I peed my pants more. I got off that block and turned down a wider street. I'd never been so happy to see an open lane. I was driving slower than my grandma, who was dead. Again Chase poked his head into the cabin.

"You're driving with lights, right? Lights, and you're taking the reds like stop signs?"

I was doing neither of these things. "Yes, absolutely. Almost there."

I sped up. My phone was dinging like crazy with incoming texts. When I finally parked in the hospital ER bay three minutes later, I felt like I'd finished a marathon. I looked at my phone. Messages of congratulations from Lexi. Thrown virtual confetti. She parked the rescue truck beside me and climbed out.

"Yes, girl!" she said, high fiving me. "You did it! You drove to the hospital with a patient and medics in the back. Woop woop! I'm so proud of you. Great job!"

"Lexi," I whispered, then I started laughing maniacally. "Girl, I hit something. I think I knocked a bunch of mirrors off some cars. It sounded like I hit a fucking mailbox. The medics thought we lost an oxygen tank."

"Let's see," she said, circling the truck. "I don't see any damage. Did anyone see you? Are you sure you hit something?"

"I mean, it was not a subtle sound. No one saw."

Lexi pumped her shoulder. "No damage, no witness, no report."

Whew.

We went inside and I dashed to the bathroom and took care of my business, which felt like bliss, then regrouped with the medics outside the trauma room. The patient's giggly husband was elated to be at the hospital. He was having fun. His wife was basically a vegetable, but he was having the time of his life.

"I love you girls," he said to me and Lexi. "Look how strong and pretty both of you are. Look how you support each other. I love seeing women like you. Thank you so much your help tonight. Where do you work? Which ambulance company? Give me your names. I'll write a thank-you letter, so your bosses know what a good job you're doing."

We told him where we worked. We gave him our names and he wrote them down.

In the hallway I stepped aside and found Chase, who'd poked his concerned head into my cabin twice. "Now, this might surprise you," I said, "but that was the first time I've driven the truck with a stroke patient and medics in the back. I think I knocked some mirrors off cars."

He grinned. "It happens. Any damage to the truck?"

"Nope, we just looked."

"I didn't see anything. I didn't hear anything, either."

The loyalty! I loved him. Love you, guy. I still felt guilty. I'm so Catholic. But what should I have done? Stop on the way to the hospital with a possible stroke patient in the back and leave flyers of apology on the cars?

Technically, we were supposed to pull over if we hit something, call another unit and wait on scene for them to take our patient, call our duty officer and explain the situation, and fill out an incident report. But in the moment? Nope. Not doing that. In the hierarchy of terrors of things that could go wrong as a driver, this was nothing. And the unspoken rule on the street was no damage, no witnesses, no report. Never happened. I know an EMT at another agency who backed an ambulance over a traffic light and nearly flattened it to the ground while cops on scene watched. “I think it was like that before,” the cops said, laughing. One team, one dream!

Sorry, chief. Sorry everyone who lived on that block. Don’t forget to turn in your mirrors.

“Do you like being a paramedic?” I asked Chase. He was always in a good mood. I thought he was probably one of those Happy Childhood types. Probably came from a service family.

“Yeah, for sure,” he said. “You can do a lot more to help people as a medic.”

“So you’re happy with your career, then?”

“Yep. I love it.”

He loved it. I loved it, too. I loved driving the ambulance. It was so exciting. So exciting that later that night, when I got home, I sat down at my desk, went online, and filled out an application to work as an EMT for the Fire Department.

8

THE CRAZIEST THING

"What's the craziest thing you've ever seen?"

It was always the first question people asked when they learned I was an EMT, just as "How tall are you?" was the first question I received from strangers for the duration of my time on earth.

For a long time, I had no clear winner when I sorted through the wet, gray oyster of my brain for a pearl from the street. I wasn't sure I'd experienced it yet, the craziest thing. Then one night the scale tipped, and suddenly every job was the craziest I'd ever worked. Are you ready? Get ready to ride!

"Are you ready for this? Are you ready? Get ready!" a cop shouted as Nina and I pulled up to an EDP job one night.

"Oh look," Nina said. "It's Larry."

The Hugger. The cop my detective ex had suggested was a virginal human broom who ate soup and wouldn't hurt a fly.

Tonight, three flashing RMPs were combat parked on the street with noses to the curb, and Larry stood with his hand on the door of his vehicle when Nina and I waltzed over. Park Slope had graduated a new class of trainees, so we had an observer riding with us that night. He was a nice, middle-aged white guy with a pregnant wife at home, and he was learning the ropes on the street.

Boy did he learn the ropes.

"Are you ready?" Larry asked, grabbing the car door handle. His face was sweaty, and he was panting. His partner that night was a short brown officer who stood dazedly to the side looking like he'd just stumbled out of a firefight. I think he might have been new. The rest of the officers were also men. Black and brown and white. "Can I open it?" Larry asked.

"Wait. Before you open the door, what's happening? Who's in there?"

"Get ready! We got a wild one for ya! Is your bus unlocked? Get the stretcher."

We got the stretcher. We unbuckled the straps and rolled it back to the RMP. Larry counted to three then opened the vehicle door and out came a short, white, balding, handcuffed little fellow who reminded me of George Costanza from *Seinfeld*. I thought, This is the guy you're all fired up about? This is why three NYPD units are here? That seems a little dramatic.

But then with superhuman strength the patient screamed and cursed and lurched at the constellation of cops with a ferociousness I'd never before witnessed, frothing at the mouth, spitting at them and kicking their legs, roaring when they came near him and trying to bite them. Yowza. The store owner who'd called 911 said the guy had punched him in the face. Not a straight EDP then, or an EDP at all. Violent criminal.

We let the cops stretcher the patient and secure him with straps, as we weren't going anywhere near that level of violence. We carried stethoscopes, not guns. And we got no bulletproof vests issued to us, although in instances like these, and others where cops searched the patient and pulled knives out of their socks, you sure wished you had a few on the truck.

It took six cops to get the patient onto the stretcher and buckle the straps. They got kneed in the chest and arms and spit on as they worked. To make a daring generalization, cops do not respond well to being spit on. You heard it here first.

The patient thrashed beneath the buckles and wiggled his feet out from under the straps and rocked the stretcher back and forth, trying to tip it over while he kicked them and called them "pigs," slurred hate, screamed racial epithets, then told them he was going to find out where they lived and show up at their houses and stab their children.

Holy shit, I thought. This is the craziest thing I've ever seen.

"Get face masks!" Larry yelled.

I told the observer to follow me and trotted to the ambulance. I flipped through the glass cabinets and showed the trainee where we kept the face masks.

"We need face masks!" Larry shouted from the street.

I was a little slow, because I was teaching. I was a teacher.

"Coming!"

Larry put a face mask on the patient, but the ones we carried were flimsy. They didn't stay on. They were cheap clear squares of plastic that went over your face and wrapped around your head with an elastic band. The patient shook his head and rendered the mask useless, and spit was again flying in Larry's face.

"Give me one, give me one," he said, wiggling his fingers.

Nina handed him a mask. "Here you go."

"Locked ER," Larry said.

And I said, "Why of course."

This night I was relieved I was driving and didn't have to ride in the back with the hostile patient. Poor Nina. Poor observer. His first night.

We'd been on scene for ten minutes and I felt like I'd just gotten back from my fourth combat tour, and I hadn't even had direct contact with Mister Costanza. The verbal assaults were enough to drain my adrenal system. Nina and the observer and Larry rode in the back as I blared lights-and-sirens to a locked psychiatric ER while Larry's partner followed behind me, using the Rumbler to go through intersections and make sure he stayed close to us.

Loved the Rumbler. Loved all the sounds of emergency vehicles on the street. "It's your mating call," a girlfriend once said to me when a fire truck sirened down the block. I felt seen.

In instances like these, if the cop on the ambulance lost control of the patient, we were supposed to pull over and the other cop stepped out and assist. That's what was supposed to happen. But I'd been on the truck when the cop lost control of a violent patient and when we pulled over, there was no RMP to be found. The officer's partner had gotten lost. "Yo, man," the lost cop said, laughing to his partner when he finally caught up with us frazzled rescuers in the ER. "Sorry, bro. I took a wrong turn."

Wrong turn. We all almost died, but no problem. Glad you could make it.

I don't remember where my phone was that night, if I'd dropped it on the truck when I was mapping the route or if I'd stuffed it in one of my leg pockets and couldn't reach it while I was swerving and air-horning my way through traffic.

"Do I turn right here?" I yelled at Nina, screaming over the patient, who had not stopped shouting profanities the entire ride.

"Right, then two blocks down, then right again!" Larry yelled.

"Ten-four! About three minutes out!"

When we got inside the locked psychiatric ER, that safe haven, I hoped things might calm down.

Psychiatric breakdowns came in waves. Patients went up and down, from combative to docile and back to combative within minutes. But I now doubted if this was a mental health crisis at all. With drugs like PCP, which often results in patients exhibiting naked violence, or designer drugs like bath salts, which I figured this guy had to be on, there were no breaks, no recesses, just a relentless flow of interminable violence.

In the locked glass psych ER box that entrapped us, we waited for a doctor to become available. I don't know how long it took. Half an hour? It felt like we were waiting for centuries.

The hurricane of ferocity continued. I'm not sure how to fully convey what it felt like to stand in that room aside from saying it was like being fire-hosed with hate. I knew intellectually that cops dealt with evil, but tonight I felt it in my bones. The patient wasn't evil, but whatever drug he was on—now there's one you want to avoid. It was the closest I'd ever stood, and hope to ever stand, to evil.

Nina and I couldn't enter the patient's sight line without having spit and profanities fly at us, and neither could the cops. There were four of them with us in the hospital. The patient rocked the stretcher again, so Larry and the other officers stood near him so it wouldn't crash to the ground. We had a power stretcher that night, a Stryker automatic. They're heavy, and bought new, they go for a pretty penny, between $15,000 and $30,000. Cheap is cheap, as they say in fashion. Medical equipment is not cheap. Break a Stryker, you put an ambulance out of service, you lose lives.

The patient kept spewing racist insults at the Black cop, and each time he screamed you could see the knife of slurs slash open the cop's face. I didn't know what to do, or how to make the hate stop. Nina stepped forward and got called a stupid whore. I stepped forward and the patient told me he was going to rape me from Tuesday to Sunday. I made a mistake and tried humor. "So Mondays I have off?" For that query I got called an ugly cracker cunt. Just your average Thursday night on the street, frankly.

In unison Nina and I looked toward the foot of the stretcher, where the observer was standing. Suddenly he was in goggles. Where'd he get the goggles? We didn't carry goggles. Did he bring them from home? Did they drop out of the ceiling like the oxygen masks on crashing airplanes? What the fuck was happening? It wasn't real. We were in a movie—a horror movie.

Then things got worse.

The patient called me by the name sewn onto my uniform and said he would remember it, Murphy, and as soon as he got released, he would find me on the street and rape me and slit my throat with a box cutter. Then he resumed spitting on the cops.

That's when it happened.

Larry put his hand on the patient's throat, the patient fell silent, and all of us held our breath. *One. Two.* Larry released his hand and the patient gasped and resumed cursing at us at full volume as if nothing had happened to him at all.

That's how I remember it. In Nina's recollection, once the patient spit, Larry lunged forward and leaned on him with his arm until he fell silent. In Larry's version of events, he put his hand over the patient's jaw to stop him from spitting. We all had different memories. Three stories. Which was true?

I was dizzy with confusion. My head ached and I was drenched in sweat, physically and mentally and spiritually roasted on a spit. Whatever happened in those two seconds, not only did I not intervene, I didn't think to intervene. I didn't want to. Those two seconds were the only break in the continuous sewage of hate we'd gotten in well over an hour. Two seconds of peace.

But still.

Even now, writing this, remembering, reliving it, makes me shiver. You tell yourself you're a good person. You have morals. You're a person who, in a crisis, makes the right call. You'll never do anything to endanger a patient, or your fellow first responders, or yourself. If you see something that turns your stomach, you'll do the right thing. Certainly, that was my view of myself before this moment. Even now, years later, I still think about that job.

I ask myself why we didn't call medics. I remember Nina and I discussed it with PD and all of us concluded the fastest way out of this was not for us to wait on scene, but to bolt to the psych ER, fast. Plus, the patient was so violent there would be no way for medics to run a line without cops holding him down and restraining him so they could start an IV, so medics weren't a cop-free solution.

I ask myself if I allowed it because it was a white cop and a white patient. Or if that's how I would want my family members to be treated if they were in this situation. But it's hard, it's genuinely impossible for me to imagine my family members in that state, spewing hatred and spitting at me, saying they wanted to rape me and slit my throat. In that moment I wanted only for the death threats to stop. For two seconds, Larry made it stop.

I don't know what else to say here. It's complicated. It's ugly. And the ugliness claws its way under your skin. It tears you apart, and it stays there. It festers inside of you. It leaves marks. And they don't go away. Mine haven't, at least.

When the ER doors finally opened it took the cops, security guard, and a fleet of doctors and nurses to hold the patient down while one of them started an IV and administered medication. Even after sedation as they rolled the patient away, he was screaming profanities.

Drugs these days.

Outside, the cold nighttime air was so cool and fresh I drank it into my lungs. We were safe. Alive. Together. All of us were fifty years older than we had been a few hours before. I was so grateful for my life. I loved every first responder I was with that night. I loved them primally, like a tiny forest animal loves the lions that save them from slaughter. It was so quiet outside. So still. Eventually I noticed the observer, who was smiling ear to ear. I'd completely forgotten he existed.

"You OK?" I thought to ask him.

He wiped his damp forehead. "That was crazy. Was that, like, a normal job?"

Nina laughed. "No. You really saw something quite special tonight."

In the parking lot we stood around with the cops for a while. Larry opened his phone and showed us old photos of himself. He had long hair. He sang in a punk rock band.

"Oh wow," I said. "You used to be cool."

"Yeah. I even did an internship at the Democratic National Convention. That was before I became a cop."

"Clearly, those days are behind you."

I shook the truck keys and we headed back to the ambulance.

"You lost your shit tonight!" I shouted across the parking lot at Larry. "You let the patient get to you! You're insane!"

"You know you liked it, Murphy! You know it turned you on!"

Turned me on? This job! The street! The craziest thing!

On the truck, Nina and I regrouped with the observer, who sat in the captain's chair in the back.

"Well," Nina said to him. "Do you still want to do EMS?"

"Oh man, yes," he said. "I loved it. I've never seen anything like that before. Jennifer, did you hear what the cop said to you in the parking lot?"

"Yes, I heard."

Nina said, "That's Larry. He's in love with Jennifer. He hugs her on scene."

"Who *is* he?" I said as I drove mind-blown back to Park Slope. "He's definitely not the fucking Broom. I'm going to kill my ex for making us think he was some dumb fumbling virgin. Lives with his mother. Eats soup."

"I had no idea the job was this violent," the observer said.

"It's not always this crazy," Nina told him. "But yeah. Welcome to the street."

So that happened. Then it happened again. Only next time, not terribly long after this night, the insanity was medical.

Let's keep driving the ambulance, shall we?

March rain fell over the city and washed the filthy winter snow into the sewers. A new season was afoot. It was time to plant flowers, by which I mean I had to change my life.

One eventless afternoon I quit responding to Tommy's texts, since he still wouldn't meet me. I didn't know why or how I did it. I just reached some sort of bottom in terms of managing my disappointment as it pertained to his refusal to appear in real life.

Suddenly I was done. My therapist and I had been doing a lot of EMDR on 9/11 these last few months, so perhaps it was that. Things had started to shift around for me internally. Perhaps letting go of Tommy was an unexpected result?

"Did you block his number?" Felice asked me one night on the phone.

"I didn't feel the need."

I knew if Tommy texted down the line, I'd want to hear what he had to say. I'd hear it, and then I'd ignore him. In the meantime I felt no temptation to text him or reply. I was OK with reality. I was done with him.

Suddenly I had a new lightness about me.

At my writer's desk, my novel was going well. And that April, Felice and I were published in a racial literacy textbook called *Tell Me Who You Are*, marketed as "an eye-opening exploration about race in America." We were mildly horrified after our interview, when the woman anthologizing us asked if we were comedians. Felice and I locked eyes. What had we said that was so funny, for a textbook about race? Um, could we see the transcript before our interview got published?

"We need media training," I said to Felice.

After our interview, outside on the street, we scratched our heads and tried to remember what we'd talked about. Did we say something offensive? We didn't think so.

We'd for sure mentioned how frustrated we felt that we were only ever asked to write about race, flattened and reduced to basic racial identifiers, a Black woman and white woman who were friends, how revolutionary, how astonishing, when we also wanted to talk about living the writer's life, pop culture, meditation, God, *90 Day Fiancé*, podcasts, recipes, Salvador Dalí, science, plays, relationships, love, words we invented ("cramazing," inspired by a combination of crazy and amazing; "torpizza," because Felice loved to make pizza on tortillas), and leading big fat messy complex lives, being women who wore a lot of hats. No one ever asked us to write about any of that.

Race. They only ever asked us to write about race.

On my birthday in May, Nina and I picked up a tour on the ambulance. How else would I celebrate turning forty-four? She gifted me a joke present before we left base. A shower curtain featuring a hideous fanged cobra wrapped around the star of life with lettering that said, EMS—IT'S NOT JUST A JOB. IT'S A MENTAL DISORDER.

I howled laughing. This was some of her finest work. I promised I would hang it up the second I got home. It took me a year to come anywhere near matching the greatness of this gift. But I did it, after I found a fitted bedsheet with a queen-sized firefighter squirting his hose at a roaring orange blaze. That present was an A+. She may never top it.

A few minutes into our tour, the sky clear and the warm weather holding, the radio served up a birthday present of its own, a pedestrian struck by a car. Hit and run. Our patient was a doughy white gentleman in his fifties laid out in the street with brief loss of consciousness and head, neck, and back pain. The usual. Nothing terribly dramatic. I'd done so many of these jobs by now I could work the emergency effortlessly. I could eat a sandwich on scene when someone was being backboarded.

Off the truck, Nina and I had started baking together. Weekly she came to my house and we baked a pie, or cake, or some kind of complex cookie. The saltier we got on the street, the sweeter we got in the kitchen. It helped us stave of gloom.

Nina liked getting out of the house, and I loved having her over. We baked and argued over how my frosting wasn't up to her ridiculous standards. Then we ordered Indian takeout and watched *90 Day Fiancé* and laughed.

One night we came up with an idea for a company we could form together, a baking business that would change and save our lives. We'd bake, then we'd deliver our desserts to our first-responder friends. We called ourselves Sweets in the Streets. Great idea, right? RIGHT?

For weeks we baked like crazy and delivered our sweets to first responders on tour. We never sold a single dessert. Not one. We couldn't even give them away for free. To our surprise, no one on the street wanted anything we baked. Everyone was suddenly healthy. Larry was gluten free. Austin didn't eat junk food. Lexi was a gym rat and always asked if there was sugar in our cookies. "Yes, girl," I said. "It's a cookie, not a bar of sand."

That summer, Nina and I kept going with the baking, even though our business was a failure. It made us happy. It made everyone happy.

"Sweets in the Streets!" Chad yelled one night when we pulled up to his ambulance with a blueberry pie. Larry let us put a cupcake on his RMP and take a picture of it on the hood.

That summer, things began to change.

Park Slope grew. One random day I got promoted to crew chief. I had no idea what that meant. Thanks? I guessed leadership thought I was a good

EMT? I felt special at first. Then I found out Chad and Raz had also been crowned chiefs. Chad's theory was that Park Slope handed out promotions like cold pizza. Everyone got a slice.

Soon I was devastated to learn the unsalaried position came with more responsibility. The agency churned out another fresh batch of new members. Those of us who'd been on the bus for a few years—the crew chiefs—now had to train the observers. I resented this. I didn't have dreams of middle management as a volunteer EMT. I just wanted to ride and go home.

That being said, training new people really helped me. Riding with Lexi and Nina I always compared myself to them and fell short. But compared to the observers, I was a medical genius. They could barely do anything on scene, just like me when I was new. Teaching new EMTs helped me see all the progress I'd made. Plus, some of the newbies at Park Slope were pretty cool.

That year—2019—I did a few tours with a relentlessly cheerful young woman with long pastel-pink hair named Soo. She worked in a walk-in medical clinic in Chinatown and was anxiously awaiting responses from PA schools. Soo loved bubble tea and pole dancing. All of us at Park Slope feasted on her sunny Instagram videos whenever we felt sad.

Soo was learning how to drive the ambulance and still ran over the curb every time she turned, or rammed into orange street dividers, and she needed help working the sirens, but she progressed fast. On the street, you have to. Learn or people die. One tour, in our downtime, Soo and I got to know each other.

"What was your first medical trauma?" she asked me. "Not on the ambulance, in real life."

I thought about it. After a while I said, "When I was five, I walked into the garage and saw my ten-year-old brother lying in a pool of blood. He'd fallen down from the rafters. And I apparently went back in the house and said, 'Mom, there's red paint pouring out of brother's head.'"

"Wow," Soo said. "That's crazy."

"Meh. Howbout choo?"

"When I was in grade school, I was in the car with my dad and we drove by this motorcycle accident, a bad one. I looked out the window and saw the motorcyclist's body in the street and then his helmet far away from him, and his face was still in it."

"What?! Your first trauma was a decapitation?"

"Yeah," Soo said, laughing. "My dad tried to speed away and I was mad at him because I wanted him to slow down so I could see it up close."

"That's when you know you're going to work in medicine. Normal people see an accident and glance at it for a second then drive off. We see an emergency and think, 'Fascinating. Let me slow down and get out of the car.'"

"The accident happened right in front of a school, too," Soo said. "I felt so bad for the kids who saw it. They must have been so traumatized."

Must have been.

Speaking of nightmarish trauma, soon I was in for some of my own. After all my itching, it was finally here. Oh, shit.

One night, Lexi and I went on a nursing home run with a pair of FDNY EMTs, two guys who lived in Staten Island. One of them had a warm, clown-around personality. He was the kind of EMT who hit a parked car on the way to a job and had to call another unit to work the emergency. How could you not love him? His partner was a young tattooed guy. I'd never seen him before.

Lexi grabbed the stretcher since this nursing home had an elevator. The four of us EMTs walked inside, expecting the usual kind of job we responded to at these senior facilities: Grandma fell down. In the elevator I asked the one of the EMTs, Mitchell was his name, what we were walking into. Just curious.

Assigned 911 units got info on their CAD, computer-aided dispatch system, which provided identifying details about the patient and their medical complaint. "Sixty-five-year-old man fell off a ladder," for instance. As vollies we often only got the call type, location, and broad description of the patient. Injury major. Diff breather. Anaphylactic. Unconscious. Sick. Woman dressed as witch wielding a broom. Some pretty amusing things flew over the air.

Mitchell told us the job had come in as a forty-something-year-old man with abdominal bleeding. I couldn't wrap my mind around the patient's age, or the call type. Abdominal bleeding? At forty? Inside a senior facility? That seemed odd.

"Internal bleed?" I asked him.

He shrugged. "I guess we'll find out. It's probably bullshit."

It was the reverse of bullshit. It was, "Oh, shit."

* * *

We walked into the patient's cramped, stuffy room, and straightway—bloodshed. We found a morbidly obese Black man in bed bleeding uncontrollably from his stomach. He was hooked up to an automatic vitals machine, and when we lifted his shirt, it looked as if he'd been attacked by a shark, the flaps of his skin ripped apart like wet newspaper. Blood gushed from every fold.

When we moved him to the side to see where it was coming from, I saw only a liter of pooled blood. I'd never seen so much blood in my life. It made the room smell metallic. I could taste his blood in my mouth. It was impossible to stop it or find its source. The patient was conscious, whimpering but alert, laying in a pool of his rapidly gathering blood. A waterfall of it. An ocean.

I looked up at Michell, whose lizard eyes bulged. "Should we call for medics?"

"No, just grab vitals and let's load and go! Load and go!"

In EMT school they used that phrase constantly for critical patients, yellow- or red-tag patients likely to die, load and go. They hammered it into our heads. If the patient was stable, stay and play. For critical patients, load and go. Protocols stated to call for backup, meaning medics, but no matter what, load and go.

Thankfully, the nearest trauma-receiving hospital was under five minutes out. In New York City, we're always about five minutes away from numerous ERs, unlike first responders who work in rural areas. Time was a-tickin', and I'd already suggested calling for medics and Mitchell had shut that shit down. From the looks on our faces I could tell we were all thinking the same thing: The patient is going to bleed out if we don't go now.

The vitals machine beeped as I wrote down the numbers, which Lexi needed to call a note to the ER to tell them what we were bringing in. We all looked at it. Suddenly the patient's pulse shot through the roof and his blood pressure plunged. A sign he was going into hypovolemic shock from intravascular loss.

"He's dropping!" Mitchell said, as if the patient weren't right there.

The patient burst into tears. "Am I dying?" he said. "Please don't let me die! I don't want to die! Please help me!"

I ran to the patient's side and hushed him. "Deep breaths, we've got you. We won't let you die." Then I said it again, this time for myself. "You're not dying. Not tonight."

We lifted him onto the stretcher, rushed him out of the room and into the elevator, raced outside, and loaded him onto our bus. It had to be our bus, because it was our stretcher.

Lexi grabbed my hand. "Do you want to tech or drive?"

There was no good position to play here. "I'll tech," I said quickly. "You drive. Fast, Lexi. You have to drive fast."

I hopped on the back of the truck. The tattooed EMT hopped on with me. He was silent. His face was a cratered moon. We opened the cabinets, the tech bag, tore open every piece of trauma dressing on the truck trying to stop the bleeding. It wasn't enough. Blood spilled over the stretcher, splashed onto the wheels, our boots. It was all over my uniform.

"Do you want my partner to go with you?" Mitchell asked.

"No, that's OK. We just need to go. Lexi! We need to go!" The stunned EMT jumped off our truck.

In my swimming head my decision not to have the other EMT ride with me made total sense. I was thinking, He's an EMT, so what good is he on the back of the truck if he's the same level as I am? The only thing this patient needs right now is fluids, and a doctor to find the source of bleeding and stop it, and we don't have that so . . . , "Lexi, let's fucking go!"

The ambulance back doors were open. Lexi gave me a thumbs-up and radioed a note to the hospital to tell them we were coming through with a critical patient who, as every second passed, was less and less likely to survive. I wasn't sure why we weren't moving. What was the fucking holdup? I peeked outside. An EMS SUV was parked behind our truck.

Mystery solved.

Bert. A short, blond, bespectacled paramedic turned EMS boss, the kind of guy you had to wonder if his diminished height activated the Napoleonic complex, with that comedic first name. His presence on scene was an indication we were on a serious job. Indeed, Bert was having a loud talk with Mitchell. I could hear him asking why no paramedics were there. Their argument probably went on for two seconds, but alone with the patient on the blood-soaked ambulance it felt like a thousand years.

"Lexi!" I yelled. "We need to go!"

Mitchell closed the truck doors for me, the saint. Sirens blared. Lexi gunned it.

The truck lurched forward and leapt over speed bumps as she blasted to the ER. I flew all around the bus, grabbing every piece of trauma gauze I could find, ripping it open with my teeth, stuffing bandages into the patient's folds of skin, each torn-open envelope of flesh spitting up blood. I hovered over the patient, fastened a non-rebreather to his face and cranked the oxygen tank up to fifteen liters. I could tell by the puffs of breath fogging his mask he was breathing for now but that wouldn't last long. His eyelids fluttered, then closed.

Oh, shit, I thought. Terrific decision I'd made on scene, not to have that EMT ride with me. Now I saw the point. I needed extra hands.

"Stay with me," I told the patient, shaking him, hovering over the stretcher like a terrified angel. "I need you to stay with me, honey. Keep talking, keep talking. Talk to me, love."

I rubbed sternum, tapped his arm, tried to keep the non-rebreather from falling off his face and sopped up blood with whatever gauze I could reach. The patient opened his eyes and stared blankly at me.

"There we go. I need you to stay with me. Keep talking."

"I don't want to die," he mumbled.

"We're almost there. Keep talking to me. You're not dying, not tonight."

But he was dying. He was in shock. His body was compensating by plunging his blood pressure and now his organs weren't getting enough oxygen. He was speeding toward the grave and I was in there with him, trying to unshovel the dirt falling over him as every second ticked on, working backward, working against death, losing.

The patient's face sheet—the nursing home printout of his medical history—was in my gloved, shaking hands, and as I worked on him, I tried to scan it so I could give the ER doctor his medical history. This man had every health problem known to humankind. There wasn't a medical condition that didn't afflict him, and I understood now why he lived in a nursing home when he was in his forties.

Within three minutes we were at the hospital and off the ambulance. Lexi was a rock star. I'd never seen her drive so fast or been so happy to race a patient into the ER.

The trauma room was aswarm with nurses and doctors when we rushed in. We transferred the patient onto the table, alert and alive. I handed the face sheet to a nurse and cleared my throat to deliver the triage report. A doctor raised his arms like an orchestra conductor and hushed everyone in the room.

"Quiet!"

Time stopped. No one moved. Everyone fixed their eyes on me. I heard myself speak.

"Patient is a forty-three-year-old male with COPD, CHF, asthma, diabetes, and ulcers. Call came over for abdominal pain, but we found him in a nursing home bed bleeding uncontrollably from his stomach with ruptured skin. Source of bleeding unlocatable. Patient has lost over a liter of blood and had brief LOC on the truck that improved with O2. Pulse 130, respirations 25, BP immeasurable. Medications are on his face sheet."

Time resumed.

The nurses and doctors moved around and furiously went to work. Lexi and I stood shoulder to shoulder in the trauma room staring at the patient. We wanted to see his vitals."Still no BP," an ER nurse said, reading the machine.

No BP, but he was alive. A miracle.

"He's alive," I said quietly.

Lexi was silent, staring at the patient. I put my hand on her shoulder and squeezed it.

Then the doctor walked up to me. He was bald. That's all I remember. He shook my hand. Lexi looked at him like he'd handed me a rose.

"Where is all the blood coming from?" he asked ponderously.

I mean—who knows, little buddy! You're the expert, right?

"We don't know," I said.

After a few minutes we rolled the bloody stretcher into the hallway. I yanked Lexi by the arm and dragged her into an empty room.

"We fucking did it, girl! You drove the shit out of that ambulance! We just saved that fucking man's life!"

I was drunk with elation and adrenaline. I felt higher than my patient on bath salts—but in a good way. It was some kind of bliss, that's for sure, and I felt for the first time the fullness of what a paramedic friend said to me after I told him I was an EMT: "There's no greater feeling than saving a life."

"You OK, girl?" I asked Lexi. "Say something. You're scaring me."

She looked up at me in silence. Then she smiled and said, with childlike sweetness, "I loved that."

I hugged her again. "Yes, girl! We're badass bitches! We did it! Holy shit, he's alive! We got him here alive!"

Lexi tilted her head and said, "Why'd that doctor shake your hand?"

"I have no idea. Maybe he saw my TED Talk."

Her phone rang. Bert. She stepped away for a moment then returned. "He wants to talk to us. He's meeting us at base."

Oh boy. We knew what that meant.

"Dad's mad," I said after we cleared the hospital and Lexi drove slowly back to base. "But we saved that patient, girl, so what's he going to say? You're in trouble for saving a man's life? You should have called medics? I suggested it, but Mitchell shut that shit down. Don't worry, honey. It's just Bert."

He met us at base. He was pensive and serious, with crinkled eyebrows. He smelled strongly of mall cologne. Drakkar Noir? Every detail I was absorbing seemed to me hilarious.

But this was no laughing matter, for Bert. With his arms crossed over his chest, he read Lexi her rights. He pretty much ignored me, but wow did he go at Lexi, since she worked 911 as a full-time EMT. He spoke only to her, but you know me by now, you know how I felt about air quotes leaders, how protective I was of my partners. They were my girls.

I kept running interference. I tried to divert Bert's attention. I snapped my fingers to get him to look at me. Nick and I used to do that to each other all the time when we worked together. Snap-snap. Clap-clap. Clack-clack, as if we were calling a horse.

Calmly I explained to Bert why no medics had been present. He listened, then said he understood. But then he kept going back to Lexi, telling her how disappointed he was in her, listing the things she should have done differently. She stood there and took it. One blow after another until her eyes looked like broken blue shells in a ravaged bird's nest, cracked and empty. I didn't know what to do, power-wise.

It seemed clear to me this scolding talk was about a boss enjoying power rather than a severe medical fuck-up. Bad bosses were a problem in EMS. And disobedient, lawless EMTs were a problem for bosses. There was nothing in our New York City BLS trauma protocols that mandated us to call paramedics for bleeds. And even if we had called medics, we got to the ER faster than they would have gotten on scene and we wouldn't have waited for them. Later, I ran this job by a dozen paramedics and doctors, and all of them said "load and go!" Furthermore, our protocols stated we could apply hemostatic dressing, or combat gauze, to uncontrolled bleeds. Hemostatic dressing was used on battlefields for hemorrhage control, utilizing the clotting properties of agents like kaolin to activate intrinsic clotting. But we didn't carry hemostatic dressing on our trucks. Neither did FDNY ambulances. Might we get some? Friendly reminder that New York City streets are a battlefield.

I never had a problem with Bert, personally. He amused me. One time he sent us on a job for a "shots," but we knew it was a false alarm. Someone had called 911 because they felt their house shaking. We went for the shots, but we got the shake. Every time I thought of Bert that's what came to mind. So I was not the right person to have around for this serious talk. I was still drunk from the rescue. That's how I was acting, drunk. It was the adrenaline. Holy shit. That rush. We saved a fucking life! My first save!

But listening to Bert lay into Lexi after we'd just been through fire and brimstone was a bit much. He kept saying how he was on his way to the gym when he heard the call come over, then he turned around and sped back to Brooklyn to "help." He must have said he was headed to the gym four times. I mean, I worked out. I did push-ups. I squatted. But this did not seem like the time to bring that up.

Lexi stood with her head bowed like a tulip being pelted by rain. My poor tulip. She had a hard time sticking up for herself. Especially if the person angry at her was a man. And a boss.

What was the point of this talk? On the street after a serious job sometimes supervisors gave you a quality assurance meeting, to go over the run. But those rarely happened immediately after the call, since rescuers were still ramped up on adrenaline.

Raising my hand. Still ramped up.

There also existed what was called a critical incident stress debriefing. To get one of those, you had to see something pretty ghastly. Dead children. Dead MOS. MCI, mass-casualty incident. I'd never had one of those. But I heard about them from Gabriel, the empath who'd taught me how to get off the ambulance quickly back when I was a sloth.

Gabriel was a paramedic now. And he had a critical incident when he was an intern. He'd responded to a job for a cop who'd shot himself in the face. He had a critical incident stress debriefing after that run. Whatever we were having with Bert, it wasn't that. Lexi looked like she was being emotionally robbed.

Suddenly I felt fangs grow in my mouth. Dad was mad, but have you met Mom? Step back.

My partners. They were young women. They worked hard. Nonstop. For nothing. No money. No respect. Totally invisible to the public. They did service. They did what some people called God's work. They saw the unspeakable, the worst of humanity, they got their hands dirty, and bloody, and unlike most of the selfie-obsessed country, they got in the game and tried to help. They suffered like I used to suffer at their age, and then some. You could mistreat me all you wanted. But do *not* mess with my partners.

"You're a match, wifey," Austin once said to me. "Thin and red and harmless. But strike you—and fire."

Austin was right. But I couldn't do much in this situation as a human match. Except interrupt Bert every two or three sentences to insert some humor into the unjust situation. Seeing that I was still bombed on hormones, that was pretty easy.

"But, Bert," I said. "Oh, man, you're so right. We fucked up by not insisting on having medics on scene and overruling the FDNY EMTs. We're so dumb. We're just girls. We're big dumb girls. We're idiots. But hey, listen. We saved that man's life, right? Pretty cool, huh?"

"Bert. Hey, Bert, I know you came all the way back for this, to help us, thanks so much for your help oh my God, you were so helpful, but are you still going to the gym?"

Again and again I interjected, until he couldn't help but grin. "We could have done better. You're so right. But, Bert, isn't it great that our patient lived?"

"Hey, Bert, Bert, Bert." Snap-snap. "Are you still going to the gym?"

EMS—it wasn't a job, like my new shower curtain said. It was a mental disorder.

And I had it.

The funniest bit, or perhaps the only funny bit, about this whole fiasco came later.

One Thursday night when I was on the truck with Nina, we ran into Mitchell outside the hospital, the tall EMT who'd been on that bloody call.

He saw me and waved me down. We ran up to each other in the middle of the nighttime street and hugged like *Titanic* survivors.

"Oh my God!" I said. "That job was crazy!"

"I know! And he fucking survived! I came back to the hospital later that night to check on him, and he was still alive. They think ulcers caused his stomach to rupture. He was in the ICU!"

"That's so great! He made it! We did it!" And then I said, "We got in trouble afterward, for not calling medics."

"I told you to call medics, and you said no."

I looked at Mitchell like he was a farm animal. "Are you nuts? I suggested you call medics, and you said no."

"I swear I told you to call medics," he said perplexedly.

"No way. I can't believe you're making yourself the hero of this call. I totally asked you to call medics and you said load and go. I did fuck up though, by not having your partner ride with me. That was dumb. I needed help in the back. I was covered in blood and his non-rebreather kept falling off."

"Yeah, I couldn't believe you didn't take an extra set of hands."

"It was a mistake."

Then Mitchell took me by the shoulders and, laughing, said of his partner, "That was his first day!"

"Oh, God! Is he OK? That's so traumatizing! Tell him he did great. Tell him he helped me a lot. And what about the part where a boss showed up and started arguing with you, and I was like, 'Um, hey, guys, sorry to bother you, but the patient is dying right now, so would you mind if we went to the ER and you can perhaps sort this all out later?'"

"I know! I didn't know who the fuck he was! I'd never seen him before!"

"That's Bert. He's a boss."

"I was talking to him like a moron, like who the fuck are you?"

"I love you so much. You're a hero. We did great."

We hugged again and congratulated each other on being lifesavers. What a ride.

I didn't care what Bert thought of me. What anyone thought of me on the white-shirt side of the street. I only cared what my patients, my partners, and other first responders we worked with thought. What mattered most was that they trusted me and knew I was medically competent. That was what mattered. EMS bosses? Shrug.

* * *

But what really happened that night? Fallible things, memories acquired in an emergency. To each their own?

I worried about Lexi after that call. She cried a lot afterward, and she was soon starting nursing school while working part-time. EMS had done a real number on her, and on me, I was starting to realize.

In one of her more famous essays, the writer Joan Didion says, "It's easy to see the beginnings of things, and harder to see the ends." My experience in EMS was the opposite. It was hard for me to pinpoint when I became a first responder. It was easier for me to see the end. I saw it that night. It was near.

9

THE END OF JOY

My problems started the summer of 2019 and snowballed from there, avalanching me in misery.

In June, Park Slope graduated another class of new EMTs. The agency sent around a chilling e-mail. Leadership informed us partners would be split up every other week. We'd now be responsible for training new members twice a month.

Fine. Seasoned EMTs had trained me, after all. And I'd still get to ride with Nina every other week. Lexi had flown the proverbial coop for nursing school, so she rarely had time to pick up tours.

Begrudgingly, Nina and I accepted our new fate. We worked tours with new people and tried to ride on the same night, at least, so we could still drive to base together. I hated my new partner, a sloppy white guy named Chuck. Mercifully, one day he disappeared from Park Slope. Maybe Beck fired him. I didn't ask. I only cared that he vanished.

Things can always get worse, as we say on the street.

And indeed, things got worse.

A few weeks later a second e-mail from Park Slope splatted bird-shit-like on my inbox, this one informing us that all partners would now be split up permanently. Here on out, we'd be training new members as well as observers every single week.

Um, what? No more tours with Nina?

A funeral commenced inside me.

Reading the announcement, I felt like I'd been drop-kicked into new era: The End of Joy. Growth for organizations was usually a positive sign. But as we were volunteers, this felt like growth at our expense.

Now, as per the latest e-mail, we'd be working harder, training new people constantly, and never get to ride with our partners. I felt enraged and taken for granted. My problems-with-authority side reared its gorgeous head. I sulked and stomped around and cursed our chiefs. How dare they! Who did they think they were? They couldn't do this. Did they know who I was?

Wait. Who was I?

I knew I was being childish and petty. But I genuinely didn't want to be on the truck if I couldn't work with one of my wives. The lure of flashing lights and finding patients in surprising pickles had worn off long ago. Now what I most looked forward to on the ambulance, the only thing I looked forward to, was spending time with my partners. No partners, no bueno.

Everyone has a shadow. My shadow met those of my coworkers—co*volunteers.*

Many of us EMTs had equally noxious reactions. Nathan became a pain in the ass to Austin, who managed the schedule. Chad, a fussy whiner who dropped his tours with zero notice. Lexi, queen of refusal when it came to riding with anyone but me, took to social media and penned a thinly veiled rant about the importance of having a good partner, how hard it was to find one, and once you found one, how crucial it was to never let them go.

Throwing a wrench into our righteous anger, Raz and Ship remained cheerful, completely unbothered by the shake-up. They were more than happy to train whoever showed up for their tours. I didn't know what to say about their reaction, or lack thereof, except they were better people than we were.

May we all be more like Raz and Ship.

"Maybe it's time for us to take a break from EMS," I said in the car as Nina drove us to base for our last tour together. "We have Sweets in the Streets to run, so we can still bake."

Just as we pondered cutting loose, things worsened.

That evening tour, we had a huge blowout with Chiefs Beck and Hartford. The drama commenced at base with a scene too dumb to dramatize here. Even relaying the story in exposition, it offers a quintessential EMS stupidity that I cherish to this day.

* * *

The scenario:

We had to reshuffle the trucks squished in the garage so we could get the ambulance we wanted to ride out on the street. Now a brief word about the aesthetics of ambulances.

Like all vehicles, which make and model of ambulance you drove communicated something about you. Picking out an ambulance to ride on the street was not unlike selecting the perfect dress for an occasion. Put simply, we wanted to ride on a good truck. Good to us (and to Lexi and Chad and Nathan) meant one of the new trucks. One of the big ones. The boxes. Those trucks were serious. They were the little black dress of ambulances. Very powerful. Very sexy.

Every EMT needs a little black dress truck, and everyone lights up when she rolls up on scene batting her flashing eyes wearing it. On the street these trucks said to our first responder peers and to our patients, We see this is a serious and important situation and we are serious and important people who have come to help you. The boxes also had power stretchers, which we preferred to manual stretchers because we had back pain. People were heavy, and America was medically overweight. Everyone go drop ten pounds for your local first responders.

Also, as volunteers, we inhabited a stigma on the street for being "loser vollies who had nothing better to do with their time," as an FDNY medic with a stick up his ass once called a Park Slope crew. Some Fire Department medics and bosses looked down on us because we were volunteers. We tried to counter negative attitudes toward us by being medically competent and helpful to other crews, and by showing up on scene in trucks that were new, with state-of-the-art equipment. Still, Nina and I were vollies, released from the reputational charge of being losers if only because we embraced our starring roles as clowntown's main feature.

Send in the clowns.

That being said, it was extremely important to us that we not look as dumb as we felt. Park Slope had one ambulance that was a van. It looked like the Mystery Machine in *Scooby-Doo*. Rolling up to an emergency in this van as volunteer EMTs was like walking into a funeral with a lampshade on your head. It was impossible for us to take this vehicle seriously, and every time we saw a crew whizz by in the van Nina and I made the *meep-meep* cartoon voice of the Road Runner and nearly wet our sexy panties laughing. So we could not under any circumstances take the van. It just could not happen.

EMS is a show. We must never underestimate the importance of glamour in emergencies. Emergencies are a performance, and how you appear onstage matters not only to the street audience, but also to your fellow first responder cast members. Why do you think everyone is so strungout on the Fire Department? I will give you a clue. It's those big, sexy, bright-red trucks. Also, red suspenders.

Back to our cartoon.

Getting ambulances out of a garage stuffed with trucks on a one-way street jammed with rush-hour traffic screaming out of the Prospect Expressway was an extremely unpleasant task.

Immediately I observed this was an unwinnable battle and consciously opted to be a pacifist in this war. I could park the busses just fine, thanks, but I did not want to hoot my driving-skills clarinet in this particular orchestra arrangement. Perhaps more than most people, because of my background I was a woman who did not respond well to being screamed at. This setup, from what I heard, from honks and curses blaring out of road ragers' vehicles and mouths, provided ample opportunity for it.

This evening Hartford was upstairs at base and had spoken to us in a curt tone before our tour about what I cannot recall, something minor, and her car was parked on the street blocking a space we needed to pull into in order to reshuffle the trucks. As I mentioned, Hartford had a commander-like personality, and because I was categorically avoidant of hot personalities, I was unwilling to ask her to move her vehicle, thereby making our parking landscape even more treacherous.

Nina stepped up. She stepped into the driver's seat because I would not. She voluntarily drafted herself in this War on Ambulance Parking.

Then, tragedy.

Nina reversed the ambulance and backed straight into a pole, trusting the backup camera to guide her instead of my screaming voice telling her to straighten out. "OK, good, now straighten out. Now straighten out. Straighten out! Straighten it! Nina you're going to hit the pole! Nina! You're going to hit the—"

After the crash, I moseyed up to my partner, still seated behind the wheel, looking a bit pale in the face, and said, "What part of straighten out did you not understand?"

"The camera said I would clear it!"

Got it. She had trusted technology over a sentient being. It happened. Only later did we discover that the backup camera was reversed. What Nina saw on screen conflicted with what I told her was true in reality and she chose the screen over me. She isn't the only person to be seduced by a screen.

Defeated, having lost the War on Ambulance Parking, we circled the truck that Nina had backed into a pole and were relieved to find no damage. That was a small victory. We found it strange, however, that Hartford was upstairs and didn't rush down after hearing my screams followed by a loud jarring crash-bang-boom. That was odd. But who cared? Neither of us. We grabbed the little black truck we wanted and went about our night. Which, remember, was our last tour together as partners.

We thought everything was fine, at first. But was everything ever fine in EMS? No. There always had to be "a problem." Things could never just be simple. An hour later, Hartford called Nina and asked what happened.

"You mean me crashing the ambulance into a pole?" Nina said.

That would be it.

Hartford said yes. She said there was damage to the truck. Paint chipped. Scratched bumper.

Oh? I didn't see that. Neither did Nina. Did bumpers matter? To someone out there, I was sure bumpers mattered. To Hartford, clearly. We had not examined the bumper. The word "bumper" to me signified that the purpose of its life was to bump into things, so I had personally only looked at the box.

But Hartford believed we saw damage to the truck, ignored it, and tried to pull a fast one on her, which I assure you was not the case.

Things spiraled from there.

Hartford called Beck. Beck got pissed. The next day, he yanked Nina's driving privileges and told her she had to retake CEVO training. Now, EMTs at Park Slope often ripped the air-conditioner unit off ambulances that didn't fit in one of the ER bays, and they weren't driver restricted. Outraged, Nina dropped all of her tours. As did I, out of loyalty, rage, this entire situation being my fault since I was unwilling to park the truck and ask Hartford to move her car, and a lack of desire to train new EMTs every week and never again work with my partners.

Nina and I were officially off the street.

That summer, my crisis caseload grew heavy. In July I got a dead-baby case, which was one of the worst types of cases an investigator could work. On Twitter, a few mothers claimed their toddlers had died after taking a novel medicine on the European market. My job was to investigate their claims and find out if that was true, or if the children had died of other causes.

Turned out the mothers were wrong. Other factors had triggered the deaths. But that could not be communicated, not on social media, where the mothers were tweeting it up. Who in their right mind would go on the Internet and suggest bereaved mothers were wrong? Their children were dead.

Let me tell you something about the anguish of parents of deceased children. The third rail of their rage could electrocute the planet. They never get over it—ever. They go to their graves with broken hearts. Right or wrong, grieving mothers deserved prayerful silence, boundless compassion, space, time, respect, and empathy, ad infinitum. So there was nothing digital to be done here.

Respectful silence and addressing the problem off-line, behind the scenes, was always extremely hard counsel for clients to swallow, as the wrongfully accused urgently wanted to speak and tell the truth, tell their side of the story, correct the record, make journalists and tweeters go back and fix the mess they created out of lies. But that crisis strategy was doomed.

The Internet is not a place for justice. It is not a place for complex narrative, thoughtful reexamination, deeper reflection, or due process. People hit the Internet when all other options and systems failed them. After the courts failed them. The media. The country. The Internet was a last resort. Defending yourself on the Internet was a beggar's language.

My clients were not beggars.

The first step in any Internet crisis was to immediately take the problem off-line and address it in the real world. Deal with it in real life, with real people, on the phone or preferably, in person.

"Do you have to look at photographs of dead children for your case?" Felice asked me one night on the phone.

We had a long-running joke in our friendship about Felice believing she was a detective because she watched *Law & Order*, and for other reasons too absurd and valid to enumerate here. I despised the show. (Sorry, I know everyone loves it, and cops and detectives consult on storylines, and Bobby starred in it. Sorry, Bobby.) But the cruelest and most violent crimes of my personal and work life fell into the unknowable pile. Heather's killing. Various mass shootings. They were unjust, chaotic, and infinitely torturous for survivors. There was no formula or satisfying emotional closure. Justice from what I saw in my life and career was the exception, not the rule. Crimes were left unsolved, and haunted survivors for as long as they breathed air. There was no law. There was no order.

"Sometimes," I told Felice. "Right now I do, yes."

"Oh, sis," she said. "I'm so sorry. I couldn't do that."

"But you must do it, because you're a detective."

"Nope. Absolutely not. I'm not looking photos of dead kids. I don't work those kinds of cases."

"Fascinating. What kinds of cases do you work? As a detective?"

"I work all the other ones," Felice said.

Because of my job I had a fraught relationship with the Internet.

"Your Twitter account makes no sense," a friend once observed. "It's all about books and writers and cool things your friends did, and the occasional EMT post."

Pretty much.

Most days, I viewed the Internet as a dumpster fire and excellent source of hilarious memes, which Felice and I exchanged constantly. In my work life the Internet was a place where things went horribly wrong and people suffered in ungodly ways. I'd seen too much. Photographs of children criminally misused. Teens bullied to the point of suicide. Elderly abuse. Revenge porn videos and hate-fueled death threats Silicon Valley moneymen refused to take down. Conspiracy theorists ranting online, threatening to kill people, then doing so in real life.

I was addicted to my phone like the rest of the Wi-Fi-connected world. But I tried to be mindful of how much time I spent online.

The connection between social media usage and poor mental health outcomes was direct. Heavy social media users were some of our society's most depressed, anxious members. The ones I worried about most were those for whom the iPhone camera was not a window but a mirror. Social media addicts—let's use that word, rather than "users," it's more accurate—trapped in a hellscape of self, posting so many pictures of their reflections their accounts looked like ripped-out pages of a highschool yearbook where they were the only student in attendance.

Those people were not doing well, mental-health-wise. Deconstruct it. What was the underlying communication of the selfie? Look at me look at me look at me. Narcissism on bath salts. These users were imprisoned in self, for life.

As for the apps themselves, they worked like Vegas slot machines. A dopamine hit. A drug. You thought you were connecting to people by sharing a bombardment of selfies and taking pictures of your salad, cat, and the day you got stuck in traffic, but you were really strung out on alienation, alone in a room. Or worse, you were with people you loved, ignoring them because you were on your phone.

As a first responder I spent a fair share of time around the sick and dying. And never once did I hear anyone say, in their final moments, they wished they'd amassed more Instagram followers or spent more time on Facebook.

And so as dispiriting as it often was on the street, being on the ambulance was a refuge from my day job, and I missed it.

There was always the possibility of riding somewhere else. But where? Park Slope was one of the best volunteer agencies in New York City. And I'm not just saying that because I rode there. They won the agency of the year award in EMS. The problem Nina and I had was an "Us Problem."

One night not long after we lost the War on Ambulance Parking, when Nina and I were baking cupcakes at my house, we surrendered to the idea of returning to the street. We didn't know who we were when we weren't on the ambulance. We felt directionless. We requested a meeting with Beck and Hartford to hash things out. They kindly agreed.

The four of us met at base a few days later. Robert was around, so he sat in on the meeting, too. I think he wanted to see if there'd be screaming. EMTs love drama.

We sat down in the crew room with Hartford and Beck and tearfully sorted things out in regard to the night of our pole accident and their decision to split up partners.

Beck explained what was going on at the agency behind the scenes. He told us that EMTs damaged the trucks so often, he felt the situation was near hopeless in terms of keeping the ambulances operational. People lied to him all the time about things that went wrong on the street, then he got stuck with the fallout. And he understood how bonded we were as partners. He loved his regular partner, too. He told us if he couldn't ride with that guy anymore, he'd probably quit his job. His partner was the only thing that made being on the ambulance enjoyable. He was an EMT just like we were, so he got it.

At the same time, he explained, Park Slope was an all-volunteer organization. People rode for a few years, then went on to do better and brighter things. He had to keep the trucks staffed, keep the ambulances in service. New members were the only way to do that. He said we could still ride together as partners, and we quickly offered to train newbies every other week.

"I know what I'm doing," I said. "I'm hiding behind Nina. When I'm training new people, even though it's exhausting, I learn a lot. I have to step up."

Nina and I promised we'd do better next time, in the instance that something went south. We apologized for not reporting the accident and said that we had indeed looked for damage, and genuinely didn't see any.

Hartford apologized, too. I appreciated her apology more than anyone else's in the room. She genuinely didn't mean to cause us any harm. She didn't know how to handle the situation and couldn't understand why two of the organization's most responsible and dedicated members would do something like that.

We understood. Nina and I agreed to get back on the truck. We even agreed to pick up a mutual-aid tour. A heatwave was in swing, so FDNY had activated all volunteer ambulance companies to assist with the increased 911 call volume. Just when we thought we'd quit, we ended up offering more.

This is what I loved about crises, even my own. Listening to Beck and Hartford tell their version of events, and how it felt to be the recipients of our behavior, I understood how upset and angry we'd made them. I saw everything that was on their plates, all the good they were trying to do for the community, and how hard it was to keep the ambulances on the street with an all-volunteer crew. I understood, and I felt terrible for adding to their troubles. They were good people. We were all the same. That's what I came away from the meeting feeling. We're all the same.

So things resolved.

That being said, I sensed that for all four of us, the fiasco left a sour taste in our already-soured mouths. A crack in the vase of our trust. I still felt somewhat beaten-down. And so I was grateful when, a week later, some good news arrived on my doorstep.

Midway through August, I got a letter from FDNY telling me to report to Fort Totten, Bayside, for a physical agility test. My reaction was, Holy shit. Am I really going to do this? Join the Fire Department? In my head I kept hearing the voices of veteran firefighters from Ladder 3, Johnny and Gonzo. "Pat would love that." "Next year, I want to see you back here in uniform."

And so, early one morning, I drove to Fort Totten. Ship had been called to take the PAT on the same day. I didn't even know he was thinking of joining the Fire Department. Yet here we were. A hundred or so of us sat at long cafeteria tables with our list numbers and waited to be called. I looked around. Men and women, Black and white and brown, mostly young. I was one of the oldest candidates present by far. I was the instructors' age, if I had to guess. But it didn't matter. We weren't individuals anymore. We were list numbers.

That morning I passed the physical tests. All of them, with flying colors. Some of the instructors running the drill booths looked amused when they saw me. What was so funny? My height? My age? I wasn't a mind reader. Everyone use your words. Your faces are communicating.

All the tests were easy to pass, except for this arm ergometer situation. That thing was brutal. It almost broke me. I kept circling the revolving pedals with my hands, pushing my arms and speaking to Pat. *Only for you. Only for you would I do this shit.*

Ship passed all the physical tests, too. Afterward, we congratulated each other.

"Listen," he said, hugging me. "Not just anyone can do this job. But we can do this. It's a calling."

There was that pesky calling thing again. When I got back to my building and lumbered upstairs, I ran into Jeremy in the hallway. He'd made pancakes and asked if I wanted one.

I said, "Sure, I'll take a pancake."

Jeremy ran inside his apartment then popped out with plated cakes. Observing I was in fitness formal, he asked if I was coming from the gym.

"No, Fort Totten," I said, eating a pancake with my hands. "I'm thinking of joining the Fire Department."

"Are you suicidal?"

"Not that I'm aware of."

Next step on the FDNY front was a background investigation and medical exam. The fire people told me they'd mail me a letter, to lock in the day and time. They were very into mailing letters.

So was Marko. He'd done some boozy reflecting on his relationship-ending behavior, and apologized. He said he had some thoughts he wanted to share and asked if it was OK to send me a letter. I said sure.

Everyone send me your letters.

I waited for what felt like forever for FDNY and Marko's letters to arrive. I checked the mail every day for two or three weeks. No letters.

Why say you were going to do something and then not do it? What did your words mean? If nothing, why speak?

End of August another work crisis struck. A biggie.

I got called into a case that involved the dark web. White supremacists and other extremist hate groups were planning to shoot up an event across the country. My job was to try to locate kill threats online and determine their validity. If the intel was actionable, I threw it to the NYPD, which threw it to the FBI and the Joint Terrorism Task Force. Then Feds knocked on doors, seized weapons, and arrested wannabe mass shooters.

I worked like crazy. Ten, twelve, sometimes sixteen hours a day every day of the week. Most of the subjects were boys. Armed suburban white boys with automatic weapons their parents bought for them. I take white mass murder personally. Some of the haters were thirteen, fourteen years old.

Children. American children.

The dark web really was dark. I found so much hate against women, gays, Blacks, and Jews, my head spun. I had to drop off the ambulance because I had no time for anything but work.

It was one thing to get called into a crisis when everyone was dead, and the worst had already happened. But this was strangely harder. Knowing people were out there planning a mass shooting and I was one of the people tasked with stopping it. The NYPD said the Feds were arresting people based on my intel. They called me asking for threat briefs, so then I started to feel shouldered with even more responsibility. I felt nervous every time I stepped away from my computer. What if I just missed an actionable kill threat when I went out to dinner? I was like one of those people on airplanes who think if they close their eyes and trust the pilot, the plane will fall out of the sky.

I tried to stay humble about it. I told myself I was just a worker among workers. But the stress was incredible. I couldn't sleep. I couldn't write. I lost weight. My hair fell out in curly red clumps. To wash my brain of hateful content I bought plants, baked pies, and watched six seasons of *The Bachelor*. I could not recall any of the reality contestants' names.

One day I woke up and told myself I had to get the hell out of town. Go somewhere. Drive upstate. Find a place to relax and unwind for a few days, if only to catch up on sleep and inhale fresh air, see some trees, maybe even some nighttime stars.

I found a writerly castle-like property in Amenia, New York, and drove as fast as I could out of town. Once I got some food in me and slept for a day, I woke up feeling lonely. I invited Nina to come up and hang. We could eat farm-to-table food, I told her. Go to a farm and pet goats. I knew what my street bride valued. I sold her the animal fantasy. "Jennifer, really?" Nina said. "Do you mean it? Can we really go to a farm?"

That afternoon she drove upstate. It was raining when she arrived. Later that night, we ate a fancy dinner at the hotel restaurant. Nina ordered wine. It was amusing, seeing my EMT partner seated beside me in a formal dining room, swilling wine around a fancy goblet. "I don't know what I'm doing," she said after the waiter told her to sniff it. "I don't drink wine."

I also did not drink wine.

The next afternoon we drove to a nearby farm. Nina skipped around a grassy meadow, talking to her friends, the cows. We met lots of nice animals. Goats. Pigs. Chickens. Nina communed with them all. There wasn't a farm animal she met that she didn't love with her whole heart. She had a special weakness for piglets. I really do think she should leave New York City at some point, for instance now. Go live upstate for a while. Work on a farm.

As for me, my relaxing escape was short-lived. When I returned to New York City, I returned to tragedy.

* * *

I checked my mailbox when I got home. Inside, a letter from FDNY. It was dated to the future, September 11, congratulating me on passing the physical agility test, and giving me an appointment for my background check and medical exam in October.

I stared at the date. It seemed otherworldly, fated to receive a letter from the Fire Department dated to that meaningful day, as if Pat were behind it. I took it as a sign.

Pat, I said as I lumbered up the stairs to my apartment. *If you want me to join the Fire Department, I'll do it. I don't see how I can afford to, but I'll do it. Whatever you want.*

On September 11, I went to Pat's firehouse and spent the day with Ylfa and Pat's brother, Mike. He made it to New York from Vegas this year for the anniversary. We went down to the memorial. In the museum, Mike stood with his head bowed and his hands in his pockets in front of his brother's glass-encased helmet and decimated fire truck smashed on the museum floor like a stomped-on Coke can. Later that evening we went to the sundown ceremony at Ground Zero.

Ylfa was so excited I'd gotten accepted to the Fire Department she shared her pride in me with a young Irish firefighter who worked at Pat's house. She thought the Fire Department was one cohesive organization. She didn't know EMS was considered a separate, lesser world within the department, looked down on by many firefighters, so I cringed when she told him.

"It's not the same," I said. "EMS isn't like Fire. It's not one department."

The firefighter nodded in agreement. "It's different. It's two different things."

At some point Tommy texted. "Do you think you would ever let me know if you're OK? I think about you all the time and I'm just checking in. I'm sorry if I'm bothering you."

I missed him terribly. It pained me to keep ignoring him, especially on 9/11, but I wrote nothing back. I hadn't responded to any of his texts in seven months and had found some kind of defeated peace with the fact that we would never meet in real life. Every other man I talked to online and went on dates with paled by comparison. They seldom asked me what I did for work. What books I'd read. What compelled me to write. They mostly wanted to know if I could cook. A handful were morons. Knowing Tommy was out there but unreachable tortured me.

Oh well.

Marko sent condolences that day, too, which was kind of him. People were starting to forget 9/11, but soldiers never forgot.

"Sending positive thoughts to you today," Marko said. "They say people die three times: the first when the soul leaves the body. The second, when they're in their final resting place. And the third time when their name is spoken the final time. Your friend, mentor, and brother figure is still alive because of the story you have shared of his life. Be well, amazing Jennifer."

Amazing Jennifer didn't feel so hot. It was a long, sad day, and when I got home, I wanted only to unwind and sleep.

Then things got even more Irish.

Around midnight, in my apartment, I had a very strange experience. I flopped down on my bed and watched a video I'd made early that morning at the firehouse. One of the kilted firemen at Ladder 3, a tall dark-haired guy, had played the bagpipes this year during the moments of silence. I could usually hold it together for a good part of the ceremony. But once the bagpipes bleated, I lost it. I'd taken a video of the bagpiper playing, and that night I listened to the music. Such a beautiful, tragic sound.

It was getting late, and I was sweaty and exhausted, so I took a shower and readied for bed. While I was standing under the rushing water, I heard bagpipes. That's strange, I thought. I must have left the video playing on my phone. When I shut the faucet off, the music stopped. In the new silence I toweled dry and went to my bedroom and looked at my phone.

Nothing was open. No apps or music. The bagpipe video hadn't been playing.

Pat. He was always around on this day. I could feel his presence. So could Ylfa. And Bobby. And Mike and Mike and Mike.

At last it was September 12. A new day, the worst day on the calendar every year, behind me once again.

I thought.

But this year, on this day, Pat's brother Mike got diagnosed with World Trade Center–related prostate cancer from digging the pile, searching for Pat.

We'd known Mike had cancer the day before, at the firehouse on 9/11, but we weren't overly concerned about it. Prostate cancer was treatable. Lots of people survived. But today Mike got the news that it was terminal. Stage four.

A death sentence.

When Ylfa called and gave me the news, a plane of terror flew into my chest.

Mike's cancer was everywhere. It started in his prostate and cannibalized his bones. Over the summer he'd reached out to several retired firefighter friends in New York to help him find a 9/11-cancer doctor, but no one got back to him. That boiled my Irish blood. But it was typical.

Anyone who's had cancer knows it offers many surprises in terms of who shows up for you and who gives you the Irish goodbye, who you pull close in your time of need and who you shield from your sickness. When I got diagnosed with cancer my mom was so ransacked with terror and grief she could barely function. She wanted to fly to New York to help me, but I wouldn't let her. I couldn't handle going to the doctor, being operated on, and seeing my beloved mom so upset at the same time. It was too hard. My diagnosis wasn't just my nightmare, it was also hers. I didn't want her to see me sick or be afraid for me.

As far as Mike's diagnosis went, firefighters were family. How many more firefighters with World Trade Center–related cancer could these first responders be expected to handle? The situation was nearing hopeless. Imagine one morning you wake up and violently lose all of your friends, the people you've spent your entire life working with, your true family, they're murdered, and somehow you survive. You survive to get cancer. To watch the rest of your friends get cancer and die. You constantly go to funerals. That's your life.

No one wanted to hear Act Two of 9/11. The act about first responders who survived, dug the pile, scoured the pit, and cleaned up the city, fell sick and died. The public preferred to believe the tragedy was behind them.

I doubted the people we launched forever wars against felt 9/11 was in the rearview, or the soldiers who volunteered to fight them. Or the families involved in the chronically stalled Guantánamo trial, still delayed twenty years later after yet another military judge stepped away.

I doubted Muslim Americans now perceived and surveilled as criminals by the intelligence community due to the terrorists' actions felt it was over, when brown became the new Black. "Where's Mohammed?" I asked a white first responder about the whereabouts of an EMT friend one day on the street. "He's at home," the guy said. "Building bombs."

And 9/11 was certainly still on the plate of first responders in New York City.

In EMT school, Nate had told us enrollment had surged after the attacks. Same thing in the fire and police departments. Everyday people signed up to become first responders.

"Tuesday's kids," children who lost parents that day and later became rescuers were called. Those 9/11 Act Two young adults were now rescuers on the street.

Everyone remembered the fallen.

The still falling were forgotten.

"Oh, nobody's doing shit about the still falling," a firefighter friend said. "That's too hard. Once they fall, you say a prayer and move on to the next memorial. These guys don't have the capacity to show weakness. And that's sad. I see it. It's a machismo thing. 'Get him a beer and let him have fun and the cancer will fall out of him.' Not how it works, slick. Cry with him. Share stories with him. Be that brother now."

Gonzo was that brother. He and a few of Pat's closest surviving firefighter friends stood by Mike and helped him get affidavits signed to prove his cancer was linked to digging the pile so he could get treated as part of the World Trade Center healthcare program.

For the most part, 9/11 Act Two rescues of the critically sick were long, slow, emotional, painful, ugly, and profoundly sad. A death marathon, not a sprint. These saves largely fell on the backs of families and friends, women and children. And Jon Stewart. He did heavy public lifting for the cancer-besieged 9/11 community, testifying with detective Luis Alvarez, who sat dying beside him, gray and riddled with cancer, and advocated for extending healthcare benefits for 9/11 first responders to an empty Congress.

I'll say it again. The way we treat servicepeople in this country is a monstrous disgrace.

Sad math was, there were too many first responders dying for survivors to bear, funerals calendared nearly every month, and cancer hit many vulnerable, grief-ravaged survivors too close to home for them to be able to assist. Cancer, suicide, drug addiction, and alcoholism plagued the first responder community, particularly survivors of 9/11—an unsurvivable event.

Ylfa had been the one who, through her friend Stephen who worked at Mount Sinai, had pulled some strings over the summer and found Mike an oncologist named Dr. Oh. Talk about being a first responder. It was hard, almost impossible, to land timely appointments with doctors who treated cancer-infested first responders, because there were so many of them. The waiting list was long.

Ylfa and Stephen made sure the doctor knew Mike's story. That he knew about Pat, and all that he'd done, and how he'd perished. Dr. Oh gave Mike an appointment right away. He'd been the one who'd staged the cancer.

"I don't know, sister," Ylfa said on the phone. "This is going to be rough. Pat's dead. Mike's wife, Janet, is dead. I'm supposed to have dinner with him tomorrow night. It's a lot."

"I've got you," I said. "See if Mike's OK with me joining you for dinner. If he is, I'll come. If not, no problem. We'll figure something out. But you don't have to do this alone, sister. I can help. We'll do it together. We'll look after Mike."

"Really?" she said. "You would do that?"

"He's Pat's brother."

"Yes."

Then we said it together, as if rehearsed: "Anything for Pat."

The three of us met up the next night for dinner in Midtown, at a loud, crowded pub Mike selected. One of those Irish joints where bartenders served pints of Guinness to patrons in sports jerseys and it smelled like there was sawdust on the floor. The kind of establishment I used to drink at, back in the day. A hole in the wall. Loved those.

We slid into a booth. Ylfa and I squeezed into a bench and sat across from Mike, who drank a few beers and ordered some kind of gamey Irish-type meat we teased him for ordering. It was strange, being with Mike. Comforting. Almost like being with Pat, since they looked so much alike. Sad as the news was, a new joy took residence in me. Another brother.

We talked for hours. Mike agreed to let Dr. Oh treat him at Mount Sinai, which was a miracle. Prior to that he'd dismissed all medical advice that had come his way. He didn't want to lose his mustache. His hair. He wanted to still be able to have sex. "You're dying of masculinity," we told him. He didn't believe it was happening or that it could possibly be this bad. Categorically, doctors made horrible patients, and Mike was no exception. This meant he'd be back in New York monthly to get treatment. That was the plan.

After dinner, Ylfa and I said goodbye to Mike, who stayed at the pub. He wanted to stay out a bit longer, keep drinking. Maybe catch up with some firefighter friends, go to another bar.

He seemed so lonely. We felt bad leaving him behind, but it was late. And Ylfa and I, let's just say our bar days were behind us.

Walking to the train together, the two of us realized it had made us both feel glum to sit in that loud, crowded pub where we had to shout just to hear what Mike was saying, which was pretty heavy. We made a pact. Whenever he was in town, Ylfa would pick the place where we had dinner. Find somewhere quiet and cozy, where we could hear each other talk. No more boozy pubs blasting rock music. And when Mike wasn't with family, we'd drop everything to spend time with him.

Soon Mike was back in Vegas, where he lived in a sprawling desert house he referred to as "the compound" with his niece Erin, who was in nursing school. After his wife died, Erin stepped in and took care of Mike. She was his true rescuer, smart and dedicated and loving and helpful, a hero in every sense of the word. Mike stayed in constant touch with me and Ylfa from Vegas. We assembled a group chat and texted and talked on the phone nonstop. A makeshift family formed in doom.

Absurdity, too.

Reality failed us, so we turned to fairy tale. We gave each other pet names after Mike and Ylfa stumbled upon some animals one day in Central Park. We were characters in a fable now. Ylfa was Duck. Mike was Turtle. And they informed me I was EMT Chick, because I worked on an ambulance and was cute. The sound I made instead of a quack was the sound of an ambulance.

Wee-woo.

If my life were a work of fiction, I'd dial this back. It was a bit much, even for a career crisis woman like me. I wasn't convinced I could handle this. Not all of it. And certainly not all at once.

When my work crises simmered down—no mass shooting, we won, the Feds arrested more naughty, felonious armed children—I returned to the street.

Measured against Mike's fate, my life and trials on the ambulance seemed comparatively minor, almost plotless. The only thing I looked forward to these melancholic days was celebrating Halloween.

One October night on the truck Nina and I brainstormed our 2019 costumes and decided to be sheriffs. My favorite uncle was a sheriff, and he was dealing with cancer, too, so it made sense to pick a spirit-boosting costume in his likeness.

We purchased mustaches, in honor of Mike. Mine was red and matched my hair color exactly. When Nina's arrived in the mail and she put it on, she looked like a crystal meth dealer.

Over the course of a week we bought matching brown felt cowboy hats. And we decided to make chocolate cupcakes slathered with orange frosting to give away to first responders. That was our plan. But as Mike Tyson says, "Everybody has a plan until they get punched in the mouth."

It seemed no time had passed and suddenly Mike was back in New York. Ylfa and I saw him every day he was here. One afternoon he and I hung out alone for the first time. We went to Central Park Zoo and had a conversation that changed my fate as an EMT. Looking back, all of this seems divinely orchestrated.

It was a beautiful fall day, the air crisp and leaves reddening, the kind of magical autumn weather that made New York City seem like the greatest city in the world. Mike and I were walking and talking, wandering around arm in arm, reminiscing about Pat.

"Did you know my brother?" he asked me.

I tripped and almost fell. I knew Pat was a legend, but until Mike asked me this, I didn't realize people who didn't know Pat at all were contacting Mike, or otherwise hanging around.

"Yes," I said. "I knew your brother. Pat and I practiced yoga together for a few years, and he helped me a lot when I was newly sober and had cancer."

"I didn't know you had cancer."

"Yeah, melanoma. Stage one, but I reacted like it was stage four because I was young and terrified and mokus. I only had a month sober when I found out, so I was basically hysterical. Pat told me I'd be OK. He said he wasn't worried about me."

Mike nodded. Walking with his head lowered, staring at the leaf-strewn path, he said, "Pat and I weren't really that close. He kinda kept his life separate."

I glanced at him. He looked afflicted.

"You know, Turtle, sometimes sober people do that. It's not that we don't like bars. But sometimes hanging out in them gets depressing for us. So sometimes, not always but sometimes, we keep our lives a little bit separate, even from people we love."

Mike said, "I understand. I never knew that."

We walked in silence for a while. Strolling around the park I told Mike I'd gotten a letter from the Fire Department and was thinking about joining FDNY. How it was torturing me a little, the decision. I felt like I wasn't a real rescuer unless I worked for the Fire Department in honor of Pat. I told him I thought it was wrong that EMS was treated like the ugly stepchild of the department while medical emergencies far outnumbered fires. That New York City was still in the dinosaur ages compared to other major cities that cross-trained firefighters as paramedics.

"You're singing to the choir," Mike said.

He was a doctor, after all. He respected street medicine. He knew what we were seeing out there, and how hard it was, and how thankless. I told him I didn't meant to slight firefighters.

"Yeah, but you're right. There aren't that many fires anymore. Buildings have sprinklers. Firefighters are sitting around eating. They get sleep."

"I know a guy who works pretty hard up in the Bronx," I said, thinking of Tommy.

"I worked in Harlem," Mike said. "I got sleep."

That made me laugh.

"You know, EMT Chick," Mike said. "I was a firefighter when I found out I got into medical school. I was working up in Harlem at the time. And I was happy being a firefighter. It was fun. I loved it. So I didn't know what to do when I got into med school. I thought maybe I'd keep being a firefighter. I told Pat, and he was so proud of me. God, he was prouder of me than I was of myself. He was prouder than anyone. And Pat said, 'Mike. You got into med school. Anyone can be a firefighter. Not anyone can be a doctor.

Go be a doctor.' So I quit the Fire Department and I went to medical school and became an ER doctor."

Just then I heard, clear as day, as if Pat were speaking to me directly, *Maximum service. We're supposed to be of maximum service to ourselves and others.* I knew exactly what he meant. He meant do the thing only you can do. You, and no one else. Do the harder thing. The thing that makes you singular. For me, that meant being a writer. I felt a new clarity wash over me.

"Were you happy with your medical career?" I asked Mike.

"Oh God, yeah. I loved it. I probably would have had an easier life if I'd stuck with being a firefighter. But I loved being an ER doctor. You can really help people."

"I love helping people. It's a sickness with me. I'm going to die from helping people."

Mike chuckled and said, "Me too. But what you're doing for work, Ylfa told me about your case, how you're trying to stop mass shootings and cops are arresting people based on your work. You're a hero. You're saving people's lives and they don't even know it. And riding on the ambulance at night, and writing. I love writers. Hemingway rode on an ambulance during the war. Not everybody can write a book. So I say if you can do that, I think that's pretty incredible."

I wanted to sob I was so relieved. Pat was gone, but he'd given me his brother, so in a way it was as if he were back. That's how I felt. Like I had a brother again. Two. Irish twins. Twin towers. The fallen and still falling. Pat and Mike.

As for Halloween, the show, as they say, did not go off as planned.

Nina and I donned our mustaches and hats, then we hopped on the ambulance and hit the streets with our beautiful cupcakes. Once again, no one wanted our baked goods. Zero. Zero first responders wanted a cupcake. This was becoming a real snag in the business model of Sweets in the Streets. EMTs claimed they had no appetites. Medics said they'd given up sugar.

However, our costumes were a raging success. We took a picture of ourselves on the truck and flung it to Vegas. Mike thought we looked hysterical. We flung it to Washington state. My sheriff uncle did, too. Later that night I pulled over to park the truck and heard a loud, awful scraping sound.

"Jennifer," Nina said. "You just hit that parked car."

"Did I? I don't think I hit anything."

"You did."

I would like to point out, for the record, I was not wearing my cowboy hat at the time of this alleged "accident," as the wide brim interfered with my field of vision and made it difficult to see. I really didn't think I hit the car. It wasn't like I was racing to a job. I was just parking. I know you're not going to believe this, but I was a pretty good driver. I got the job done.

But Nina was convinced I'd hit the car. Fine. I pulled over and we climbed off the truck. Some people standing outside a restaurant where the car I'd supposedly hit was parked looked at us like criminals. We're not criminals, I thought. We're sheriffs.

We found no damage to the car, or to our ambulance. The car had some cat scratches by the driver's side doorhandle, but those looked old. Again I told Nina I really didn't think I hit the car. Maybe the plastic flap thingy-bop that went over our tire hit the other car's tire flap? It didn't matter. People were watching. Witnessed "accident." We'd been down this rotten road before and done the wrong thing. Now we did the right thing and called our duty officer. That night our DO was Lexi, thank God.

"Hey, girl," I said, calling her from scene. "So I just hit a parked car. Nina thinks I hit a parked car. I'm not so sure. But either way, there's no damage to our truck or the other vehicle."

"Did anyone see?" Lexi asked.

"Yep. They're staring at us right now. We're sheriffs, but they can't tell because we don't have our hats and mustaches on. They think we're EMTs."

"Is the driver of the car you hit there?"

"Negative. Car's empty."

"OK. stay there. I'll be there in twenty minutes."

"Ten-four."

On the ambulance, Nina fumed about the fact that we had to wait for a DO on Halloween, our dream tour. Then I got mad at her for getting mad, because I was the one who'd just supposedly had an accident, which, by the way, I'd never had before (and still hadn't), and we'd just gotten out of trouble and now we were going straight back in.

Wonderful. Just wonderful. I could feel Chief Beck's eyeballs rolling from across the city. My dream above all dreams was that the driver of the car I'd supposedly hit would appear on the street, get in his car, and drive away as if nothing had happened. I closed my eyes and tried to visualize what I wanted. I prayed and prayed.

When I raised my head off the steering wheel, I told Nina what I'd done. A long time ago we'd agreed I had psychic powers. Once, when we were bored on the truck, I told her I could manifest things. I was joking, but then I actually did it. I was eating gummy bears, and I said, "Now tell me what gummy bear flavor is your favorite, and I'll close my eyes and pull that exact flavor out of the pack. I'll do magic." Nina picked orange. Excellent choice. Lots of reds in gummy bear packages, too many if you ask me, but very few orange bears. I closed my eyes and pulled out an orange gummy bear on the very first try. "Jennifer you did it!" Nina said. "You manifested your vision."

Yes. That was correct. And Halloween night, I did it again.

Soon, a man walking at a fast clip appeared out of nowhere. I saw him in the rearview mirror heading toward the car I'd supposedly hit. He didn't blink or pause when he got inside it. He saw nothing, because there was no damage, friends.

Before we could get off the truck to talk to him and explain what had happened, he sped away. He drove right past us. I felt a mountain slide off my back.

"I did it," I said breathlessly. "I manifested my fantasy."

"Wow," Nina said. "That was your wildest dream, and it happened."

"This night is a dream!" I shouted. "I love Halloween!"

By the time Lexi rolled up, there was nothing corrective for her to do. She confirmed what we'd told her: No damage to our truck. No damage to the other vehicle, which was no longer on scene. No driver. No report.

Happy Halloween.

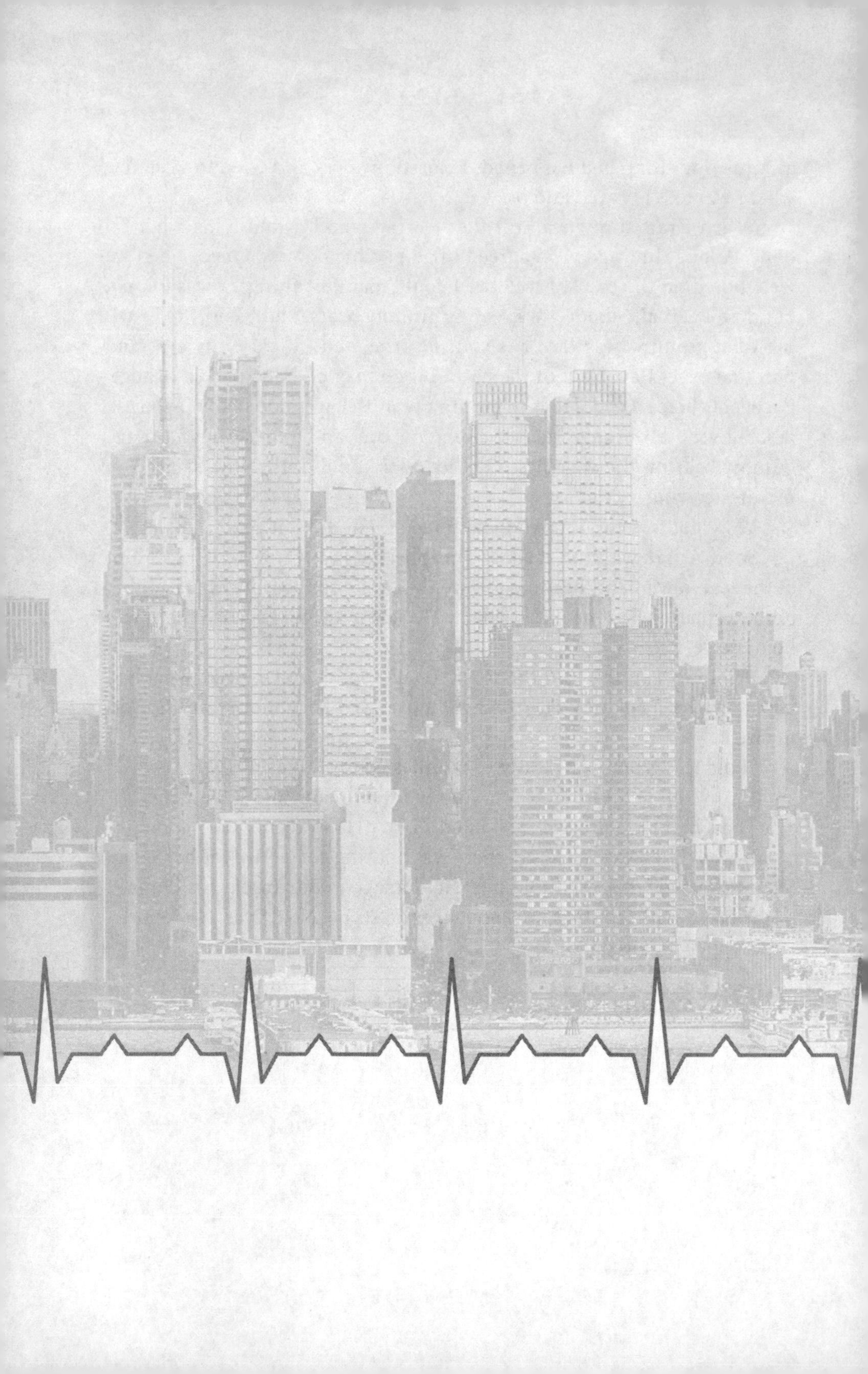

PART THREE

MUTUAL AID

10

TWO WIVES

By November I'd let the date of my FDNY background check and medical exam lapse without regret, thanks to that fate-changing conversation I had at the zoo with Mike. Instead of progressing as a full-time Fire Department EMT, I flew to Louisiana and met my mother in New Orleans. She'd never been.

My mom was in her seventies. And lately we'd been having conversations about things she wanted to see and do while she was still healthy. It was important to do these things before it was too late. The street never let me forget that life went fast, and we were really here for a very short time.

In New Orleans, my mom and I had a blast. For a week we strolled around the French Quarter and Garden District, clapped for street musicians, ate our faces off. Shrimp with grits. Crawfish. Sacks of warm beignets from Café du Monde.

Nights, we talked about everything under the sun, except for my brother. He was a sore subject. I guessed he always would be.

Being an EMT helped me let go of my pervasive, lifelong need to try to save him. Working on the ambulance, I understood that dispatchers were never going to send us on a job to do CPR on our family members, since we'd be so tormented with emotion, we wouldn't be able to function. To the contrary, we'd get in the way and potentially jeopardize a rescue.

In serious emergencies, a conditions boss was always on scene with us to manage devastated family members—an emergency of its own—so the families didn't interfere while we were working, trying to save a life.

As first responders we save strangers. Rare exceptions aside, we do not rescue our own families, or people we love, because emotion takes hold and makes us unable to perform our job.

In New Orleans one night I told my mom about Mike being sick. She said she would pray for him. She understood how much he meant to me, how badly I needed a brother.

"Yours has never really been present in your life," she said. "But God gave you Mike. You're blessed to have him. And he's blessed to have you. You're a beautiful person."

"You're being generous, because you're my mother."

"No, I'm not. I couldn't be prouder of you. You've worked so hard on yourself. Everything you have in your life you've worked for. Your job. Your writing. Being an EMT. You didn't get anything from me. You did it all on your own. And you have an incredible life."

That really touched me, that my mom was proud of me. And what she said before, about Mike, I felt it, too. I felt blessed.

We talked about the happier aspects of my childhood. For generations, my family had cabins in the Sequoia National Forest, in a tiny mountain town called Camp Nelson. My dad and brother never liked it up there. Too rustic. Nothing to do. But my mom and I loved the mountains. That forest was our church. Giant redwoods and ancient sequoias, the ground covered in bear grass, the smell of pine and firewood during night walks with beamed flashlights. Just me and my mom walking through the moonlit forest, beneath a sky pebbled in stars. Heaven.

I thanked my mom for everything she did for me growing up. She did so much. There was no fire she wouldn't walk through, once she got off all that Valium the doctors put her on.

"I was a nightmare as a teenager. If I had a kid who acted like I did, I'd lock myself in an institution."

"You were angry," my mother said.

"And drunk. I was awful. Grandma called me an asshole once."

My mom giggled. "Did she? She was quite a woman."

"Quite a woman."

Our last day we packed and flew separate ways. I left New Orleans sad to say goodbye to my mom. On the plane I thought about how much I loved and missed her, more than I allowed myself to feel. Her marriage to my father had been a failure, my childhood a shitshow. She stayed married way too long. Twenty-five years. She stayed because she was afraid to leave. She was ashamed to be a divorced woman. She didn't want to disappoint her parents. She was Catholic.

But in the end, she got out. Six or so years after she divorced, my mom found a man who truly loved her and now enjoyed a happy second marriage.

In life there existed the person you were supposed to marry, the person your parents approved of, the right choice on paper, the person who made you feel safe but never stirred your soul or made your heart pound with fear and wonder. The appropriate choice. For her that was my father. He wasn't a bad person. And he certainly wasn't a murderer like Heather's dad. He just had an anger problem. My mom only knew him six months when they got engaged.

I almost married that guy, too. The wrong guy. Jim, the architect I was dating back when I had that seizure. He was a safe choice. There was nothing wrong. But there was nothing right, either. He saw parts of me but not all of me, not even close. Something vital was missing. My mom corrected her error with her second husband and married someone she was crazy about. Someone who, in her seventies, made her giggle like a schoolgirl, who she ran across the room to kiss. She married the guy who treated her well and also thrilled her.

May we all be so lucky—blessed.

My mom saved her money and bought a cabin in the Sequoias, in a little town called Alpine Village, just above Camp Nelson. It was her dream in life to own a cabin in those mountains, and she accomplished it. She had a magical place to go and escape the god-awful Bakersfield heat.

She did her best in that western house of my girlhood. Better than I probably would have done in her position. She gave me this beautiful life. And for that, I was truly grateful.

Back in New York that fall, Mike went from being my brother to my veritable husband—co-husband.

Mid-November he returned to New York with family. His cousin Jay, a retired California firefighter, and Jay's wife, Judie, a tall beauty. They were great. Very solid, very loving. They came along to accompany Mike to the doctor. Chaperone. Chaperone was a better word.

Mike was having chest pain as of late. In the exam room with Dr. Oh, Jay made Mike fess up about his symptoms. The doctor requested an EKG, which meant Mike had to go to the ER.

Waiting for his EKG in the hospital, he grew anxious. He didn't like sitting among patients, lines of stretchered sick people waiting to be triaged, full hospital beds, the steady mechanical beeping that created the ambient pulse of emergency rooms. It was too much for him.

He and Jay had been separated inside the ER, so Mike was momentarily on his own. Defiant to the core, he found the tech who ran his EKG and insisted on reading it himself. Seeing it was normal, he decided he didn't need to wait around to speak to a doctor. He was a doctor. So he asked a nurse for directions to the bathroom, then sneaked out of the hospital. He called Jay from the street. Then he called me.

"Turtle," I said. "What's happening? Did you get your EKG? Why are you out of breath?"

"I just escaped the ER," Mike said. "I ran out, EMT Chick. It's a fucking war zone in there. I can't be in there with those people."

"Oh, Jesus. It's a hospital. It has doctors and patients."

"It was fucking crazy. You have no idea."

"I do have an idea, I'm an EMT. It's New York City. All ERs are like that. Did you at least get your EKG?"

"EKG was normal, I read it myself. Probably anxiety. Now I'm waiting for Jay to find me."

"You're whispering like a convict."

"I'm out of breath, because I ran."

"Do you still have EKG stickers on your chest?"

"Yeah," Mike said, laughing. "I still got the stickers."

"You're bonkers. But I'm glad your EKG was normal. Think it might have been a panic attack, honey? I think maybe we need to have a little talk about feelings."

"Yeah. Oh, there's Jay. Jay!" he yelled. "Listen, EMT Chick. I don't know if I'm going to make Ylfa's opening tonight. I'm kinda upset."

Ylfa was in a short film called *You Can Kiss Me* opening at a festival that night. We were all supposed to go see it together.

"Take care of yourself, Turtle. Duck will understand. Deep breaths. Nice and easy. Hang out with Jay and Judie and see if you can relax, OK?"

"OK. Hey, listen. Jay's here, I gotta run. Love you."

"Love you more."

We said that to each other now, all three of us: I love you.

Mike made the film opening. Upset as he might have been about his visit to the ER, he didn't want to miss seeing Ylfa on the big screen.

All through the fall, Mike had a terrible crush on Ylfa, which unsettled her, since she was essentially Pat's posthumous bride. "If Pat had survived 9/11, he probably would have married Ylfa," Mike often said. "She'd be my sister-in-law."

But that didn't stop him from being bedazzled by her.

You couldn't blame him. Ylfa was gorgeous, talented, and so spiritual she'd almost entered some kind of fairy-tale realm. Tragedy had that impact on some people. They lived in thin places. They were thin people. They straddled the line between this world and the next. That was Ylfa.

Still, she was Pat's girl. I worked tirelessly on her behalf, for months, to snuff out the idea of a romance forming between she and Mike. It took a lot of energy to keep pushing that cat off the kitchen table.

"I'm so in love with Duck," Mike confessed one day as we strolled around Central Park.

I had to muffle laughter, the way he phrased it. Talking to Mike about his feelings for Ylfa was like talking to someone who'd just micro-dosed at a ZZ Top concert.

"I'm in love with you, too," he declared.

"Stop it. You are not."

"Yes, I am," he said strongly. "Ylfa saved my life. She's the one who found me Dr. Oh and got me in to see him. Her friend Stephen did that for me. Not the firefighters. And you're saving my life, too. Just by spending all this time with me. You guys are really helping me. I look forward to coming to New York see you. I get kinda lonely out in Vegas. So I'm in love with you, too. I'm in love with both of you."

"You're a firefighter. You're in love with everyone."

Mike stomped his foot. "No, I'm an ER doctor. And I'm only in love with you and Ylfa, Duck and EMT Chick. No one else."

I knew what was happening here. Mike thought he was falling for us because we were helping him at the critical hour, just as Pat had helped me. You fall in love with the people who help you in your darkest moment. It happens to newly sober people when they meet old-timers in sobriety.

It happens to first responders and rescued patients. It's not romantic love. It's sacred.

"OK, Turtle," I said. "You can be in love with both of us if you want. We can be your wives."

"I would love that," Mike said. "I've got cancer. So I get two wives."

"At least."

So now I was married.

That night before the film opening, after his great escape from the ER, I picked Mike and Jay and Judie up at a bar in Chelsea, then we met up with Ylfa at the theater.

My sister-wife had talked to me earlier that week about Mike seeing the film. It included a scene with her kissing a woman, so she was worried about how he'd react. Mike didn't know the film contained an erotic scene. "He's going to lose his mind," I said. "He has no idea what's in store for him. He's about to experience life beyond his wildest dreams. His goddess on the big screen, kissing a woman. He'll collapse with pleasure. We'll have to roll him out in a wheelchair."

In the crowded lobby of the theater I chatted with Jay and Judie, who were lovingly exasperated by Mike and his man-child escape from the ER. Jay and I had a long talk about being first responders and trying to assist patients like Mike. How hard it was, on scene, when patients who really needed to go to the hospital refused go. How worried you got that they would die if you left them behind. How powerless you felt.

Soon the film started. I sat between Jay and Ylfa. Mike sat beside his one true love, Duck. I was making some progress demolishing his romantic dreams, but this forthcoming kissing scene was going to send me a lot more than two steps back.

A few films aired before we got to Ylfa's movie. It was a great short. The plot worked and the end was "surprising, yet inevitable," as Aristotle says made the best endings. The kissing scene was tastefully done. I was proud of my sister.

Afterward, when the lights came on and I looked at Mike—he looked like the guy in that old Maxell ad that showed a man sitting in a chair with his hair and tie blown back by the incredible sound of the music. That was Mike, after seeing Ylfa's film. He was the blown-away man. I couldn't look at him with a straight face.

"How ya feeling, Turtle?" I asked him later, when the group of us went to dinner.

Mike said, "Oh, wow. Wow. I'm so glad I saw Ylfa's movie. I almost didn't make it, after being in the hospital earlier, but I'm so glad I did. I thought it was the best movie in the festival. Ylfa's a great actor. She's up there with James and Bobby."

James Remar, and I already told you about Bobby Burke—both actors and two of Pat's closest friends. Mike's, too. After Pat died on 9/11, they also became first responders. An EMT and firefighter, respectively. Pat had that impact on people. He created rescuers.

"Our Duck is really talented," Mike said.

"She sure is. She's our star."

"I think she was magical," he continued, staring enraptured at his water glass. "And I'm not just saying that because I'm in love with her. Don't forget, I'm in love with you, too."

"Never forget."

I couldn't stop laughing. I laughed all through dinner. I laughed on the subway ride home. On the phone later, with Ylfa. When I turned the lights out that night, I was still laughing.

God bless Mike Brown.

In December I flew to Paris to relax for a few weeks. Being with my mom had been wonderful. But I needed to flit around Europe. Do some of that relaxing the French were so good at. Speak broken French. Get catcalled by men on Vespas wearing pink cashmere sweaters who called me jolie, drôle, Zheniffer.

I'd meant to go to Paris in September, back when the weather was fair. But I'd gotten slammed with crisis cases. Then Mike got diagnosed with cancer, and I didn't want to miss any of his visits.

America and its armed hate groups had really worn me out these last few months. It had worn out the NYPD's intelligence arm, too, which in December announced the formation of a new unit focused on racially and ethnically motivated extremism. For two decades, the intel community's focus had been on Islamic State terrorist groups. Now it was on domestic terrorism coming from far-right and neo-Nazi organizations like the Proud Boys.

Finally I timed it right and took a break from my country. Au revoir. I'd finished my novel, so there was nothing to do in France but unwind.

I took a trip to Brussels to see an investigator colleague who used to work kidnap and ransom cases in Mexico, so that was nice. She'd met her new boyfriend, a bilingual diplomat, on Tinder. I met jack shit. I met guys who said things like, "Good morning," and after I said, "Good morning" back, they said, "I'd like you on all fours by midnight."

Thanks. Thanks, everyone on Tinder. Very romantic. I look forward to seeing you on the sex offender registry.

I Eurorailed back to France. Paris was drizzly and gray by winter, the air so cold my teeth clattered no matter how much I bundled up. But Paris worked. I always found the beauty of France renewing. I returned to New York City a new woman. Or an old woman with new eye cream.

That December of 2019, nights on the ambulance were slow. Patients climbed on our truck with the usual winter maladies. Flu, pneumonia. If COVID-19 was in circulation in Brooklyn at the time, which it very possibly was, I didn't know anything about the virus yet, and I didn't see anything noteworthy on the street.

At some point that winter Nina called out sick because she came down with what we assumed was sudden onset flu, complete with a high fever that left her exhausted and bedridden. After a few days it passed. Was it a cold? The flu? Coronavirus? God alone knows, though four months later, when New York City exploded with COVID and became the epicenter of the virus in the United States, I teased Nina that she was patient zero.

Mid-month, Mike returned to New York to see Dr. Oh. He was here so much these days it seemed he lived on the East Coast. It was nice to have him around. There was no one like Pat Brown. But let me tell you—there was no one like Mike Brown, either.

Where Pat was intense and fast-talking, Mike was relaxed and measured. Where you could imagine Pat forcing a door and standing in your burning apartment with his eyes darting all around, you could see Mike standing behind him with a ponderous expression on his face, considering things.

If Pat was action, Mike was thought. You could feel Mike thinking. Pat was serious and protective. Mike, sweet and goofy, almost childlike. Pat was wound tight and ringing with life whereas Mike carried an air of melancholic defeat, even when he was laughing. He made you want to throw your arms around him and pull him close. Pat was shorter than Mike but presented to the eye a towering grandeur. Mike was approachable. Human-scaled. A guy.

"I'm just a guy," he said whenever Ylfa and I asked why he did certain things. It always made us laugh. "Mike, your jeans have holes in them. You're a doctor. Why are you walking around looking like you just got out of rehab?" "I don't know. I'm just a guy." We took him to the store and insisted he buy new jeans. "Mike, is that a comb in your back pocket? Are we in a time warp? Did you just go to the bathroom and comb your hair, is that why it's wet? "Quit teasing me. I'm a guy." "Mike, I'm in the middle of telling you a story about my life and you interrupt to make me look at guitars in the store window. Why do you do shit like that?" "Cause I'm a guy?"

Lately we'd been teasing him somewhat mercilessly about giving away piles of money to barflies. He gave this guy a loan. That guy a loan. Ylfa and I made a lot of jokes about Mike walking into a bar.

"Mike walks into a bar and says, 'Hey, everyone. I'm Mike and I'm rich. Anyone need any money?'" "Mike walks into a bar with his routing number on his FDNY T-shirt. #RoutingNumber." "Put your wallet away and get some self-esteem," we told him. "People asking you for loans aren't your friends. They're robbing you and you're letting them. They're rats."

"Hey, my friends aren't rats," Mike said.

"Rats!" we yelled at him.

This visit, he and I met for coffee one gray rainy afternoon at Maison Kayser, a French bakery up by Central Park. We got cappuccinos. I ordered a coffee éclair and told Mike to get one, too.

"I've never had an éclair before," he said.

"Get one, Turtle. You'll like it."

The cappuccinos arrived. Mike ripped open a half-dozen sugar packets and doused his coffee with a landfill of sweetness. He demolished his éclair and said, "Hey, I liked that." Then, out of nowhere, he started talking to me about his drinking.

The conversation turned serious.

In the café, Mike said that most nights after Ylfa and I left him after dinner, he stayed out and went to bars all by himself. He got drunk. He'd gone out the night before and drank so much he couldn't walk.

"I thought maybe that wasn't good, that I lost use of my legs."

I nodded. "Legs are kind of important."

"Let me ask you something."

"Shoot."

"Do you think I'm an alcoholic?"

I almost choked on my éclair. Oh boy. There it was. The million-dollar question. I thought he'd never ask. Ylfa and I had been praying for Mike to get sober for months. Years? A long time. Ylfa had planted a seed in the summer, suggesting Mike quit drinking while getting treatment and maybe check out sobriety, as Pat had done. But there was nothing any of us could do until Mike tapped out. You get there when you get there, and some people never get there at all. I supposed Mike was Pat's unfinished business in a way. Last wishes. We wished for it, too. We knew Pat wanted his brother to get sober.

"The answer's in the question," I told Mike at the café. "If you're asking the question, you've got the answer."

"Yeah, but I'm asking you. What do you think?"

"You were drunk the first time I met you at the firehouse on 9/11. At eight o'clock in the morning."

"But do you think I'm an alcoholic?"

"Alcoholism is a self-diagnosed disease."

"But what do you think?"

"Pat was sober. And all your closest friends are sober. You love sober people. You're surrounded by them."

"Yeah, but what do *you* think?"

"You want my opinion?"

"Yes, I do."

I took a deep breath. Then I leaned over the table and said, "Mike. I think you're a raging alcoholic."

He balked and slapped his hand over his face in shame. I squealed and took a picture of him and sent it to Duck. Then Mike took a photo of me with my hand on my face, and we sent her that, too. Then Ylfa sent us one of her face-palmed.

"I don't think I'm an alcoholic," Mike said. "I don't know. I'm all mixed up. But I've been thinking— "

Some part of me stopped listening when I heard that word, "thinking." Alcoholics were always thinking. Talk with an alcoholic about their drinking, and you'll get that response almost every time: "I don't think I'm an alcoholic. Let me think about it. I just need to figure it out." But alcoholism was a disease of the body and mind, medically and clinically, so the mind was not the place to solve alcoholism. It got solved in the gut and heart and spirit. Alcoholics died alone in their rooms or on barstools, thinking and drinking, thinking and drinking. Figuring it all out.

But I was wrong. That was not what Mike was talking about at Maison Kayser. "Seeing that I have cancer," he said, "I was thinking I want to get ready."

"Ready for what?"

"You know."

"Death?"

"Yeah. I'd like to be present and awake, if this is all the time I got left. Like, really present. I'd like to have a spiritual life. I don't want to be at the bar all by myself. And since I'm getting treated now, thanks to Duck finding me Dr. Oh, I think maybe it's not good to be drinking so much I can't use my legs."

"Yeah, that's no good. Your poor body's working so hard to fight the cancer. And you've got a great doctor thanks to Duck, and you're taking your medicine. Half your medicine."

Ylfa and I had nicknamed him Fifty-Percent Mike, because he did half of what Dr. Oh suggested. Sometimes less.

"I'm Fifty-Percent Mike!" he said in the café.

"Yes, you are, and it's not a compliment. And I think that's a great idea, Turtle, to be awake for life. You've spent enough time at the bar."

"I've spent practically my whole life in bars."

"Right. Maybe it's time to try something different. I think Pat would be so happy."

"I'm supposed to go out with a doctor friend after this, for dinner. And I know we'll drink."

"Drink away. Is he a rat? You gonna give him your routing number?"

Mike laughed. "He'll probably expect me to pay for dinner and stuff."

"Listen to me," I said seriously. "If you ever want to stop drinking, the only thing I insist is that you not do it alone. Let us help you. Don't be a dry guy. Don't white knuckle it, it's not a good look. It doesn't work, and it's very painful. I'll do anything I can to help you get sober, and so will Ylfa. Pat helped me when I was getting sober, and I never got to thank him before he died, so it would be really nice for me to have a chance to thank him by helping you. Same goes for Ylfa. Nothing would make her happier. We love you so much."

"Well, I love you guys, too," Mike said. "That's why you're my wives."

* * *

After we parted, I texted Ylfa and told her it was happening. "Sister. It's a fucking miracle. Mike just asked me about his drinking." I told her the deal and she was on it.

When Mike called Ylfa later that night, after dinner, she acted as if she had no idea what was happening. She told him we were meeting up the next morning for breakfast, with some sober friends, to have a little meditation. Mike asked if he could come along. He sure could.

He drank that night, of course. First with his friend. Then alone at his hotel. Those sad little liquor bottles.

Next morning in downtown Manhattan, Mike met up with me and Ylfa. We introduced him to Pat's old sober crew. It was Mike's first day sober. He asked for help, and Pat heard his prayers and answered. I believed that. Most alcoholics had a moment of clarity about their drinking just before they got sober. Mike had a moment of éclairity. We did a little meditation together that morning. Not for long. Five minutes. Afterward, Mike had a look of bewitchment on his face. He was shaking his head back and forth, fast, as if in ravishment, like he was trying to shoo away a bee. Ylfa and I went up to him.

"You OK, Turtle?" we asked.

"Pat was here," he said, his eyes transfixed on us.

Ylfa and I said, "What did he say?"

"He pushed me on the shoulder and said, 'What took you so long?'"

Mike never drank again.

It was the season of miracles. Christmas morning, I woke up like it was any other day. I lay in bed sipping coffee and reading, then stumbled to my desk and wrote for a few hours.

I was getting ready to send my novel out to try to secure a literary agent. I prayed it would work this time. My writer dreams had been interrupted by tragedy for so long I felt very behind. My friends were lapping me, pushing out beautiful and important books every other year. I was nowhere. It was unbelievably hard to get an agent, and as my writer friend Rosecrans once said to me in passing, publishing a novel was like having a meteor land in your backyard.

Meanwhile, EMT life. Austin and Nina and I planned to ride three on the truck this frosty Christmas night, and Park Slope let us. They knew we were street wives. We bought festive getups to spread holiday cheer. Austin wore a Santa hat, Nina had a reindeer antler headband, and I got stuck being Mrs. Claus, with a ridiculous red felt shower cap contraption on my head that had some holly around the edges.

When I showed up at base that evening, my wives were overjoyed to see me, which was the way I wanted to feel about people I spent time with on Christmas. Austin fell in love with me a few years back, after I declined a call from an FBI agent because she and I were on the truck, talking about boys. "Wifey, did you just hang up on the FBI?" she asked. "Yes," I told her. "We're in the middle of a very important conversation. The FBI can wait. That's literally their job. Waiting." Austin loved me after that.

That night we sat on the truck in our holiday hats and got festive beverages from Starbucks. Toward the end of our tour we went on a job for an injury major. When we pulled up, an ambulance was parked on the corner with the doors flung open, a bad sign. That meant the EMTs had flown off the bus to help someone before they had time to shut the doors.

Across the street we saw two EMTs hovering over a downed body, the tattooed guy I'd worked the uncontrolled bleeder with and his dark-haired partner. They were treating someone lying on the sidewalk on the other side of a parked car. Damn. Not on Christmas. It looked bad. Nina and Austin and I ripped off our holiday hats, gloved up, and trotted toward them.

On the ground we saw an elderly man who looked like my grandpa splayed in the gutter next to a tipped-over wheelchair. His white hair was combed off his bright, open face and his body was round and soft. He was so cute I wanted to cry that he was lying in the gutter on Christmas. This fucking world!

On the sidewalk the patient's daughter explained that when she'd tried to move him into the car, he'd fallen and gotten stuck. His pants were caught in the seat of the wheelchair. We tried to wiggle him free, but his paralyzed legs were heavy, and we couldn't unhook him from the contraption. It was freezing outside. I worried the sweet, old patient was getting cold. He kept apologizing for wasting our time, which sank my heart.

I hated it when people genuinely needed help and felt bad for needing help and apologized. That always ripped me apart. On the street people who desperately needed medical care often didn't call 911 soon enough, while the "worried well" who didn't need anything from us called constantly. It wore us out.

Austin or one of the guys—my memory is fuzzy—smartly pulled out trauma shears and cut the patient free. Now we just had to lift him. Nina stepped back and Austin and I helped the two guys on scene get the patient onto his feet, then eased him into his car. I reached over and put his seatbelt on for him. Click.

"Thank you so much for helping me," he said. "I got stuck. Merry Christmas."

"Merry Christmas!" we said.

We asked if he wanted to go to the hospital, but he assured us he was unharmed. Nothing hurt. Lift assist only. Someone grabbed a Toughbook to type up an RMA.

"What's your date of birth, sir?" Austin asked.

The patient said a month, a day, "1915."

What?

"When did you say your birthday was again?" I asked.

The patient's daughter looked at me. "You heard him right. He was born in 1915. He's 104 years old."

"Oh my God!" we shouted. "Sir, you look wonderful! You're so cute and happy. What's your secret?"

"Oh," the patient said, giggling. "I don't know."

"Wow," I mumbled after we said goodbye to everyone and loped back to the truck. "I've never met a person that old before. He looked great, too. That's amazing."

Next thing I knew Nina was at my side, tugging on my sleeve with a frantic look on her face, her eyes alight with panic. "Jennifer," she said beggingly, and immediately I knew where this was going. Nina's worst nightmare was prolonged life. "Jennifer, listen to me. If I ever live that long, if I get to be a 104 and you happen to still be alive . . ."

I tore her hands off me. "Nina! Stop it! Get off me. First of all, I will not be alive at 124. I'll be dead."

"But Jennifer, if somehow, if by chance there's some miracle of science . . ."

"There will not be a miracle of science, and even if there is, I'm not killing you. It's Christmas. Get back in the truck right now. Put your antlers on."

It was a magical holiday with my wives. Probably the sweetest Christmas I'd ever had. Our patient was unharmed, we first responders were together, and no loneliness could touch me.

The ambulance was a refuge. So was my writing life.

* * *

Last week of January, a literary agent I'd e-mailed wrote me back and requested I send her my entire novel. Then another agent replied and requested the same. I was at the gym when I received the e-mails. I was so excited I fell off the treadmill.

"Congratulations, sis!" Felice said. "You're in the game."

A week or so later Felice and I did a story-exchange workshop at Pratt through an organization called Narrative 4. Felice worked for Narrative 4, and I'd been trained by them a year or so earlier as a facilitator in empathetic storytelling. My downstairs neighbor, a writer named Ellery, headed the creative writing program at Pratt. I'd told him about Narrative 4 one day over coffee, and he brought Felice and me in to lead a workshop.

We had a blast. There was nothing I loved more than being in a classroom or on stage with my sister. I was always amazed, listening to her speak about writing. And the students were incredible. So much open-hearted storytelling it could melt a glacier. I loved the writer's life.

The rest of life, not so much.

The second I got home from Pratt sorrow rushed back to me. These last few months had been so brutal and heavy. I was worried about Mike. I missed talking to Tommy. I used to talk to him a lot about Pat, and all that he'd meant to me. I could use some support now that Mike was sick. I thought about texting him and asking him to have coffee. But I couldn't get myself to do it. He'd never once in all these years come through for me in the real world, and I couldn't bear any more disappointment.

Overall, I was glad the year was over. Enough with 2019. Devil be gone. On New Year's Day I embraced the arrival of 2020. I had no idea what lay ahead of me—ahead of us all. I thought it was going to be an easier, softer year.

In early January 2020, the World Health Organization tweeted about spate of strange "viral pneumonia" cases in Wuhan, China. No deaths. COVID wasn't taking up real estate in my head. Nor was it flagging that it might turn into, oh, I don't know, the biggest global health emergency of our time. So fatal that when I did a second draft of this book, I had to do a "find and replace" search to tone down my overuse of the phrase "everyone died."

At the start of the year, life in New York went on as usual. Lexi and I picked up a tour together, our first in a while. Nothing eventful happened. One snowy Saturday, we took a CrossFit class together, then spent the afternoon at Spa Castle in Queens.

Soon Mike returned to New York and I focused on being one of his two wives. We went on so many dates, the three of us. And we shared so much joy and wonder. As time passed, Mike, newly sober, with stage four cancer, began to speak of his visits to New York as the happiest time of his life.

Same for me.

One night Mike took me and Ylfa to see David Byrne, and we rose from our seats and sang "One Fine Day" together and wept. We walked all over the city. By the rivers and through the parks. We introduced Mike to Paul, a sober Vietnam veteran and one of Pat's closest friends. Those two hit it off, and Paul became Mike's spiritual advisor. We gobbled up hot dogs at McSorley's, where the Irish firefighter from Pat's firehouse bartended. He served us seltzers and fed us for free.

When Mike's whole body ached with pain, Ylfa suggested we get massages at one of those walk-in places. "Hey, guys!" he shouted across the dead-silent room. "How long are we doing? An hour? Do I take my clothes off?"

Please do not take your clothes off.

One afternoon Mike and I went to the Museum of Natural History. He let me pay, for once. "Yes, can I get the senior citizen discount?" I asked the desk lady. "My husband's in his mid-sixties. Don't let the mustache fool you, he dyes it." Mike gasped and scurried away in laughter and shame.

Ours was a happy marriage. So happy that that riding on the ambulance started to feel like a dreadful chore.

Not since I was a toddler had I gotten in trouble as much as I had since I'd become a volunteer, I repeat, volunteer, EMT. These January nights, it seemed not a tour went by that I didn't get corrected, reprimanded, or screamed at by someone, somewhere, for something.

I forgot to switch off the ambulance lights when I parked in the hospital bay. I stayed on scene too long. Wrote my patient chart wrong. Didn't give dispatch a status update to let them know I wasn't dead. I blocked a street to respond to a child hit by a car and honking drivers stepped out of their

BMWs and cursed at me for backing up traffic. I deposited a violent EDP into the nearest 911-receiving facility when the nurse didn't have time for this shit. "Why'd you bring him here?" she asked me. *Oh sorry. I thought this was a hospital. Is this a bank? Can I get some cash?* I grabbed a cold pack out of the hospital restock cabinet without asking for permission. The fall-down-drunk who Austin and I lifted out of a pool of his own spilled blood called me an idiot for insisting he go to the hospital to get staples in his split-open scalp. The homeless lady hearing voices that told her to stab people didn't want my help, and ranted at me for being a stupid bitch, dumb cunt, and my personal favorite—the White Whore. (Title of my next book.)

I got spat on. Lied to. Grabbed at. Kicked. Humiliated beyond comprehension. "Everyone, stop what you're doing!" one of my patients, a sick prisoner, screamed as we rolled into the ER. Everyone turned and stared at me. "Do you see this woman?" he said, pointing at me. "This woman needs to be fucked! That's why she's an angry bitch! Can someone here come fuck her?"

Patients. Nurses. Civilians. Bosses. It was like being kicked to death by rabbits. On and on the grievances against me went until the Irish milk of my attitude soured. Inside me blossomed fresh hatred for everyone around me, including the people I was supposed to help. Whenever I ran into other rescuers on the street who lumbered up to my window to confess that they hated people, I nodded my agreeing head.

"Oh, Jennifer," Nina said when we climbed on the truck one night, cold wind rocking the ambulance. "We're miserable. Should we go open schedule?"

I didn't know. Open schedule meant we'd quit riding our weekly tours and pick up shifts whenever we felt like it. Which lately, was never.

In my mind, we had no defensible excuse for our saltiness. We hadn't even been on the street that long. Nina four or so years. Me, approaching three. As volunteers, no less. A few nights a week. No time at all in the grand scheme of things and nothing compared to the full-time folks. And yet our tours were crammed with enough bullshit and disaster and naked human wreckage to make us feel abused and bitter.

We weren't alone in this, either. The median career expectancy for EMTs and paramedics is only five years. Maybe for full-time first responders it was the insulting pay that broke them. EMTs rank fourth from the bottom in salary of all jobs in the country, outpacing preschool teachers, meatpackers, and dishwashers. The national average yearly income for EMTs is only $29,924 a year. As previously stated, in New York City garbage collectors make more money than EMTs, though the last time I checked they weren't making life-or-death decisions on the job or being verbally assaulted by people who called them White Whores.

Winter nights on the Brooklyn streets remained painfully slow. Being on the ambulance started to feel like a waste of time. Lately it seemed like most of what Nina and I did was sit on the truck and complain. Between jobs we killed time talking about the ill-starred couples on *90 Day Fiancé*. We bought each other joke coffee mugs with quotes from the show. One of them said, THINGS ARE ABOUT TO GET A LITTLE BIT MORE STUPIDER. We looked up recipes for desserts we wanted to bake for first responders and ran emergency scenarios to entertain ourselves.

One tour I asked Nina what it was like to respond to a cardiac arrest, then made her reenact it on the truck. I'd developed a looming fear I'd forget what to do when I finally got sent to that particular emergency. We talked constantly about dropping our regular weekly tours and going open schedule, riding whenever we wanted, but we couldn't seem to release ourselves from the prison of our own design.

"Why don't you just take a little break?" Mike suggested one day on the phone. "You don't have to quit, but it sounds like you're getting pretty burned out. This open schedule thing sounds like a good idea."

I guessed. I was too depressed when I thought about it to make a decision.

By the end of the month, January 2020, COVID-19 was bubbling in the news. But the story was still largely focused on China and various travel restrictions. One US citizen who'd visited Wuhan had been confirmed positive for the virus.

On the last day of the month, when the World Health Organization declared a public health emergency, I paid the news no significant attention. My mind was on Mike, the novel I'd finished that a few literary agents were now reading, and what to do about my dissatisfaction with my EMT life. To go open schedule, or not to go open schedule, that was the question.

11

DON'T BE A HERO

One bleak February evening Nina came over to my house and we baked chocolate chip cookies and talked about our future as EMTs, and what to do about being unhappy. I'd gotten us fluffy white baker's hats, so we put those on and stood in my kitchen covered in flour, laughing our heads off. Later that night Nathan swung by and plopped down on my couch.

"Hey, these are pretty good," he said, trying a cookie. "Sweets in the Streets! I think you guys might be onto something. How's business?"

"No one wants our baked goods," I said dismally.

Nina said, "We literally can't give them away."

"What do we do about our EMS misery?" I asked them.

"Man, I don't know," Nathan said, lifting his hat and scratching his head. "I miss Chad and MJ. It's not the same, riding with new people. I think I'll go open schedule soon."

"Nathan," Nina said. "You've been saying that for a year."

We all said it—soon. Mañana, mañana. But none of us did it.

Why?

Clearly, our first responder honeymoon was over, and the marriage needed work. Yet we were still sitting in the ceremonious church with thrown rice in our hair staring transfixed at the empty altar. Did we think someone might wander over and help us? Rub our sternums to see if we were still alive? Who would do that? No deities or politicians watched over us. No civilians, either. People waved at firefighters and flipped off cops. They didn't even see us EMTs. We were invisible. Uniformed ghosts. Sometimes when we rolled up on scene, I heard my inner Lionel Richie sing, *Hello? Is it me you're looking for?*

And while the street was unforgiving, wearing our boots down to the soles, it was part of us, this world. For all its worn-down atrocities, painfully slow nights, and unspeakable tragedies, the radio also dispatched magic. That's what people didn't understand about the street. The horrific was wed to the wondrous. They were attached.

It was sacred to me, being out there. Being with my partners and patients. Being with everyone at Park Slope, service-minded people who did unimaginable good for the community and asked for nothing back. Even the people I didn't like at the agency I loved. The ambulance infused my life with meaning. It meant the world to be part of a tribe of rescuers who went out each night to chariot the sick and injured to hospitals and act in defense of life. I felt proud, assisting people in need. And quiet nights weren't truly a waste of time, since I got to hang out with my partners.

Every time I fell asleep after a night of working on the truck, I woke up the next morning feeling groggily at peace with who I was in the world. The kind of bioluminescent peace you feel after you've accomplished something impossible. I felt rich. Useful. Blessed. Like if I died right then I'd be fine with it. I'd die a satisfied woman who'd done something purposeful with her life. Who'd gotten her hands dirty. Who'd really lived. I guessed that was why they called this kind of hard, high-risk work "a calling." They called it a calling because it made no sense.

Nina and Nathan felt that way too, I suspected. They didn't say it that cookie-scented night at my house. But I knew we all asked ourselves the same question:

Where in the screen-drunk world of iPhones and Amazon Prime were people like us going to find that awestruck feeling, experience direct contact with the sacredness of humanity, interfere with death, witness and embody astonishing acts of tenderness, see ghosts and crack jokes and shake with gallows laughter, if we went off the ambulance?

Contagion-wise, in early February the number of COVID-19 cases in the United States still wasn't alarming. Though twenty-five countries had confirmed patients, news continued to focus on the outbreak in Wuhan. There, one whistleblower doctor died from coronavirus. An American citizen perished in China as well. According to timelines published by various health organizations, there were 638 confirmed COVID-19 deaths worldwide by February 7, 2020, but only two of them outside of China.

On the ambulance that February I still wasn't seeing or even looking for anything especially peculiar. I lapsed into a cringingly American mindset: COVID was an "over there" problem. Healthcare workers were dying in Wuhan, not here. China announced via state news channels that nurses and doctors who died trying to save COVID-19 patients would be designated as martyrs. Cruise ship infections were a problem. Japan saw an uptick. Italy reported one death. But compared to Mike's cancer and the epidemic of hate-fueled mass shootings, one death in Italy from COVID seemed somewhat bearable.

That February visit to New York, Mike got us tickets to see *West Side Story* on Broadway. It had been his and Pat's favorite musical as kids. His mother loved musicals, and she'd died when Pat was in Vietnam.

Sitting in the theater beside Ylfa and Mike, I felt Pat was with us, watching the show. Outside afterward, huddled together on the billboard-lit street, all three of us looked at each other and whispered it, "Pat was there."

Afterward, we went out for Korean. Ylfa had a surprise for Mike. She'd invited Bobby to dinner, but she didn't tell Mike he was coming. She knew how much Bobby meant to him, and she wanted it to be a surprise. Bobby had taken care of Mike after 9/11. Made it his sacred duty to look after Pat's brother.

We stood outside the restaurant and lingered. When Bobby walked up and Mike saw him, he fell into Bobby's arms, buried his face in his neck, and wept. My eyes welled. Ylfa and I smiled at each other, our hands flagged over our hearts.

Brotherhood.

I never tired of seeing it. One tough guy embracing another. So much history and loss and love between these men it could light up Times Square. It could keep you alive.

At Mount Sinai a few days later, Mike got bad news from Dr. Oh. I went to the hospital with him, and he spiraled after seeing his bone scan and learning the shots he'd been taking had stopped working. He had to try a new treatment. He didn't want to take the pills Dr. Oh suggested as a next step, because the side effects were hideous. He didn't want to do chemo or radiation and die like his wife, Janet. He missed her and talked about her often. In his hotel room he fell apart.

Our poor husband.

Ylfa was in Iceland that week, but Pat's sober Vietnam buddy Paul and I were around. We ran to Mike and held him close. Devastated, he flew back to Vegas the next morning. A day or two later, he had an epiphanic moment. He realized he wanted to live, and he was willing to do whatever it took to extend his life.

First, he tried to get into a clinical trial in Seattle. Pat's actor friend James flew to Washington and met him there. James had gone with Mike to his first doctor's appointment here, too. But a week later Mike found out he didn't get into the trial. Crushed, he decided to consider giving the pills Dr. Oh suggested a try.

He also decided to move to New York.

We all thought it was a great idea. This way, he'd be close to his family, friends, doctors, and wives. We could all watch over him. Make sure he was never lonely. When he returned in March, we would look for apartments for him. Find him a nice place.

For now we conjured hope. We had a plan, at least. We didn't know back then, not yet, COVID-19 would destroy it.

Soon thereafter, I took a much-needed break and went to Costa Rica to surf, and, feeling revived after a week abroad, was getting ready to fly home to New York, then do laundry and zip out to LA. A producer friend had read my unpublished novel and wanted to introduce me to TV people. I still couldn't wrap my head around what I was hearing about COVID. It sounded like people were gearing up for World War II, and given everything Mike had going on with 9/11-related cancer, I was still rather preoccupied with World War I. I had a hard time accepting the arrival of a new war.

At the same time, I knew from experience that when it came to disasters, sickness, and death, denial could be fatal. When I got diagnosed with cancer, I couldn't believe it. And yet it was true. When I stood in the street and watched the North Tower collapse with Pat inside it, I couldn't believe it. And yet.

Then my mind journeyed back in time to something an FBI agent had said to a lawyer I worked with on a mass shooting.

The lawyer had season tickets in the orchestra pit of a theater that were smack in the middle of the auditorium. It made him nervous, to have middle seats. We all got weird after working a shooting. Personally, I didn't attend many events that involved huge crowds. I'd seen too much of the aftermath. Not a great scene.

One day, the attorney asked the FBI agent, "What's the one piece of advice you would give someone in terms of how to survive if there was a mass shooting in a place like that?"

"*When* there's a shooting," the agent said. "Not if. *When* there's a shooting. And the single most important thing to do is believe that it's happening. Believe it's happening, and your instincts will kick in. Your body will go into survival mode and you'll run or hide or fight. Most people die because when the shooter starts firing, they can't believe it's happening. They don't think it's real, so they freeze. Believe it, and your chances of surviving skyrocket."

I wasn't alone in my disbelief about the gravity of COVID at this point. I was frozen. Mike didn't believe the virus was a problem yet, either. First of March, he texted me with alarming news:

"James told me coronavirus was found in the hospital we went to in Seattle."

"Oh, God," I said. "People are obsessed with the virus."

"The flu is worse. They'll push this as far as they can, then finally people will go out again and say, 'Hey, I'm not dead.'"

Chilling, for me to write that sentence now, in late 2020. We were all frozen then. But people who'd been studying pandemics like I did for mass shootings, they also knew it was a matter of when, not if.

On Wednesday, March 4, I flew from New York to Los Angeles for my fancy Hollywood meetings.

I saw nothing unusual by way of COVID at the airport in New York flying out. Not that I noticed, at least. No people in masks. No mention of coronavirus at the airport or on the plane. Just me and my long legs folded painfully into an economy-class aisle seat on a packed flight from JFK to LAX.

However, when I was wheels down in Los Angeles, California declared a state of emergency. That was a shocker. The news still didn't land for me.

At the time, COVID infections in California were attributed to the cruise ship *Grand Princess*, which had a confirmed case in an elderly traveler who was critically sick. Public officials ordered the cruise ship to stay offshore after eleven passengers and ten crew members exhibited potential symptoms of coronavirus.

I wasn't elderly, or on a cruise ship. I was in Hollywood.

That was my thinking at the time.

I stayed with my writer friends Rachel and Rosecrans in LA. Next two days I took meetings with my producer friend to discuss potential TV projects. I was psyched.

Mike suggested that while I was in California, I meet his and Pat's actor friend James, so I did that one morning. James and I grabbed coffee and talked about the tragedy of Mike.

The trip went well, I thought. The TV people seemed to like me and my writing. But then Rosecrans and Rachel told me that was the deal with TV people in LA. They always gave writers the sense that things were sunshiny, but that didn't often result in a deal. "There are no bad meetings in Hollywood," they said.

Two days later, on Friday, when I returned to LAX to fly home, I got to the airport two hours early. I saw a flight attendant swiping boarding tickets for a flight that was leaving five minutes from then and asked if by chance I could hop on that plane rather than wait? I assumed she would say no, since flights between LA and New York were always full. But instead she said, "Sure, you can hop on this flight, it's empty. It's only 30 percent booked."

Empty flight from LAX to JFK?

That's when it hit me that COVID was here. It was real. I believed it.

Had I known what the future would hold, I would have stayed in California longer, and driven two hours north to Bakersfield to see my mom. I thought I was just hopping out west for a quick business trip, which I was. But later, when the world went on lockdown, and I thought about this LA trip, it tortured me to know I could have seen my mother, and I didn't.

New York reported its first COVID-19 case on the first of March, a few days before Mike's return to the city. I was in bed that evening wasting my life on my phone talking to this fire marshal I was barely dating, and had my news-reading eye on Italy, where the virus was exploding. New York

City seemed OK for now. It was still an "over there" problem. China, Italy, Washington, California. Nothing worrisome here.

When Mike arrived in March, Ylfa and I met up with him and went to see a bunch of apartments. A real estate lady wearing pearls was very confused when Mike introduced us as his wives.

After he'd received such terrible news last month, Ylfa and I decided on a plan to lift our co-husband's spirits and give him something to look forward to in the future.

Over lunch, we told Mike we'd marry him. Not for real, of course, since legally he couldn't have two wives. But we could have a little ceremony, we said. A spiritual wedding to formalize our bond. A sacred ceremony.

Our Turtle was so excited he immediately spread the news of our forthcoming union to everyone who had a pulse. He alerted half the Fire Department. "I'm getting married!" he told his friends. "I got two wives!"

Whatever it took. That's what Ylfa and I said to each other. "Whatever it takes. Anything for Pat."

Anything within reason.

Mike's ultimate fantasy was for the three of us take a road trip in his RV. He talked about it constantly. He wanted me and Ylfa to wear Daisy Dukes and drive cross-country. We shut the RV idea down every time he brought it up.

"Turtle, we'll marry you," Ylfa said. "But I don't know about the RV."

I said, "An RV road trip is not on my bucket list. I know you think it's romantic to travel the West in an RV, since you're from Queens. But I'm from Bakersfield. Winding up in a trailer is not my idea of victory."

Mike ignored us. "Hey, guys, I just told Mike Daly we're getting married, and he said that's a great idea. He thinks its genius. Maybe he can be our minister."

That made sense. In addition to being close with Pat and Mike, Michael Daly had written a book, *The Book of Mychal*, about his beloved friend Mychal Judge, the sober Franciscan friar and Catholic priest who served as the Fire Department chaplain and was the first certified fatality of September 11. So to us, Michael Daly came from holy FDNY lineage.

"We can ask him at dinner tonight," Ylfa said.

Then we went with Mike to his doctor's appointment.

Finally, at last, our husband agreed to take the pills Dr. Oh suggested. He tried to wiggle out of it at first, but then he was hoist on his own petard by telling the doctor, "The pills are in my pocket." Grinning, Dr. Oh said, "The pills don't work if they're in your pocket."

Ylfa and I shrieked with laughter and applauded. Mike surrendered to following doctor's orders.

Sweet relief.

Later, the three of us went to Central Park and visited Pat's tree. Firefighters illegally planted it in the park after he died, and it stood guard there, where Mike's late wife's ashes were scattered. We said hello to the tree. Gave it a hug. Ylfa took a beautiful, mystical photo of Mike embracing his lost brother, the tree. His eyes were closed in reverence, the sun shined down on him, and a band of green-gold light encircled his hands.

When you die, you often get a tree.

Many of my friends are trees.

Walking in Central Park, when Mike's shoelaces came undone, I knelt and tied them, since his stomach hurt from the shot so he couldn't bend down. He helped Ylfa memorize lines to a play about Ernest Shackleton, an Irish Antarctic explorer. The play was going up at a theater the next week.

We listened to our wife read from the script as we strolled around Central Park and Mike performed beside Ylfa, pretending to be her costar in a video I recorded that still makes me laugh. The three of us watched the video three hundred times. We decided that when Mike moved to New York, we would get a dog and name him Fifty, short for Fifty-Percent Mike.

In his hotel room later that day, my husband and I lounged in bed and talked, as couples do. We were both exhausted and tried to nap. Every time I closed my eyes Mike pulled me closer, and I giggled and slapped his arm and scootched away.

"You're my wife," he said. "So I can do that."

"It's not that kind of marriage."

Tommy had recently texted me again. "Why. Do. You. Hate. Me? I keep trying."

I'd had enough. He was going to text me for eternity unless I blocked him. The thought of doing that deflated me. I asked Mike for advice.

"I don't like this guy," he said.

"You don't like anyone for me."

I'd recently told him about the fire marshal—Felice called him "the fire cop" because as an arson investigator he carried a gun—and that was Mike's same response: "I don't like him."

"He never showed up to meet you?" Mike said about Tommy. "Not even for coffee? After you helped him? That's not very nice. I say block him."

I stared disconsolately at the ceiling.

"Or," he said. "Or, what you can say is, 'Listen. I don't hate you. Let's get coffee next week. If you can't do it, I understand. But I can't keep texting, so I'm going to block you."

"Thanks, Turtle," I said. "You're a good brother."

"I'm your husband."

"You're a good brother-husband."

"I can tell you really like this guy."

"Yeah, I love him. I know it sounds crazy, but I do."

"It doesn't sound crazy. You guys have a strong connection. You really helped each other. I think he's probably intimidated by you. Firefighters aren't the bravest when they're off the truck. They can be shy and some of them are cowards, especially with women."

"I guess. I think you might be blowing smoke up my ass."

"No. I'm not," Mike said strongly. Then he put his arm around me and said, "You know, EMT Chick, if we ever really did get married, for real? And you were off the market? The whole Fire Department would be depressed. All the firefighters would be suicidal."

I laughed. "That's not true."

"Oh, I think it is."

Mike flew home to Vegas the next day. We didn't know it then, but soon COVID became a global pandemic, travel restrictions went into effect, New York City locked down, and Mike was stuck in Vegas, unable to get treated at Mount Sinai.

He never returned to New York.

That same night, when I got home, I sent Tommy a text with the exact phrasing Mike had suggested. He replied and said yes, absolutely, we could meet for coffee this coming week.

I was shocked. Was it true? Were we really going to meet each other for the first time, in real life, after texting for three years? I couldn't believe it. But now we had a date, place, time. Maison Kayser. Harlem. Friday the 13. Two o'clock.

Maison Kayser was becoming a strangely important place for me, by way of meeting up with firemen.

Meanwhile, coronavirus. Over the next few days headlines grew worrisome. Iran announced nine hundred new cases. New York surpassed the state of Washington in infections. We now had the largest number of confirmed COVID cases in the nation—142 cases as of March 9. That week, New Rochelle became a containment zone. Italy expanded its quarantine to cover the entire country, which sparked prison riots.

In New York City things got eerie. Broadway shut down. Events got postponed, then canceled.

We're sorry to inform you; we're sad to say; out of an abundance of caution; we hope the show will resume next month. City officials said to avoid busses, trains, crowds.

Um, crowds? New York was the most densely populated major city in America, with 27,000 people per square mile. How were we supposed to avoid crowds?

Friday afternoon I took the train into Manhattan to meet Tommy. I was so nervous I couldn't eat. I didn't notice anything markedly different on the subway in terms of COVID. No one was in masks. The train wasn't as packed as usual. But then again, it was Friday afternoon. Sometimes the city emptied out before the weekend, when New Yorkers headed out of town.

Overexcited, I got into Manhattan far too early, and wasted time downtown wandering in and out of stores. All of them were empty. No shoppers. None. I was the only one around. An hour before we were supposed to meet, my phone buzzed in my pocket. Tommy. A text. Seeing his name I braced for him to cancel and felt dizzy and nauseous.

"Talk to me," he said. "Are you good?"

My stomach dropped. "I'm good. Heading uptown momentarily. You?"

"Just woke up from a nap. Worked last night. I'm good. I have coronavirus but I'm good."

I couldn't tell if he was joking. I started to panic.

"Just kidding," he texted. "Maybe. I don't know."

I still didn't understand. I didn't know if I was about to be crushed. I held my breath and leaned against a clothing rack to steady myself. "You're not meeting me, then?"

"I am. 2:30, OK?"

"OK."

I stumbled out of the store in a daze and wiped my eyes with my fingertips, then dried them on my pants.

In Harlem, Maison Kayser was empty, too.

A quarter past two o'clock I walked into the café and sat down at a two-top that faced the street. I was the only person there. Typical me. The city was emptying out, everybody got the memo, and there I was, just going about my day, don't mind me, I'm just having coffee with a firefighter at a café situated on what appears to be the edge of the end of the world.

I ordered coffee and waited. Tommy texted and said he was running a few minutes late. I silenced my phone and braced for him to cancel. My expectations could not have been lower. I was prepared to be disappointed in Real Life Tommy, who couldn't possibly compare to Virtual Fantasy Tommy. On terrific reality TV shows like *Catfish*, *90 Day Fiancé*, and *Love After Lockup*, the entire plot turned around the fact that the virtual was incomparable to the real. In general, people were much worse in real life. Not as handsome. Not as sexy or charming. Sometimes, not even the same person you thought you were texting.

I knew Tommy was who he said he was, since we'd FaceTimed once. But I expected to be hugely disappointed in his three-dimensional presence. Real life required the X factor. Chemistry. The tone of a person's voice and the way they smelled and treated waiters. I was looking forward to being let down so I could move on, and we could move forward and be friends. I missed our helpful talks. I ached to tell him about Mike.

I drank coffee and stared out the window, and there he was.

Finally, Tommy.

I couldn't believe my eyes. He was so handsome. Like virtual Tommy, only better. He smiled at me and glided inside, did a funny balletic spin to amuse me, and came to the table. I stood up and we hugged hard and for a long time. Emotion pooled in my eyes and I swallowed tears of joy and relief. I couldn't remember the last time I'd felt so lucky.

He was wearing a thin heather-gray sweater and jeans and nice shoes. Did he do that for me? I didn't know. But he had nice style. He smelled incredible. Better than a bonfire on a nighttime beach, a moonlit walk in my girlhood forest, a day at the sea. Fireworks exploded in different neighborhoods of my body and I felt overheated and sick. He was five foot nine but seemed towering. Like Pat, he possessed a certain grandeur.

"You showed up," I said squeezing his arms. "I'm shocked. And look at you, you're so handsome. And you're huge. Your arms are the size of my legs. You're even better in real life."

"You're fucking beautiful," Tommy said. "I knew you'd be beautiful."

He excused himself to use the bathroom.

At the table I sat down and smoothed my napkin on my lap. My hands were shaking. I wanted time to slow down. I breathed in and drank down coffee and feelings of bliss and hope, and the fact that this was really happening. By some tender grace Tommy had finally appeared in my life at the very moment I needed him most, when Mike was sick, and COVID was zeroing in on New York. He wasn't just a fantasy anymore. Some ideal guy I'd created in my head. He was real. His presence felt like one of those gifts in life whose arrival signals higher meaning and the possibility of better days ahead. I couldn't help but leap into an imagined future where we were single and finally got to be together.

But also, where was he? He was taking an awful long time in the bathroom. Did he get stuck in there? Meh. He was a fireman. If he got stuck, he'd get himself out.

He came back ten or so minutes later with an iced coffee in a to-go cup and a big bottle of seltzer, apologizing for the wait.

"It's table service," I said as he sat down.

"Oh," he said, laughing. "I didn't know that."

I asked if he was nervous to meet me and he said no. Then I spilled my entire glass of water on his leg. A waitress standing at the ready handed us fresh napkins.

"Sorry," I said.

For over an hour we caught up. We started off light. Talked about work stuff, mainly. A dash of acknowledgment that a pandemic seemed to be eyeballing New York, and the city was emptying out. Tommy had an incredible voice, and I loved listening to him talk. He thanked me again for saving his life by introducing him to Headstrong. I brushed it off. He'd gotten rid of his last girlfriend, he said, who had a drinking problem. If a firefighter says you have a drinking problem—run to Betty Ford.

Tommy was out of therapy now, though he missed it. His therapist had released him since he was doing so well. I was proud of him. I told him about Mike. He listened and said he was so sorry, he knew how hard that must be for me, and he was here if I needed anything, I didn't have to do this alone.

That meant so much. I wanted to stay in the café forever. Time was going too fast. The date had just started but soon it would be five o'clock and then he'd have to rush off to work and it would be over, and I didn't want that to happen. I didn't know how to slow things down.

We approached the subject of love, and I held my breath. Clung to the fraying rope that he was single, and we would finally get to be together, now that he was doing so well.

Then a surprise.

Tommy said three or four months ago, after he'd gone on some bad dates and given up on finding someone, he lucked out and met a woman who was truly wonderful. She was smart and sane and kind. He felt like he'd finally met his person.

The rope slipped out of my hands and I plunged like a doomed woman to the ground. I stared funereally at the table so I wouldn't cry. Then after a moment I looked up, and smiling, said, "I'm so happy for you. That's great."

"What about you?" Tommy said. "Are you dating anyone?"

I couldn't think straight. My head hurt. He was so much better in real life than I anticipated, he made the fire marshal I'd been dating seem ridiculous. I just wanted to go home. I was embarrassed by my feelings.

"Not really," I said.

After a while longer, Tommy had to go to work.

When we said goodbye outside, we hugged for a long time and said, "I love you." Then he looked at me, his eyes sloshing with regret, or maybe it was recognition. He opened his mouth to speak but sunlight seemed to fill it. I sensed he had something to say. I didn't know what it was, but suspected it had to do with the cost of admission to the events that made us luminous, and all we'd been through and lost.

"Thank you for meeting me," I said, and my voice cracked when I spoke.

I always knew we'd get to meet one day. I'd looked forward to it for years. I thought maybe he was my person.

Oh well.

At home three days later, staring at my phone, I happened upon a video called "10 Days" directed by Olmo Parenti that changed my view of COVID, and how seriously I took the virus.

In the video, quarantined Italians recorded messages to themselves about things they wished they'd known ten days ago, before the pandemic infected 24,000 people in their country and killed 1,809 Italians. "It is believed the US, England and France are 9 to 10 days behind Italy in COVID-19 progression," the title card said.

"Are you afraid?" one of them asked.

"I am you in ten days," said another.

And another: "I am speaking to you from the future."

The Italians spoke from locked-down cities, spoke in second person, using direct address, a desperate point of view, presumptive and insistent; they spoke to me directly about things they wished they'd known, a chorus of impending horror.

They said the worst-case scenario was about to happen here. Infections would increase. It wasn't bullshit like we thought. Ten days ago they had 2,000 people infected. Now they had 18,000. They'd already passed 1,000 deaths. An Italian nurse said she was working deadly shifts at the hospital. They were in a surreal situation, they said. Nobody could leave their house. A whole nation stuck at home. Hospitals blowing up with patients. Lots of infections, even among young people. Kids intubated. In intensive care.

They took it lightly, they said. Mistook it for the flu. "We should always be light in spirit, but not with our gestures," one woman said. "Because what you're risking is not a regular flu." They said they'd seen worrisome videos from the US and France, of people not taking this thing seriously. They said the issue was more serious than the world believed. Theirs was not "unfounded pessimism." They knew China was far away. "But this virus was faster than we thought." "Start doing your part," they said. "Don't fuck up." "Stay at home." "You're not the only person in this world." "We underestimated this," they said. "You don't have to do the same. Stay at home."

I watched the video a dozen times. I shot it to my closest friends. Felice. Ellery. Rachel, in LA. I was an experience-based wisdom person. I read the news, like everyone else. I saw the swelling numbers and bar charts. But when I heard the quarantined Italians speak from experience, people who'd seen the virus and tried to warn us—I believed them. I believed it was happening. And my chances of surviving skyrocketed.

Now I wanted only to hear from the New York streets.

Nina came over the next night and we baked lemon bars and cookies, then drove to Park Slope to talk with Austin. She was on the truck with an EMT named Friedland, a big lumbering white guy who loved Sweets in the Streets. He'd eat anything, that guy. He was a two-donut-at-a-time first responder. We found their parked ambulance and handed Friedland a container of cookies.

Then Nina and I bombarded them with questions. Are you seeing COVID patients? How do they present? What are their symptoms? How old are they? How sick? How do those runs come over the radio? Do we have enough personal protective equipment? How contagious is this thing? Do you think we're going to get it? Is it safe for us to ride? What about our families?

Austin and Friedland were seeing COVID patients. They presented with fevers and coughs. Their symptoms ranged from flu-like exhaustion to difficulty breathing. Doctors believed the virus attacked the lungs. They were mainly elderly. Some of them were very sick. The runs came over as a new call type: "fever cough" and "sick fever cough." Some crews had ample N95s and surgical masks. Others had limited supplies and what they had was being tracked and rationed. Park Slope had enough PPE for now. The virus was highly contagious. It was presumed we'd all get sick. It wasn't safe for us to work, but what else was new? High risk was our baseline, our norm as first responders. But our families could get COVID.

Driving home that night, Nina and I had a serious talk and tried to figure out what to do. We were volunteer EMTs. It was a global health pandemic. Was volunteering in a lethal contagion the stupidest thing we could do? Or the most self-sacrificing?

Nina was terrified to ride because she lived with her parents, and they took care of her grandmother. If she got sick, she could potentially infect them all. She was fine risking her own health, but not that of her family. I lived alone, so I didn't share the burden of infecting anyone I loved. I could avoid people. Isolate.

"Didn't you think when you first signed up to be an EMT," Nina said before I dropped her off at home, "that if there was going to be a disaster in New York and we got called to work as first responders, it would be for another terrorist attack like 9/11?"

"Yes. That's absolutely what I thought."

"And instead it's the flu."

"Well, it seems a bit stronger than the flu. Italy's got so many dead they can't bury them."

"So what do we do?"

We decided to think about it. Give it a few days.

That week, my friends grew worried about me. They weighed in with advice. I wasn't mandated as an EMT, they reminded me. I didn't have to be on the street. I could easily opt out. Felice: "Sister, I know you love riding on the ambulance, but do you think maybe you could sit this one out? Since you're a volunteer?" My mom: "I understand if you want to work as an EMT, Jenny, but could you maybe do it a bit less often?" Rachel: "You just finished your novel and have a potential TV offer coming in. This would be a really bad time for you to die."

One afternoon, Ylfa called crying, begging me not to ride. She didn't want to lose another rescuer. COVID was dredging up her grief over losing Pat. Bringing back haunting memories of September 11. When she said that I scanned my body to see if I felt the same. If I felt like COVID was dovetailing with 9/11 and bringing that nightmare back to life for me. I was amazed to find my nervous system returned no significant results by way of distressing memories. In EMDR therapy, I'd worked hard on 9/11 for a year. The work appeared to have paid off. There were notable similarities between the events. But my body didn't send me reeling into catastrophic grief. Not yet.

Mike called that same day. He knew I was going to work on the ambulance before I did. He was trying to work in some capacity, too. He was an ER doctor, designed for emergencies. It frustrated him that he couldn't rush back to New York and work in a hospital because of the pandemic, and because he was sick.

"Listen to me," Mike said sternly. "If Pat were alive, he'd say, 'Jennifer, my little brother is suffering, and he needs you. Don't be a hero. Work on the ambulance, but stay balanced, and take care of yourself. Wear all the PPE they give you, and if they run out, you have to stop.'"

I promised him I would do all of that.

"Fuck it," Nina and I decided within days. People were sick and needed help. This was why we became first responders. To be of service when people needed it most. Not to sit on the bench during what was rapidly escalating into the most fatal pandemic the modern world had ever known. Turning our beloved city into a hot zone. We had to help. New York City was our home. We'd do anything we could to assist. No one beat New York.

The next week, on my way to my first COVID tour, Jeremy saw me heading out of my apartment in uniform. Shaking his head, he said, "I knew it. I knew you weren't going to stop riding on the ambulance because of this. You're a hero Jennifer. You know that, right? You're a hero."

"I'm not a hero."

"Then you're my hero."

"OK. You're my hero, too."

12

FEVER COUGH

I remember exactly where we were standing when I thought, *This is it. This is the moment we're getting sick.*

Nina and I had just brought a teenaged boy into the pediatric ER in Park Slope. When we rolled into the hospital, we observed with alarm we were the only people in view who were naked-faced, unmasked. We felt like canaries in the coal mine, sheep going to slaughter. Around us, doctors and nurses, EMTs and paramedics, all of them dawned surgical masks or N95s—except us. I froze upon realizing this while Nina briefed the pediatric nurse. Gave her the story about what we'd found twenty minutes earlier when we'd arrived on scene, meaning why we'd brought our patient to the hospital.

It was Saturday, mid-March. After the World Health Organization declared coronavirus a global pandemic on March 11. After then President Trump declared a national emergency two days later, on March 13. After the New York City mayor told New Yorkers to brace for a quarantine. After the governor of New York state went on TV to stomp out mayoral rumors that New York City was going to quarantine like Italy and China. After 1,700 people were infected with COVID and a dozen people perished across the state.

"New Yorkers should be prepared right now for the possibility of a shelter-in-place order," Mayor de Blasio declared in a City Hall press conference on Tuesday, March 17.

"No city in this state can quarantine itself without state approval and I have no interest whatsoever, and no plan whatsoever, to quarantine any city," Governor Cuomo declared, also on March 17.

All the men in power had declared something. The president, governor, and mayor. Daily, the three of them tussled on TV, schoolboys in suits, playing dodgeball with power, with thousands of lives on the line, mouthing off about one another on camera, verbally shoving each other on the playground of the hounding media, a dick-wagging contest. "The Bermuda Triangle of Incompetence," I referred to them at the time.

Send in the crisis manager, I thought. Bring in the woman—because the nation's top players in the crisis space were women—bring in the woman who will stand invisibly off-camera and quietly, expertly, meticulously manage one of these not-doing-so-hot-communicating politicians. The woman who will mute the baseline personality of whoever becomes the leading man. Starve his hostility and tendency to run his mouth on camera, and spoon-feed him statements of tenderness, love, and hope that will nourish and focus not only New York, but the whole country. The woman who will choose which stories he tells.

One of these men must step up and speak directly from the heart of COVID. Which would it be? Three contestants stood before me on reality TV. Let's watch.

But first, let's see what's on the history channel.

In the aftermath of 9/11, it was Rudy Giuliani.

The crisis communication I shaped my career around, the words that informed the way I spoke to people when they called me for help on the worst day of their lives, the words that made me who I was on and off the ambulance, as a crisis manager, an EMT, and writer, came from the city's then mayor after 9/11. Leaders who communicate in a standout manner during a crisis are doing so while being suspended in the amber of disaster, under the careful guidance of a crisis manager. When the tragedy passes, the amber falls away, the crisis manager departs, and leaders return to their baseline personalities. To whoever they were before.

Almost immediately after the attacks, reporters hounded Giuliani for the death toll. They wanted the number. Reporters shoved cameras and microphones in his face. Demanded he speak. They needed to know yesterday. Today. Right now. Immediately. How many were lost? What was the number?

He could not get this wrong. Not with the towers leveled, the world watching, first responders buried in rubble, the city enshrined in candles, flowers, missing posters, bereaved, terrified, dangling-from-the-ledge New Yorkers clutching onto the balcony of his words, trying not to fall, waiting for him to tell us how bad it was by giving us the number. We needed to know.

Giuliani didn't have the number yet. It was too soon, in the chaos of the immediate aftermath, while we were being waterboarded by images of the planes crashing into the towers. What could he possibly say? How could he reassure people who'd lost so much? Who were waiting for the number he didn't have?

"The number of casualties," he said somberly, "will be more than any of us can bear, ultimately."

A perfect communication.

And with those words, an oft-despised politician rose to the occasion, spoke in the decimated voice of the unimaginable, and was crowned America's Mayor.

Who would communicate from the suffocated heart of COVID? I wondered this often during these fatal mid-March days as I watched the news. Prayed one of my favorite crisis management colleagues would step in. A woman I looked up to as a mentor, who I believed in and trusted with my life—and yours.

New York City public schools closed that week, on March 15. Next day, bars and restaurants followed suit, shuttering their doors except for deliveries. It sure seemed like we were doing some of that locking down we were never going to do.

That Saturday I realized we were going to get sick, Nina and I drove to base in anxious silence, afraid to work our first coronavirus tour. "The Rona," everyone called it on the street.

All first responders were afraid.

"Come ride on the ambulance with me," I told a firefighter friend.

"I don't want the Rona," he said.

Gentlemen. You vest out at $100K a year. People call you "the Bravest." Locate your balls.

Chad had asthma, so he pulled himself off the truck and stuck to his desk job at a hospital. Lexi was riding her usual hospital ambulance tours. Gabriel, now a paramedic, was on the street. Aaron had left Park Slope and was now an FDNY EMT. On Instagram he posted a photo of himself kissing the bursting stomach of his pregnant wife. "Kiss 'em both before leaving for the front lines," he wrote.

"How are you holding up in all this?" Tommy asked.

"Not bad," I said. "I used the pandemic to extricate myself from the fire marshal I was dating. How are you?"

"Extricate!" Tommy said. "I'm OK. Just busy. Work was insane last night. There were fires everywhere."

"I didn't know there were still fires," I joked. "And yeah, EMS has been nuts, too. A few of my partners said they had the new call 'fever cough' today."

Confusion about symptoms and how to determine which patients were infected with COVID reigned among us. The virus was novel, this was not in our textbooks. A meme of three captioned spidermen pointing at each other circulated between first responders: "Coronavirus!" "Spring allergies!" "Seasonal flu!" the spidermen said. How were we supposed to tell?

A chart flew around the EMT community, too, to help triage patients. Do you have a fever? If yes, are you experiencing shortness of breath? If yes, you may have coronavirus. Other symptoms: cough, fatigue, weakness, exhaustion.

If you have a fever but aren't short of breath, you may have the flu. Other symptoms: cough, fatigue, weakness, exhaustion. If you don't have a fever, do you have itchy eyes? If yes, you may have allergies. Other symptoms: sneezing, runny nose. If your eyes aren't itchy, you may have the common cold. Other symptoms: sneezing, runny nose, mild chest discomfort.

Oof.

When Nina and I got to base, Chiefs Beck and Hartford and a few duty officers buzzed around the garage, stocking trucks with sealed plastic bags of PPE and decontaminating equipment. Each sealed bag contained two N95 masks, goggles, and gowns for us EMTs, and a surgical mask for the patient if they could tolerate it. One young new EMT lingered in the garage. His day tour had been canceled and he'd been taken out of service because he hadn't shaved, and N95s didn't fit properly on hairy faces.

When I'd first become an EMT at Park Slope, I had to get a "fit test" to make sure my N95 mask fit my face. I ignorantly assumed that "fit" was short for fitness. I was in pretty good shape, so I wasn't worried. Imagine my surprise when I walked into a health clinic and a nurse put an N95 on my face and a beekeeper-type box over my head, then sprayed a mysterious aerosol in the room and asked if I could smell or taste anything. She adjusted the size of my mask until my answer was "No."

EMS organizations were supposed to carry N95s in your size, in case of a viral or chemical emergency. The masks were made of two outer layers of fabric with a thin filter sandwiched in between. The inner filter was made of nonwoven fibers fused together in a process called melt-blown extrusion, which made the mask medical-grade. Due to COVID, supply-chain shortages of that magical inner filter material that stopped 95 percent of microbes from entering the mask caused a global scarcity.

Due to the worldwide shortage of PPE, we were lucky to have any N95 masks at all—let alone ones that fit. EMS organizations citywide handed out whatever N95s they had. Forget about what size you wore, or if it created a strong seal. I had a small head and could happily wear children's sunglasses, so my N95 had gaps around my chin and poked my eyes. Not exactly virus-proof.

Nina and I were eight-hundreding our truck when Chief Beck came up to me while he was on the phone—he was always on the phone these days, all of us first responders were always on the phone—and handed me a roll of winter sealant tape. He told me to seal the front of the truck from the back. Tape off the dividing partition between the two compartments so it was airtight. That way, if we had a COVID patient, the virus wouldn't travel to the front of the truck. That was the theory. Like a lot of theories, there were some holes in it.

As we knelt in the ambulance and fitted the tape around the partition, I said to Nina, "What happens if you're in the back with a violent patient and you need help, and I can't hear you?"

"Well, if we have a violent patient, we'll have PD with us."

"True. But what if I get lost on the way to the hospital and have to scream for you to give me directions?"

"I guess you'll call me on my cell in that case. And you won't get lost."

"I don't know. This isn't good. I don't like being cut off from you in the back. We can't communicate with each other at all. We'll both be totally alone."

Just then Robert called and asked if we were 98 yet, available for a job. I told him we were not. That Beck was having us seal the truck. He said that was too bad, as there was a serious job nearby. A construction worker had fallen three stories off a scaffolding a few blocks away. Injury major. "Sorry," I said as the sound of sirens filled the air. A moment later I saw a flaring red smudge that appeared to be a fire rig streak across the landscape.

"There goes the injury major," I said to Nina.

Ship appeared before us, looking relaxed and chewing gum.

"Let me ask you something," I said without bothering to say hello. My brain was manufacturing questions. "Say we took that job for the injury major. Guy who fell off the scaffold. That's not a COVID patient, so we don't open a PPE bag and wear a mask for that? Not even if he can't breathe and we have to bag him?"

"I wouldn't," he said. "Not for trauma. Only open the PPE bag for COVID patients."

But wasn't everyone presumed positive, asymptomatic, and infectious? Wasn't that why everyone in the city who wasn't us, who wasn't essential, who wasn't a first responder, was told not to go outside or touch or gather?

I couldn't wrap my mind around the new protocols and how they played out on the street when it came to us doing close-contact rescues, which involved an awful lot of touching, not to mention firehose levels of respiratory droplets and more fluids and pus and goop than one could imagine.

Before we left base, I found Hartford in the garage and pestered her with more of my bafflement. That's what bosses were for at the time, afflicting with our on-the-ground confusion.

"Sorry to ask so many questions," I said before I slammed her with a scenario.

"It's not a problem. It's a dynamic environment. Shoot."

"We keep the sealed PPE bags with our N95 masks on the truck? Not in the tech bag? We don't bring them with us on scene?"

"Correct."

"So what happens if we go inside an apartment for a diff breather, and it turns out the patient is having difficulty breathing because of COVID? Then what?"

"Then you go back to the truck and open the PPE bag and put on an N95 mask and gown up, then go back to the patient. I know it doesn't make a ton of sense, but we're following the Fire Department's protocols for now, and they're keeping all PPE on the trucks, not in the bags, so that's what we're doing."

If we opened a sealed PPE bag, Hartford added, we had to scan the bar code on the front, as it was tracked due to the supply-chain shortage. Every time I heard that constantly repeated phrase it was like being pitched into a void of terror.

Nina and I sucked it up and, minutes later, hopped on the ambulance and radioed dispatch that we were available. We pulled out of base, naked-faced and worried for ourselves.

It was a warm spring evening in Brooklyn, the March sky clear and bright. Not quite time for our long-sleeved duty shirts yet, so Nina and I were still wearing our faded winter work sweatshirts.

Most of the runs pouring over the radio were "fever cough." Listening to these calls was listening to panic. Once the job hit the air it sank into our psyches, we couldn't just shoo it away or push it out of sight. I was still baffled by the protocols. I texted Lexi to see what she was doing on the hospital truck.

"Girl, for diff breathers—are you in gloves, gown, goggles, and N95?"

"Nope. Not for fever coughs."

"Oh my God."

"You can't use PPE for everything."

"Do you wear an N95 at all?"

"Nope, surgical mask. We only wear the N95s for arrests. Jennifer, you need an arrest. This is your time."

Was it?

After a while we got sent to an EDP, our favorite type of emergency—and gratefully, non-COVID, to boot. Nina told dispatch we were en route, and I hit the sirens and gunned it to a brownstone near Prospect Park. It was much easier to drive the ambulance without Ubers and UPS trucks double-parked every other block, so that was a perk.

When we arrived on scene with an FDNY ambulance, cops were already inside the apartment. "Always happy to see 93 King," one of the FDNY EMTs said as he grabbed his tech bag, referring to us by our unit number. He looked exhausted.

"We're here for you in your hour of need," I said. And restating political blather, "We're in this together."

For psych emergencies, assaults, and other runs where there was often violence in progress, our protocols in New York City dictated that EMTs and medics did not enter a building or even get off the ambulance until police had secured the scene. "BSI scene safety" was the first thing they taught us in medical training. Body substance isolation meant put your gloves on before you touch anyone. Scene safety meant try not to die. Unlike many rules, this one had a lot of common sense in it.

On scene, the four of us EMTs grabbed our AEDs, tech bags, and stair chairs, and strode into the building. Inside a well-kept apartment, two beleaguered brown male cops were writing a report. From what we could understand, which was not a lot, the mother of a teenaged boy had called 911 because they'd gotten into a fight after she refused give her son his phone back, so he could play video games, and he'd reportedly shoved her. The boy sat on the stairs holding his head in his hands, pulling his hair and telling us his mother had overreacted. He'd only tried to make her give his phone back. I believed him. So did Nina, who asked the teenager if he had any diagnosed mental illness.

"Not really," he said. "Just ADHD."

"Do you take medication for it?" she asked.

"No, because I don't like the way it makes me feel."

All of this seemed understandable. The teenager didn't seem clinically insane or even mildly distressed. He seemed quite rational. But the livid mother insisted we take her son to the hospital for evaluation, since he'd shoved her.

My mind exploded with anger, as it often did on scene. I couldn't believe a parent would make their child get evaluated during a pandemic or tie up first responders, nurses, and doctors with a domestic squabble that was so minor. Perhaps it wasn't minor, and I'd missed something. But I couldn't see what, and neither could the other EMTs or the cops. He was a small teenager, waifish and timid. Sizing him up, he didn't look like he could injure his mother. Who knows.

The cops drove the insistent mother to the hospital, and we transported the teenager in our truck. Nina and I were terrified to walk into the ER without masks. The day before, Nathan had told me not to worry. He said the hospital security guards were standing at the ER entrance, giving everyone surgical masks when they walked in. This evening the hospital was a ghost town. One ambulance in the bay. No one in the ER triage line.

"Do you have masks for us?" I asked the security guard when we walked in.

"No," he said. "Yesterday we had masks. Today we don't."

I looked around. Doctors in gowns and goggles, nurses in respirators, other EMTs in surgical masks and N95s. Nina and I were the only people in view who weren't wearing any PPE beyond gloves. We felt vulnerable and stupid as we escorted our patient to the pediatric ER. Nina gave the triage nurse our report, and I heard the nurse laughing about the story.

"I'd be pissed too if someone took my phone and wouldn't give it back," she said. "It's a pandemic. The phone is all we have!"

While they talked, I stood with my back against a wall, overhearing a bonneted doctor geared up in full PPE begging a sick nurse to go home. "You have to go home," he told her. "If you stay here, you could infect patients."

And first responders, I thought. For instance, me and Nina. Right now. I understood in that moment that there was no way for us to stay safe. Not in the hospital and certainly not on the street. We were bathed in the virus.

I slathered my hands with disinfectant from a dispenser on the wall. Outside, we cleaned the stretcher, wiped down the truck, and cleared the hospital, telling our dispatcher we were 97, available for another run.

Not long after that job we got hungry and looked for somewhere to eat. All the restaurants were closed. Starbucks was closed. We went to 7-Eleven and loaded up on snacks. An hour or so later one of our duty officers sent us to a motor vehicle accident on Atlantic Avenue.

We rolled up late on scene, just as a fire engine pulled away. It was embarrassing to show up late, when the emergency was wrapping up. "We look so stupid," Nina said. She was grouchy that night. She was grouchy most nights, as was I. We were frightened and cranky and what you might call "on edge."

The hospital EMS unit already had a patient in the back of their ambulance. I knocked on their truck door to make sure they were cool and didn't need a hand. The EMT on the bus said he was all good, the patient wasn't injured, he was signing an RMA. Nothing to do.

A food delivery guy stood on the sidewalk next to his mangled bike and a few cops. It appeared to be that type of call: car versus bike, which happened all the time in New York City, and rarely ended well. But in this instance, the delivery guy was also unharmed. I climbed back on the truck.

Nicholas, our DO that night, appeared out of nowhere and came up to our window. He said he was in the area and just wanted to check on us, make sure we had everything we needed, that we were OK. Nina and I loved Nicholas. He was our favorite DO. On the street we told him how moronic we'd felt on that last job walking into the hospital without masks, when everyone in the ER was bedecked in PPE.

"Was your patient COVID?" he asked.

"No," I said. "But would you walk into a hospital right now without a mask?"

After a reflective moment he said, "Probably not."

Nicolas confessed he had a box of surgical masks in his car. His wife had gotten them somewhere. He offered to give us one each—as long as we kept it a secret. "Don't tell anyone I gave these to you," he said. We agreed. It felt like a drug deal. We were overjoyed when he handed them to us. PPE was the best present a first responder could receive at the time.

Meanwhile, the hospital-based EMTs had finished their paperwork. One of them came up to our ambulance and shook Nicholas's hand. Neither man was wearing gloves. That's it, I thought. Now you guys have the Rona, too. You just gave it to each other with that handshake. The EMT had magically acquired a box of chicken nuggets after the motor vehicle accident and now offered one to Nina. She accepted it. I couldn't believe it. What was she thinking?

"If you didn't just get infected with the Rona from the sick nurse in the hospital, you're getting it now from that chicken," I told her in a scolding tone. "That's COVID chicken."

"What do you want me to do?" she said. "I'm hungry."

A few minutes later a homeless man in tattered clothes wearing a sagging, dirty neck brace locked eyes with me. He was in the middle of the street, and I could see he was going to amble up to my side of the ambulance, wanting to chat.

This happened a lot. People constantly walked up to us when we were sitting on the bus and asked us for things. Did we have aspirin? Yes, but only if you were having an MI, a myocardial infarction, or heart attack. If you had a headache then no, we did not have aspirin. Did we have water? Yes, if it was summer and you had heatstroke, we often carried bottled water on the truck. However, if you'd just been shot and lost a liter of blood and were begging us for water, then no, we did not have water. Because your thirst was a bad sign, it meant you were dying, suffering from intervascular loss, so your kidneys were screaming for water. You thought you needed water, but what you needed was a tourniquet, bags of blood, and a surgeon.

As the homeless man got closer, I made sure the doors were locked. Nina often teased me because whenever people walked by our ambulance, if the doors were unlocked—which they never should be—I immediately locked them. The locks on our trucks made a loud clacking sound, so sometimes passersby heard me suddenly lock the doors and looked at us, offended.

But I locked the doors because I was thinking of Yadira Arroyo, the FDNY EMT in the Bronx who got dragged to her death and run over by her own ambulance by a schizophrenic man who came up to her truck. So that's what was on my mind as a first responder whenever someone approached the ambulance to ask us a question. If someone came up to the truck to interact with me, I'd roll down the window one inch. One inch, that's what you got if you wanted to talk to me or my partner. Pandemic or not, we were always vulnerable on the street. We were sitting out in the open, in a world where violence toward EMTs was constant, and where injury and tragedy were the norm.

I rolled my window down an inch and the homeless man spoke. He wanted directions to the nearest hospital. I felt bad for him. The homeless and the emotionally distressed were getting a bad hand in the pandemic. The cops pretty much ignored them unless they were actively suicidal or homicidal, since the police were overextended on other jobs.

I gave the man some flimsy directions and he wandered away. When I rolled up the window I thought: He just gave me the Rona, too. And I gave it to him. As first responders, we were presumed positive and asymptomatic.

The rest of the night on the ambulance, Nina and I mulled over what we'd been through and reached a heart-sinking conclusion about our first Rona tour: We're screwed.

The next day the governor went on TV and declared a state of emergency. He said all nonessential workers in New York must stay home. He played hot potato with language to avoid being injured by his previous statement. New York wasn't "locking down," he said. We were going on "pause."

* * *

Days later, with New York paused statewide and nonessential workers stuck at home, Nina and I geared up in our uniforms and braced for our second Rona tour.

The uniform set us free. Brought us together. Allowed us to stay close to each other and do something to assist when the rest of the city was forced indoors. New Yorkers who had no medical part to play in the unfolding disaster were trapped at home, bored, anxious, and unemployed, gorging on news and numbers. As for me, I felt lifted. Blessed to be able to help. Act.

These fatal spring days, New York City became the epicenter of the coronavirus pandemic, accounting for 5 percent of the world's infections, half the COVID cases in the country, with 15,000 people testing positive across the state. New Yorkers were quarantined, sheltering in place, and Times Square and Citi Field, the Oculus and Yankee Stadium, the Brooklyn Bridge and Holland Tunnel, all of them were deserted. The only people on the street were first responders and public servants. The sound of sirens was the only sound that filled the air. Day and night, Brooklyn and Queens, Manhattan and the Bronx, Staten Island, sirens and sirens and sirens nonstop.

A colleague at the Centers for Disease Control who knew I was a first responder working on the street wrote to me one afternoon, to thank me for my service. He said, "The sound of sirens will be how we all remember this for the rest of our lives."

For many, for my sweet sister-wife Ylfa, who called nightly, weeping, begging me not ride on the ambulance, New York City becoming a COVID hot zone conjured horrifying memories of September 11, when the cityscape was wiped of towers, and white tents went up as makeshift field hospitals, when emergency rooms braced for a flood of patients, and none came.

For me, COVID was not like 9/11. The sound of 9/11 was silence. There were no bodies after 9/11. There was no hope.

The sound of COVID was sirens. Where there were sirens, there were bodies, first responders en route to help. There were people to assist and save, patients who might survive. There was a chance. And those white tents went up again.

* * *

In September 2001, when those tents went up after that god-awful Tuesday morning, I prayed Pat was in one of them. I begged God. Petitioned. I said, Please, please. Anyone but him. Not him. I can't do this without him. I don't know how.

I told myself he wasn't dead—he was missing. I just had to wait a little longer. Just wait, I said. Tomorrow they'll find him. He's probably in one of those voids. He has to be. He's Pat. That guy could survive anything. He's not dead, he's missing. Just put up a poster of his face. Maybe someone will see him today and recognize him. Then it will all be over. Just wait.

My therapist defined me as a woman chronically drawn to the waiting room. I could wait longer than anyone I knew.

I am still waiting.

So COVID was for me not like 9/11. Not yet. And yes, Mike was sick. Critically ill. As were the gasping COVID patients calling 911, filling the air with sirens, but Mike was in Vegas, safe and alive, for now, and here in New York, we were being waterboarded with sirens, but sirens meant some patients were alive, for now, so there was hope.

One of the most shattering aspects of September 11 for me was my total inability to help. I felt so powerless. I was a civilian back then. A young, newly sober woman living in downtown Manhattan, unemployed and recovering from cancer. Now, almost twenty years later, I was a strong, healthy, middle-aged woman deep into sobriety, a crisis manager and writer, a first responder, an EMT. That made all the difference for me, in terms of how I was registering this event, horrific as it was. To be able to do something, to be of service. It changed everything.

Late March, for the first time since I'd become a first responder, I felt acknowledged and respected by the public. Finally, people saw us. They cared. The sirens forced them to see what we were doing out on the street. What we'd been doing all along, for years, invisible and alone. Suddenly people thought we were important. Deserving of respect, gratitude, praise.

What a feeling, to be invisible for so long, and then to suddenly be seen.

13

DIFFICULTY BREATHING

Good news. Our second Rona tour, Robert texted as Nina and I drove to Park Slope and said there were two N95s waiting for us at base. We were overjoyed.

We'd heard a rumor from a few first responders that the FDNY EMS station in our area had heaps of N95s at the time, while we were grateful to get one measly mask each. That was the way it always worked in terms of donations. Because the Fire Department was so pervasively well known, perceived as the gold standard in EMS, the public gave them supplies while the rest of the EMS community—hospital and commercial and volunteer crews—received comparatively little, if anything at all, simply because people didn't know we existed.

In late March, that started to change. Suddenly friends who knew I was an EMT texted and asked where I worked, where to donate masks and money. I sent them to Park Slope.

As Nina and I climbed on the ambulance and pulled out of base, we gave ourselves a secret mission for the night: acquire more PPE from our first responder pals. All of us looked out for each other on the street. Not just during the pandemic—always.

EMS was a family.

That night, the calls coming over the radio were more serious. If four days ago "fever cough" had been the norm, now every other call was a "diff breather" and "respir," short for respiratory emergency. It seemed all of New York City couldn't breathe.

While Nina and I habitually filled the ambulance cabin with gallows laughter and giddy excitement most nights, eager to see what kind of extraordinary scenes the street would throw at us, this tour we sat staring out the windows in locked silence. We were afraid for ourselves. For our families. Our friends.

As first responders, we'd consciously signed away our rights to a safe life and agreed to dive headfirst into the sea of infectious diseases and death. We worked directly in the realm others denied and repressed. The ugly, unpleasant world of critical illness and injury most affluently healthful people swept under the rug. COVID ripped the rug out from under them, from under the world. Finally, everyone was on the same page as we were in terms of what we'd been acutely aware of since the invention of time. Namely, the uncertainty of the world, the persistence of sickness and death, the fragility of life, the truism that it was indeed precious and very short, it could go at any second, tomorrow was not promised, and no one got out of this alive.

While we'd volunteered to lead high-risk lives as EMTs and paramedics, our families hadn't signed up for this level of risk, nor had our friends, who suffered just by loving us. My phone turned into a hellscape of messages from dearly beloveds, friends trapped at home with an awful lot of time, anxiety, and children on their hands. It seemed they had little to do aside from feast on grim news and fear for my life as a first responder.

On the ambulance I ignored a bombardment of incoming messages from panicked friends, which raised my already accelerated pulse and served no useful purpose in terms of helping me keep my shit together long enough to function as an EMT. To the contrary, the messages gaslit my terror. Snarfed up whatever dregs of peace I'd managed to scrape together to drive the ambulance and respond to jobs.

It wasn't just close friends checking in. There were fleets of stragglers. Acquaintances and veritable strangers. People I'd had one conversation with in ten years who knew I was an EMT suddenly found this to be a great time to inquire about my welfare and get a pulse check from the street, calling me a healthcare hero, posting photos of me on Instagram without my knowledge or consent, sending more texts my way if I didn't reply to their messages in what they felt was a timely fashion.

Incoming questions were numerous and repetitious. How was I doing? Was I OK? What was it like on the front lines? Did I have a second to talk so I could fill them in? Was what they were reading in the news true? Were all of my patients dying? Did I know I was a hero? Could I answer their last text, just heart it or send them a read receipt so they'd know I was alive?

Ahh, I knew they meant well, but I just needed to be left alone.

It was a part-time job, fielding these questions. Managing everyone's stress. It created more work for me.

In the driver's seat I pocketed my chiming phone and stared out the scummed ambulance windows. Emergencies were coming over one after another. Just listening to dispatchers spew out petitions for help was so exhausting that sitting on the truck creamed my psyche.

Nina and I got sent on a job for a diff breather. We couldn't get through to update our dispatcher with our status, as he was fielding calls from other units. That was a first.

"PS-5, we're 63 to the diff breather." "PS-5 to dispatch, do you copy?" "PS-5 we're 84 with EMS." "PS-5 to dispatch, how do you show us?"

No response.

Dispatchers were inundated with other units, they had no bandwidth to respond to us. Our duty officer came over the air and gave dispatch an update while we went on the job.

We arrived on scene with an FDNY EMT unit staffed with two guys we knew and liked. "Remember our mission," Nina said. Get masks. If the rumor was true and FDNY had a bounty, that was our goal. The four of us EMTs put on N95s and lumbered up a fifth-story walk-up. When we got to the top of the stairs, I was breathless and sweating from every pore. It was hard to breathe in the N95s. Sweat ran down my face and chest, it poured down my back.

Inside a stuffy apartment a frantic elderly white man in pajamas answered the door. He said his bedridden wife had pneumonia and couldn't breathe, she wouldn't eat, and she had a fever. He handed one of the FDNY EMTs what appeared to be hospital paperwork. A tiny dog appeared at our feet and yapped. Nina bent over and scratched its head.

"This says she's positive for COVID-19," the FDNY EMT said, handing the paperwork back. He stepped away from the husband, after hearing this.

We were inside the apartment already and had been told to try to stay six feet back from COVID patients. So much for that. The other FDNY EMT was at the patient's bedside, taking her vitals. There was no six-feet-back for him, either, not while taking blood pressure and measuring the patient's oxygen saturation levels, then hopping his stethoscope around the patient's chest and back, listening to see if her lung sounds were clear.

In the apartment, the husband rushed up to me with a frantic look on his face and tried to explain the situation.

"Sir," I said, though it pained me to say it. "I need you to take a step back."

"I don't know what to do!" he screamed. "My wife was in the hospital on Saturday. They gave her antibiotics and released her. She won't eat or drink anything, not even a smoothie."

What we were seeing on scene confirmed what I'd read in the news: ER doctors were aggressively discharging patients to make room in overflowing hospitals for people who needed ventilators. Patients they would have otherwise kept they now sent home. These patients fell on us.

"She's satting at 94," the EMT said from the bedside. He took out a nasal cannula and gave the patient a bit of O2 to see if her oxygen saturation went up. Ninety-four was decent in terms of the body's intake of oxygen. We started worrying when it dropped into the eighties.

The husband said he wanted to take his wife to see her doctor at a hospital that was fifteen or so minutes away. The FDNY EMTs explained that due to the virus, protocols had changed. There was no more "patient's choice" in terms of where we could transport patients. We had to go to the nearest hospital. We said we could do that easily, transport her to an ER three blocks away.

The husband refused. He didn't want his wife to go there, he only wanted her to see her doctor at the hospital that was farther away. In a normal world, we had some wiggle room as volunteers to transport patients to their hospital of choice. But this was not the normal world. This was a pandemic. All hospitals in New York City were now overwhelmed with COVID patients, many of them starting to run out of beds.

The FDNY EMT said, "Sir, if the doctor released her four days ago, and her vitals are stable, which they are, he's just going to release her again."

From bed, the wife said, "I don't want to go to the hospital. Any hospital. I'm not going."

"She doesn't seem to want to go," the EMT told the husband.

"But she has to go! I've never seen her this sick. She won't eat, she won't drink anything, not even a smoothie. Can you test her for COVID? Can you see if she has it?"

"She has it," we said. "She's positive. It's on her paperwork."

"But I didn't see them test her at the hospital! How could they have done it if I didn't see?"

"We don't know, sir," I said. "But they tested her. Her discharge papers say she's positive."

The longer we stayed there, locked in the apartment with the virus, the longer we were exposed, too. The higher chance we were all getting sick.

"Can you call our doctor and get him to come over and see her?" the husband asked.

"No, sir," I said. "We don't have that kind of power."

"I'm not going to the hospital!" the patient yelled from bed. She was speaking in full sentences, quite loudly I might add, so she was definitely getting adequate oxygen.

"Are you sure, ma'am?" Nina asked her. "We can take you if you'd like to go. If you're not feeling well it might help to get checked out. We're close to a hospital."

"I'm sure, I'm sure. I want to stay here."

Again the husband rushed up to me in fright of the future, his wife died in his eyes, I could see it, I could see her body-bagged in his pupils. It was all there.

"Sir," I said. "I'm sorry but I really need you to stay back."

"But she won't eat! You have to help me! Please! Tell her to drink the smoothie."

I could smell fear on this man, terror radiating off his body like he'd been nuked. The news and body count had gotten into his head; anything bad that happened to someone in the papers happened to his COVID-infested wife, who the doctors had discharged, sent home, and I couldn't blame him for being lit up like Mike's bone scan with metastasized pain.

"What's her name?" I asked him.

"Sarah."

From the hallway I said, "Drink the smoothie, Sarah. You have to eat."

"Sarah, did you hear that?" the husband said. "She said you have to drink the smoothie."

I ran downstairs and grabbed our Toughbook from the truck and ran back upstairs and gave it to Nina, so the patient could sign an RMA. Nina explained the risks to the patient. That if we left her behind, she could get sicker and die. Nina asked her for the third or fourth time if she was sure she didn't want to go to the hospital. She refused. She signed the paperwork and we packed up our tech bag and clomped downstairs. We were all drenched, our faces raining sweat, dripping with it, and probably now infected with the virus.

Outside, Nina and I returned to our truck. The FDNY EMTs followed us. The guys walked up to our ambulance. As for our secret mission, I asked them if the PPE rumor was true. Indeed. They had six N95s each per tour and if they ran out, they could restock and get more. We told them in cute voices, eyelashes batted, we only got one mask each. Nina gave me the look she always gave me when it was time for me to ask someone for something.

I pumped my shoulder and said in a forcedly girlish voice, "Do you maybe have extra masks for us?"

"Yeah, sure," one of the EMTs said. "But you guys have to take two more of my jobs—and call me Daddy."

We clapped and snorted with laughter. "You got it, Daddy."

He went to his truck and returned with two N95s, flattened, folded, and sealed in clear, crisp plastic bags. Beautiful.

"Wow," Nina said, staring mesmerized at hers. "These are the good ones."

"Thank you so much," I said. "This is the best present a girl can receive. Even though I'm not a girl, I'm a woman. I'm old enough to be your mother, Daddy."

The EMT laughed and asked if we were on Instagram. Nina was not—she stalked people through our joke business account—but I was, so he followed me, and I followed him back. Then we told him about Sweets in the Streets and encouraged him to follow our failure of a baking company.

"Of course," he said.

Satisfied with our night so far, we drove by Prospect Park to give a box of gloves to Larry. The NYPD had even less PPE than we did at the time, so earlier in the week I'd gone by the drugstore and bought a few boxes of gloves for him.

"Pornhub gave FDNY masks and free porn," Nina said as I drove to the park. "I think that's why they have more than everyone else."

Nina was dating an FDNY EMT, so she usually had good intel. I liked the guy, but he'd hurt her once, badly, so while they'd recovered and recommenced their romance, I told Nina I was happy for her, but I was also prepared to hate him at a moment's notice.

"Well, that makes sense," I said, "because I'm sure the Fire Department sends considerable traffic to Pornhub. They probably singlehandedly keep the site in business."

"Pornhub does a lot of good in the world. They're very supportive of first responders."

"Do you think that patient we just RMAed is going to die?"

"I don't know," Nina said. "Probably."

Ten or so minutes later, we circled around inside Prospect Park and found Larry. He was sitting alone inside his lit-up RMP, parked on some wet grass. He stepped out of his car in a mask.

I slid off the ambulance and gave him a box of gloves. We chatted for a bit. Someone had been stabbed in this spot the night before, and the uncaught perp promised to do it again, so Larry had to sit here all night and make sure no one got stabbed. What a job. He thanked us for stopping by. He said seeing us was the best part of his tour. I took that as a compliment, even though compared to waiting alone in the dark for someone to get stabbed, the bar was pretty low.

Not long after we left the park, we drove by the hospital to see how busy it was. We were shocked when we saw the ER bay that had been empty just days before was now clotted with emergency vehicles. Lines of ambulances waited to get into the bay. There was nowhere to park anywhere near the ER entrance.

As we crept around the hospital, the radio continued firing off nonstop with jobs for the "sick," "fever cough," and "difficulty breathers." That was all we heard very minute of every hour all night long. Sick. Fever cough. Diff breather, diff breather, diff breather. It got into me, the radio. I heard it later, when I stepped off the truck. The dispatcher's voice stuck in my head, played in a loop, I could hear it ringing in my ears, people all across the city having difficulty breathing, gasping for air.

* * *

We were worried we might get it.

When she got home that night, Nina's parents told her she could no longer ride. It was too risky, too dangerous. If she got infected, they would, too. They didn't want her going anywhere near COVID.

"I'm so sorry, baby love Jennifer," she texted me the next morning, using a pet name one of the *90 Day Fiancé* characters called his girlfriend. "But I'm also terrified of giving it to them, so I think this is best."

"I understand, baby love Nina. I'll find a new partner."

"Ask Nathan," she suggested. "I'm sure he'll pick up tours with you. He'll be your Rona partner."

I told her I'd call him.

That week, as the media released piece after piece about dwindling PPE, Nick called and said he had four N95s for me, from the NYPD. Beautiful. I drove into the city and met him on a pier along the East River. We sat together for an hour or so, masked and socially distanced, on the sun-warmed wooden planks, and caught up with each other as water lapped beneath us.

Nick was working a lot. Too much, as usual. I always teased him about his destructive relationship to work. He was the kind of person who was constantly sleepless, constantly canceling lunch with me because he had too much work, constantly doing PowerPoints in the car while someone shuttled him between business meetings. Unlike me, he was always late. I joked that the epitaph on his tombstone would someday say, "Here rests Nick. He should be here any minute."

In the pandemic, Nick's company was doing contact-tracing contracts, so he was even busier than usual.

I was not. My crisis consultancy got eerily slow. I was scared I was about to be in the Russian bread line, as one of my friends phrased it, with the rest of the country—world.

Nick had high hopes that since I was a crisis manager, the pandemic would eventually generate work for me. "You specialize in mass-casualty incidents," he said. "You're going to be a fucking funeral director after this."

Possibly.

When I got home, Mike rang in a panic from Vegas. He was going stir-crazy at home, reading the news. He wanted to fly to New York. Volunteer as an ER doctor. He said he'd made some calls. I listened, then gently explained there was no way in hell any hospital in hot-zone New

York City was going to let a doctor with stage four 9/11-related cancer work a lethal contagion.

"Imagine the headline," I told him. "'Brother of legendary firefighter who perished on 9/11 gets World Trade Center–related cancer then dies of COVID-19.' No one wants that headline, honey. It's not going to happen."

"But you're working, and you had cancer," Mike said.

"I had stage one cancer twenty years ago. And I'm not immunocompromised."

"But you could still catch it."

"Yes."

Mike paused. Then he said, in a voice torn with grief, "I don't want you to ride on the ambulance right now. I know what you're going to say. You're going to say you're working and there's nothing I can say or do to stop you."

"I'm working. And there's nothing you can say or do to stop me."

"But I want you to listen to me. I need to say something. Are you listening?"

"I'm listening."

"Nothing can happen to you, Jennifer. Do you understand? Nothing can happen to you. You can't get sick. I need you. I can't do this without you. I can't get through it. You're the only person who speaks to me in a way I can understand."

I was so touched I couldn't speak. That was how I felt once, about Pat. My whole body was covered in chills.

"Did you hear me?" Mike asked.

"Yes, Turtle."

"So if you've got to work on the ambulance, I understand. You're EMT Chick. But you have to be safe. Don't catch this thing, OK? I love you and I really need you. You're my wife. One of my wives."

"I love you, too, honey. You're my Turtle husband. Nothing is going to happen to me. I promise I'll be safe."

But I wasn't sure when we hung up if that was true.

Last days of March, New York City COVID infections skyrocketed to over 30,000 cases. A tsunami of calls flooded the already-overwhelmed 911 system and turned the streets into a war zone. Ambulances and hospitals became inundated with critically sick COVID patients. The New York City 911 system typically fielded around 4,000 calls a day. On March 31, emergency dispatchers received 7,253 calls, an almost 50 percent surge in volume, a record-breaking number of cries for help not seen since the terrorist attacks.

"This is worse than September 11," veteran first responders now said on the street at the end of March. "I worked 9/11, and this is worse."

A field hospital opened in Central Park.

"These bougie Fifth Avenue people are in for a real corona treat," Lexi texted me one night.

City officials tried to get control of the mass panic, get call volumes down by releasing public announcements. "Help first responders assist those most in need: Only call 911 during a real emergency."

It didn't work. Dispatchers answered nonstop calls.

Now that Nina was off the truck, I rode one Saturday night with Nathan, my newly acquired Rona partner. I missed Nina tremendously, but I would have ridden with anyone at this point, as the city was engulfed in COVID and I wanted only to be of service. All my petty grievances against Park Slope and anger toward EMS more broadly for being a thankless job flew out the window. The pandemic did what all crises do—it served as a bullshit eliminator. My minor complaints vanished. A new purpose revealed itself. I was grateful for that. Disasters were spiritually slenderizing.

Half Persian, half French, Nathan was in his late twenties, but everyone who met him assumed he was my age. One night a year back we'd worked together and had a pediatric emergency with a super cute gurgling baby, the kind of baby that made your ovaries hurt, made you want to reproduce immediately.

I was holding the cooing baby in the pediatric ER and said to Nathan, "I wish I had baby."

He looked at me, confused. "But Jen, you can have one."

"Negative. I'm dead single and I'm forty-three."

Nathan ripped his hat off and screamed, "*What*?"

The baby cried. I bounced her in my arms and said, "Nathan, you scared the baby."

"I thought you were in your thirties!"

What can I say? Clean living. Aside from the crow's feet around my eyes, I looked—and acted—younger than I was. Whenever I complained about my face being prematurely aged and raisined by the Bakersfield sun, Tommy came down hard on me. "You have face dysmorphia," he often said.

Nathan never ate meals on the truck and subsisted solely on snacks. Coffee, potato chips, ice cream. He had a weakness for geriatric patients and was crazy about the elderly. "Jen, they got the wisdom," he said to me tonight on the truck, our first Rona tour together. "We have to listen to them, because they have stuff to teach. And we have to take care of them, because they're fragile."

He had loads of experience in the field, and he was addicted to working cardiac arrests, whereas after three years on the street I still hadn't seen that fucking job. "We're going to get you an arrest tonight," he said. "Tonight's the night."

He was almost right.

That tour, the radio went nuts. There were no breaks between jobs, which ranged from abdominal pain to minor injuries to the gravely sick. Dispatchers fired out runs nonstop. Everyone and their mother called 911: "worried well" patients terrified by COVID symptoms reported by the media and medical authorities. "Sick fever cough" patients who'd turned into "difficulty breathers" the week before. "Difficulty breathers" who were now going into cardiac arrest.

Arrests were flying over the air every ten, fifteen seconds. The new thinking from medical professionals was that COVID didn't just attack the lungs, it also attacked the blood, the brain, it stopped the heart. That was the only song playing on the radio, the song of the cardiac arrested; sick people doctors had aggressively discharged from overflowing ERs were now arresting at home, dying in the field, on the streets, on us.

I couldn't stop thinking about the patient Nina and I and those FDNY EMTs had let sign an RMA, the one I'd told to drink the smoothie, Sarah; her name played on repeat in my head. She'd probably arrested at home, she had to be dead by now. Her husband had been right all along. He saw it that night, and we hadn't been able to help him at all; he wouldn't let us take her to the nearest hospital, and she didn't want to go to the ER. I felt like we failed her.

I became an EMT because I wanted to save lives. Not to let people die in the street.

It was all dispatchers said tonight—the whole city in arrest. "48 Dave, you're going to the arrest." "32 King, I need you for the arrest." "44 Ida for the arrest. 32 George, 48 Boy."

On the ambulance with Nathan, listening to radio for two minutes was enough to trigger more anxiety than I could bear. It's wasn't just COVID patients flooding the system. There were more DOAs. More members of service getting sick. More suicides as unemployment surged.

"The other day I had a jumper down," Nathan said. "He didn't even open the window. He went right through it."

On top of the new chaos, the old chaos continued: medical emergencies pouring in for motor vehicle accidents and strokes, allergic reactions and heart attacks. Every fifteen seconds the dispatcher sent a unit on another job.

"Arrest, arrest, arrest."

Worse still, paramedics repeatedly told dispatchers they were extended, meaning they were a long way out from jobs. They were getting killed on the streets, intubating people in the field, working a bombardment of arrests.

In EMS, response times mean everything. They mean life.

With cardiac arrests the first five minutes were crucial; you had to get the heart pumping, blood circulating, breathe air into the dead patient's lungs until they could do it themselves. Survival rates dropped 10 percent every minute that went by without defibrillation. Take much longer than that to start working them up and the patient had no chance of surviving at all.

"We're fifteen minutes out to the arrest," paramedics said. Fifteen minutes out meant the medics would not be responding to a savable arrested patient, they'd be responding to a DOA. Things worsened. Fifteen minutes turned into twenty minutes for paramedics to get to jobs in Brooklyn and Queens. Ambulances were reportedly taking over thirty minutes in some parts of the Bronx. Tonight in Brooklyn, units staffed with medics became unavailable, tied up intubating patients and working arrests and waiting hours to triage patients at overwhelmed hospitals.

"I have no medics!" the panicked dispatcher said. "No ALS! I have no medics available! Do your best! Everyone do your best!"

I looked at Nathan. "No medics. Holy shit."

I'd never heard a dispatcher say that in all my years as an EMT.

"It's a war zone," Nathan said.

In Queens, Gabriel, my precious lamb, was getting slaughtered as a new paramedic. His mother was in the hospital with cancer. On the ambulance, he worked nonstop, back-to-back arrests, five, six, seven, one after another. He lost all of his patients. Everyone died. There weren't enough cops to get to the bodies.

The medical examiner was so backed up with corpses it took them forever to get on scene. Cops were waiting with DOAs their entire tours. Gabriel worked one arrest at two o'clock in the afternoon and pronounced the patient dead on scene, and when he returned to the patient's house twelve hours later, at two o'clock in the morning, to pick up a piece of equipment he'd forgotten, the same cop was still there, standing with the body.

Gabriel said he remembered the faces of all the patients he intubated during COVID. Their faces were in his head. Swimming on repeat, just as Sarah's name did for me. *Drink the smoothie, Sarah. You have to drink the smoothie.*

Luna was losing it with fear as a dispatcher. People kept calling her with jobs, but when she tried to triage for COVID, callers said the patient didn't have a fever, then they called back later, after she'd sent a crew, and told her the patient did have a fever, and a cough. It tortured her. "I'm sending my units out there to get infected," she said. "I feel horrible. This is fucking awful."

Cops were getting sick, dropping dead. Eleven cops wiped out from COVID so far, and 19 percent of uniformed police officers out sick.

"I don't want to die," Larry texted.

"Hopefully we'll all be OK," I said. "Wear your mask, honey."

Nathan pulled up to a hospital to assess the situation. In the darkness a white tent fluttered in the ER bay and sent chills down my spine. Ambulances lined the block. A big rig we recognized as a refrigerator truck used as a makeshift morgue for the deceased was sloped on the ramp. Just seeing it turned my stomach and haunted me, flung me back to the aftermath of September 11, when hospitals waited for patients who never came because everyone was dead.

The radio rained patients. More people than we could save. Dying in the street. These nights EMTs and paramedics riding on commercial, hospital, volunteer, and Fire Department ambulances in New York City worked tirelessly, relentlessly, to respond to the surge in calls. It was impossible. An unwinnable landscape. No one could survive this. The call volume was just too high. There weren't enough of us to respond. Not in a time frame to save lives. Not with this many arrests and no paramedics or paramedics extended, fifteen minutes out to jobs.

Nathan and I heard FEMA was sending 250 ambulances, 500 EMTs and paramedics, and 85 more refrigerator trucks to serve as temporary morgues to New York City, since our morgues were overflowing. The military was likewise doing its part, sending forty-two people to the medical examiner's office, as the situation in Queens was dire. We hoped and prayed the FEMA trucks would arrive soon and save us.

We rescuers needed rescuing. We needed help. Urgently. Now. Yesterday.

Due to the skyrocketing call volume, we were burdened with making life-and-death decisions on the street. What were we supposed to do with the frail ninety-eight-year-old lady who fell down and broke her ribs? Transport her to COVID-infested hospitals, where if she caught the virus she would undoubtedly die? What about the patients going into respiratory arrest at home, who couldn't breathe, who now needed intubation in the field when all night the dispatchers told us there were no medics available?

On the truck I got a message from the fire marshal I'd cut loose. He got in touch tonight to tell me he was sick. Fever cough.

Oh, wonderful.

Just after I received his message, Nathan and I went on a run for a difficulty breather.

We arrived on scene with an FDNY unit of EMTs. When we got inside the house, a man with a relaxed air about him led us inside a cramped, dark apartment to help his mother. We followed him into the living room and found an elderly Black woman slumped in a wooden chair, barely alive.

My eyes darted up and down her neglected body. The buttons on her filthy blouse were undone. Spittle dribbled down her chin. The zipper of her pants was open, and she'd pissed in them. Flies buzzed around her, around us. In the kitchen, dirty dishes and empty takeout containers.

I felt so angry at her son, the man who'd let us in. It broke me, to find someone living like this, in total neglect.

"How long has she been like this?" I asked him.

"A few days."

"A few *days*?" Nathan said.

"Yeah," he said casually. "My father's in the hospital, too."

Rapidly, the four of us EMTs took the patient's vitals, one of us checked her lungs, another took her blood pressure, another checked her oxygen saturation. It was low, 47, she was going to arrest at this level, she needed to be intubated—now.

There were no medics available.

That's all we'd heard all night. We were alone.

"Can you hear me, sweetheart?" I asked the patient. Then her son: "What's her name?"

"Margarite."

"Margarite, can you hear me, sweetheart?"

She nodded to say yes. She wasn't getting enough oxygen to speak. We put her on a non-rebreather and cranked up the O2 to fifteen liters per minute. When we asked for her medical history, her son said she had a host of conditions. Diabetes. Asthma. CHF, congestive heart failure.

"Is that better, my love?" I asked the oxygenated patient.

"Yes," she whispered. "Thank you."

So sick, dying of COVID, minutes away from going into respiratory or cardiac arrest, in desperate need of intubation and a vent, and that was what she said: "Thank you."

I felt a thousand things at once. I wanted to sob and run out of the apartment into the dark, desolate street. I wanted to quit and never work again as an EMT. I wanted to work every night on the ambulance and treat every sick, dying patient I could find. I wanted to become a paramedic, so I could intubate.

We packaged our patient in a sheet and quickly stair-chaired her outside. It was raining now. The sky had opened up. We loaded her onto our stretcher. The FDNY EMTs thanked us and said farewell. On the street, Nathan must have asked me five times if I'd be OK in the back while he got ready to gun it to the hospital.

I wouldn't be OK. I wasn't the first responder this woman needed. I was an EMT and she needed medics. But I was all she had. I was terrified she would arrest on the back of the truck.

"I'll be OK," I said. "Just go, go. Just get there fast."

I heard the ambulance doors close with a woosh and soon Nathan was in the driver's seat, and we were blasting lights-and-sirens to the hospital, swerving crazily, I swear at one point we were on two wheels. Nathan floored it. I caught air on the bench in the back, holding Margarite's hand, squeezing it though I wasn't supposed to touch her, I didn't have my gown on, no goggles either, we hadn't known she was COVID until it was too late. I was asking if she was OK, telling her we were almost there. "Almost there, sweetie," I said. "Almost there. Are you breathing a little better?"

She nodded and her eyelids fluttered. Again she thanked me for helping her, which broke my already-broken heart.

It was agony, this job. This virus, and what it did to people. To the body. Watching people suffocate to death. Our city's oldest and Blackest and poorest, most vulnerable residents. That's what this was—agony. A horror show. War. The sky was pouring bodies. People we couldn't save. A hailstorm of DOAs. Corpses.

I'd been wrong. There was no hope for these patients at all. Or for us.

Nathan got to the hospital in under five minutes. The second we blew into the ER we pushed Margarite into the hands of an ER nurse expecting our arrival who shouted, "Bring her in here! In here!" We raced the stretcher into a tiny room.

Nathan and I transferred her onto the hospital bed while a chaos of gowned and goggled nurses and doctors swooped in and surrounded her. They prepared to intubate. I swallowed tears.

Was she going to die, my patient? This sweet, neglected woman? Was my mom? Felice? Ylfa? Mike? Were we? Who was going to survive this virus?

We weren't supposed to stay in close contact with COVID patients, and by the way Margarite was presenting—fever, with difficulty breathing—we knew she was positive for it. But we couldn't leave her. We couldn't stay six feet away. We stayed at her bedside. I stood at her feet and Nathan stayed at her head, watching as the nurses kept an eye on her vitals and unsealed their bags of intubation tools. Endotracheal tube that went through the mouth. Curved blade of the laryngoscope that looked like something out of a medieval horror show.

I couldn't watch. I didn't want to. The tools were gut-wrenching to see. Just being in the room with them and knowing that was soon going down Margarite's throat rocketed me out of New York City, onto another planet of pain.

Nathan stood by her side for a long time while I dragged the stretcher toward the hospital entrance and searched all around for disinfectant wipes. They were scarce. I found one purple-lidded container hidden beneath a lab coat by a nurse's station.

"Murphy!" I heard.

I turned and saw Votter, my favorite ER nurse. I hadn't seen him in some time, and tonight I nearly doubled over with relief when we locked eyes.

"Oh, thank God," I said. "Are you OK? You healthy?"

"So far. It's fucking crazy in here."

"It's crazy on the street, too. We have no medics. They're all on jobs. Everyone is arresting. The whole city is in arrest. We just brought in a patient who needed to be intubated."

"They all need to be intubated. Every patient is COVID. You be safe out there."

"You be safe in here. We'll be back."

"I know you will. See you later, Murphy," he said, zipping off, trotting down the hallway. "Stay safe."

Soon Nathan wandered dazedly toward me, fussing with his hat, scratching his head. He looked shattered. "Jen," he said as I wiped down the stretcher. "This is so sad."

In silence we rolled the stretcher outside, feeling like failures. In the ER bay, we peeked inside the tented white field hospital. It was empty.

"Who goes in here?" we asked one another.

A nurse in pink scrubs wandered outside with a cigarette and said, "It's for non-COVID patients who aren't that sick, but they aren't using it yet. It's too cold. They'll use it when it warms up."

"Got it," I said.

We took our time cleaning the back of the truck. Disinfecting everything Margarite had touched. Then slowly, silently, we lumbered back to the front seats.

When I took off my mask and looked at my face, it was mangled and carved with deep red marks. My hair was frizzy and sweaty, stuck to my forehead. I looked like I felt—wrecked. An FDNY unit of women EMTs pulled up to our ambulance in the street and rolled their windows down.

"Hey, guys, crazy out here, right?"

"Nuts," Nathan said.

"What have we gotten ourselves into?" I asked them.

"I don't know," the EMT behind the wheel said. "It's crazy. We're crazy for doing this."

"Crazy," I said.

Then Nathan drove slowly back to base.

"Do you think Margarite is going to survive?" I asked him. "Or do you think she'll wind up inside the refrigerator truck?"

"Jen," Nathan said. "This is really sad."

Before we went home, we stood on street outside of base for a bit. Nathan apologized for racing to the hospital, as my knee was sore from banging it on the stretcher. I told him he did a perfect job. He got Margarite to the ER alive, in time to be intubated. He said he was sorry for being so quiet all night. He wasn't feeling well. He had a pounding headache.

"Oh no," I said. "When did your headache start?"

"Earlier today."

When I got home, I disrobed before setting foot in my apartment. In the hallway, I peeled off my boots and socks, pants and tactical shirt, and left my uniform puddled on the floor.

Inside, standing naked in the kitchen, I got a garbage bag out and trashed my uniform. Then I Lysoled my boots and put them in the hallway. My uniform wasn't allowed in my apartment. That wasn't new. I never let my boots or EMS clothes go further into my apartment than the front door, where I sprayed down my equipment and bagged my pants and shirt.

In the shower, I lathered up and wept for Margarite, for all the patients in respiratory and cardiac arrest, suffocating at home, dying on the street, streams of terrified people flooding 911 in need of rescue, who had no one to save them. I wept for Lexi and Nathan, Luna and Gabriel, Nina, stuck at home, Ylfa having nightmares, and Mike, trapped in Vegas. I wept for myself.

This is worse than 9/11, I thought as I went to bed.

"My God," Mike said on the phone the next morning, when I cried and told him what I'd seen. "You're in a war zone."

14

GETTING SICK

In April, as news rippled across the country about the COVID outbreak in New York City, I received a radiance of support. Friends. Neighbors. Ex-boyfriends. Practically everyone who knew me, and knew I was an EMT, offered me an outpouring of gifts. People sent flowers, brownies, tea, plants, cards, gloves, goggles, hand-sewn and medical-grade masks. Everything counted. Almost daily I had a package in the mail. Some of them from people I barely knew.

One day Marko messaged me. "Thinking of you while you're on the front lines. You're amazing, so please stay safe and healthy." He apologized if he was bothering me. To the contrary, I appreciated his concern.

"I'll talk to any ex who may have an N95 mask," I said. Then I told him what I was seeing in the field.

"I see every day on screen what you're seeing with your own eyes," he said. "This is a monumental task we're facing. But you're the one who's fighting it. I'm so sorry, Jennifer."

Later that same day, Marko wrote again, to tell me he'd gotten his hands on some masks to send me. The next week they arrived, a gigantic box of them, hundreds of masks, and I let him know how grateful I was. These days off the truck were easier, though washed in sorrow.

But then things took quite a turn.

One afternoon, Tommy texted to say he had the Rona. He'd been out sick for two weeks. Fever, achy, chest pain, tired.

Welp. That made two firefighters and two COVID patients I'd been in close contact with these last two weeks, all of them now infected with the virus. It seemed every time a firefighter got sick the media attributed it to "community transmission." What community might that be? Firefighters weren't responding to the majority of COVID jobs inundating the 911 system. I joked with Tommy that for firefighters, coronavirus was a sexually transmitted disease.

After that last tour with Margarite and the news of Tommy having COVID, I popped some vitamin C and relaxed. Drank tea. Lounged. Took myself on meandering walks around the neighborhood. Nightly I talked on the phone to Felice, Ylfa, and Mike. Daily, I checked on my first responder friends. That's what helped the most when I was holed up at home. Talking with EMTs and medics who were seeing what I'd seen on the street. We really were in this together.

"I think I have it," Nathan texted me a few days later.

Oh, great.

A day after that, I was struck blind with exhaustion, more tired than I'd ever felt. I lay down for a nap and couldn't stop coughing. It was a deep, dry cough that made my chest burn and hurt. I heard echoing from my throat the same hollow, guttural sound that came from COVID patients hacking in the ERs. I told Lexi, who was also out sick.

"Oh no, Jennifer," she said. "That's how it starts."

That was how it started, alright.

The first day I had that awful cough. A headache that no pain killer diminished. A heavy, leaden feeling in my chest as if a vicious animal were sitting on my heart. The chest pain worsened when I lay down and made sleeping impossible. I had insomnia. Achiness. Shortness of breath that made staggering from my bed to the bathroom an athletic event. Red, swollen sore throat. Bounding pulse. Disabling exhaustion. I couldn't keep my eyes open for longer than an hour at a time. Then I'd have bursts of feeling A-OK, nothing wrong at all. Then pow! I'd be bombed with tiredness and bed-bound. Up and down, this virus. COVID was wavy. Fine one second, dead in the bed the next.

No fever. At least not according to the cheap digital thermometer I kept in my medicine cabinet. Still, I knew from Margarite and other COVID patients that a fever wasn't the sole indicator of the virus. The COVID fever was low. Or inextant.

"You gave me the Rona," I teased Nathan on my third or fourth day out sick. He'd lost his sense of smell and taste. He was bedridden, hot, exhausted, achy. "You're patient zero," I said.

"Jen, that's not true! You can't prove it. Margarite gave you the Rona."

"Both of you gave it to me. I was sealed in the back of the truck with her and sealed in the front with you. That tour was 100 percent chance of me getting the Rona."

"It's not going to be pretty for a while, but we'll get through it together. And hopefully not die."

Hopefully. Nathan and I joked a lot when we were out sick. Tried to laugh. Keep our spirits high. But we were frightened, too. We'd seen the medical tools paramedics and nurses used to perform emergency intubations. We'd seen the white tents and refrigerator trucks. The suffocating patients, gasping for air. We feared we might wind up like them. Dead.

There was no shortage of COVID patients in the ERs these April days. A doctor at the hospital where we'd taken Margarite reported treating seven COVID-19 patients one Tuesday afternoon, ranging in ages from twenty-five to seventy-two. EMT friends on the streets said they were waiting an hour, sometimes two hours just to triage patients, standing in lines outside hospitals. What world were we in?

In EMS, emotions ran high. First responders were tired. Sick. Depressed. One paramedic blasted government officials on social media about how medical first responders were being treated during the peaking virus:

"Each EMT and paramedic understands what we signed up for every time we go to work, every time we put on our boots and log on for assignments. We are being treated like an immune, immeasurable resource. But clearly, we are not. We have not been acknowledged by the city we work for, our mayor, our governor. We have been left to respond to calls alone, without the protection of the NYPD or the assistance of Suppression, who are Certified First Responders. Yes, I said it, when so many people won't.

"We're working back-to-back tours. We're run-down and getting sick ourselves. We're rationing what PPE we have because it's getting to the point that we'll run out in a few weeks, if not sooner. Think of Christell right now," the medic said. Christell Cadet was a Black FDNY paramedic who was currently intubated and hospitalized, in a coronavirus coma. "And think of every member of the Bureau of Emergency Medical Services in New York City—us, and our barely spoken-about brothers and sisters in the voluntary agencies who work with us.

"Something is going to give, and as you can see—it is us."

It was us.

Now it was our turn go from being first responders to COVID patients. Our number was up. We got hit hard and first.

Early April, one out of every four FDNY EMS workers were out sick. Of the 4,000 EMTs and paramedics in the Fire Department, 25 percent had COVID. Nina's boyfriend was off the truck. "Not just him," she said. "His whole unit is out sick."

On the suppression side of the house, 17 percent of firefighters called out sick. One in six cops were out, with 1,500 others in the NYPD infected. Cops fell ill tending to DOAs and when the city mandated them to enforce social distancing.

Despite the lockdown and rising death toll, I was astounded to learn some New Yorkers still weren't taking the virus seriously while first responders and patients were dropping like flies. What would it take for people to generate concern for others?

One afternoon I found and saved this tweet from a woman named Kimberly Dinaro: "Everyone in NYC who is saying they're 'not worried' abt #coronavirus bc they're young & healthy has lived on nothing but cigarettes, cocaine & bodega meat for 9 years, shares a moldy shower w/7 internet strangers & is in an open relationship w/ an anti-vax couple & 2 park rats."

Now that was an appropriate use of the Internet.

Just as first responders dropped out of service in New York for two or three weeks at a time, since COVID was a long, slow virus, 911 call volumes continued to spike. There was no manpower left on the street to address the record-breaking surge in emergency calls. There weren't enough first responders to respond to jobs, the fatal crush of bodies.

One night in bed, my eyes welled when I saw a photograph online of fleets of ambulances from all over the country, crews from Indiana, Ohio, Nebraska, you name it, driving down a dark mountain road, heading to New York City.

FEMA.

They were coming to save us. There was no way they'd get here fast enough to rescue us, respond to scores of COVID-stricken patients calling 911 now, tonight, this week, going into respiratory and cardiac arrest on the street, dying in the field, in the arms of EMTs and paramedics, since hospitals were blowing up just like the Italians warned us they would, isolation rooms and hallways overflowing with vented patients. People afflicted with COVID calling 911 right now would perish. Die in the lurch.

But eventually, eventually these FEMA trucks staffed with first responders would get here and help. When they arrived, we learned, they'd be dispatched from staging areas scattered across the boroughs. One of them, at the Bronx Zoo—a detail that generated chuckles and gallows laughter among us city EMTs and medics, since this whole pandemic was quite a circus.

We needed FEMA to get here now. New York City hot-zone disaster, and COVID Wave I frontliners were out of service.

All of us, it seemed, but a few.

As a new paramedic, Gabriel was still working, out there drowning in cardiac arrests. At this time, some hospitals in the city ran out of beds and ventilators.

Gabriel transported an arrested patient to an ER in Queens, and a panicked nurse ran up to him and told him to pronounce the patient on the stretcher, in the triage line. *My God.* That was someone's mother, father, child, grandparent, friend. Dead because the hospital ran out of life-saving equipment.

"You have to call it! You have to pronounce! We have no beds!" the nurse said.

He saw another nurse staggering around crying. She looked so exhausted he pulled her aside. Told her to let it out, he was there, she could talk to him. "I can go out of service," he said.

"We're out of beds," she sobbed. "We're out of ventilators. We don't have enough PPE. It's all COVID. I can't take it. It's death after death after death."

As for those of us out sick, we were in near-constant touch, desperate to get tested.

* * *

"Get tested. Get tested. Get tested," Nick said when I told him I was out sick.

He was a post-9/11 cop. He knew the importance of having paperwork in case there were long-term ramifications from the virus. You had to prove you got sick on the job. No one knew shit about how long COVID lasted. Or what it did to the body over time. The virus was novel, unknown to medical mankind. If I wanted to get insurance coverage for medical conditions that, God forbid, I developed from COVID down the line, I had to have paperwork. Nick kept insisting. "Get tested, Lioness. Get tested."

I knew it was important. When Mike got diagnosed with cancer, he had to get signed affidavits from firefighters verifying he'd worked the pile, proving he'd dug, searching for Pat, in order to qualify for World Trade Center–related treatment. Testing mattered tremendously for our future. Yet no one was testing EMS members of service at this point.

No one.

It was impossible to find a hospital or walk-in clinic that would see me as a first responder. For a week I sat at my desk feeling like trash, calling this or that clinic that various cops said they'd heard were doing tests for MOS. They sent me names of clinics in Westchester, New Jersey, Staten Island. But when I called, the lines were busy or dead. Then their websites crashed. One clinic that opened at eight o'clock in the morning ran out of tests by noon. I spent hours online booking time slots for appointments only to be greeted by pop-up windows telling me the clinic had run out of tests, and the next appointment was in two weeks.

Two weeks?

It was enraging, how impossible it was for us in EMS to get tested, those of us on the front line, risking our lives to save others, sick because we volunteered to help. Many days I fell apart at my desk, weeping with frustration and exhaustion. Talk about the disposability of first responders. The way we treat servicepeople in this country is a monstrous disgrace.

I kept trying to find a clinic. Nathan stopped.

"I give up on America when it comes to testing," he said.

Sick and tired, weight sliding off my frame like clods of dirt, I grew enraged. I had to take my anger out on someone. Who better than Larry? It was his buddy, the guy in the White House, minimizing the virus cratering my health, killing thousands of people, turning my city into a morgue.

One day, Larry made the mistake of sending me a photo of himself from the street. He was wearing an American flag mask.

"Must you wear the flag as fashion?" I asked him.

"It's fashionable protection. I'm a proud American."

"Oh, fuck this piece of shit country right now. Your president is killing us with his stupidity. If I'm on a ventilator it will be because of him."

"Trump didn't give you COVID."

"He is COVID."

Facepalm emoji.

"I'm your street wife," I said. "Deal with it."

He dealt with it, Larry. Two days later, he tiptoed back to my phone. "How are you feeling, dear? Not talking to me?"

"No, I love you. I'm sick. But I'm still extremely pretty. Stay healthy. I'll be back on the bus later this week, I hope."

"Don't worry about the bus. Get better first. Love you, too."

I wasn't the only one coming undone.

Stuck at home in Bakersfield, my mother grew bored. She discovered a bounty of apps on her phone. One afternoon, she FaceTimed me. That was a first. She'd never FaceTimed me in my life. I declined, because I was on a call when she rang. But then I got paranoid something was wrong. Maybe she was sick with COVID. I called her right back.

"Mom, are you OK? Did someone die?"

"Oh!" she said, giggling. "I'm just learning how to use these new things on my phone and calling to check on you."

Exasperated, I told her I'd call her later.

Weariness sent me to the couch. I flopped down and watched TV. I wanted to watch only absolute trash. Nothing highbrow. Nothing serious. No plot. Life had enough of a plot for now.

Later, I called my mother again.

"Mom," I said. "What is happening over there?"

"What do you mean?" she said innocently.

"I see you've joined Instagram and posted a thousand pictures of me online. On your public account. You know how I feel about social media." I was very private when it came to being online, given my day job, but philosophically, too. I hated being hashtagged a healthcare hero. More dollars in Mark Zuckerberg's pockets, and no real impact where it counted.

"Is that bad?" my mom asked. "Am I not supposed to do that? I don't know how these things work."

"Clearly."

I explained I was trying to move a mountain over here and get tested, and I was sick, and half of New York City was body-bagged. I told her she needed to tone it down with her giddy discovery of social media then walked her through steps to privatize her account. Explained I was conservative about posting photos of myself online, on account of my job—jobs.

As soon as we hung up, my mother deleted all of the photos of me. Wiped them clean. It only took two or three seconds for me to descend into regret.

I was so tired, and sick. I hadn't asked my mom to delete every picture of me. I just wanted her to make the account private. But I'd come down so hard on her. Been a real pandemic bitch. It was my terror masquerading as rage. I was so scared she was going to get sick, and then I'd lose her. She was all I had, in terms of real family. And she was so far away. I made myself cry, remembering how I didn't visit her when I flew to California for those stupid meetings. Then she sent me the kindest e-mail.

"Jenny, I changed my Instagram account. I'm sorry about posting pictures of you. I understand, but I didn't know how you felt. I only joined it because of my sister who's on it, so we could keep in touch. I really miss my sisters. I didn't mean you any harm. Take care of yourself. Rest as you see fit. I'm praying you're able to get well. Love, Mom."

I missed my mom.

I apologized profusely for being so hard on her. I thanked her for dialing back the photographs of me. I was her only daughter, and she was proud of me, that's all.

"Thanks, Mom," I said. "I accepted your friend request on Instagram. And I sent you one, too, so you can see my account."

It was all we had now. The Internet. Mother-daughter content.

Next few days I hid out in bed with my nose in a book. I read *Columbine* by Dave Cullen. Just a little lighthearted reading about one of the grimmest mass murders in American history. Wow, what a masterful, powerful book. I devoured it.

* * *

My first responder family took such good care of me while I was out sick. Robert and Chief Suzy were in constant touch. They checked on me night and day.

"Ginger, do you need anything?" Suzy asked one afternoon. "I can bring it for you. Seriously."

I told her I felt like shit and had an extra N95 mask for her. Suzy was working as a nurse in the ER, and all hospitals citywide were short of PPE. Robert had told me she only had one mask, which she had to reuse.

"You're a healthcare hero!" I said.

"Hello! You're MOS too!"

"I'm an MOS hobbyist, Suzy. You're the real thing. My Rona Queen!"

"Hobbyist! You have me laughing. It's even more admirable that you do it in your free time. So kick this out of your system! We have to stay healthy. Rest up and let me know if you need anything. Keep eating, even if you aren't hungry."

As they say, not all heroes wear capes. My civilian beloveds stepped up, too. My friend Clara, who'd found me this apartment, brought me sacks of groceries. Soups and kale and bone broths galore. So did my friend Ben, from writers group. In my building, Ellery checked on me via text to see if I needed anything from the grocery store whenever he went. Jeremy ran to CVS for me and got me aspirin. I spent hours on the phone each night with Mike and Ylfa and Felice.

My sweet heroes.

Everyone wanted to help me, and everyone did. I was so loved. What a life I had. I was one of the lucky ones.

After a week of beleaguered attempts, Larry sent me the name of yet another walk-in medical clinic in Park Slope, which he heard was testing symptomatic MOS. One afternoon I dragged myself out of bed and landed a virtual intake appointment with a nurse, who told me I could come to the clinic at seven o'clock that evening. Finally. I felt like I'd won the lotto.

"I found a place," I told Nathan. But by the time he tried to book an appointment, they were all gone. "Keep trying," I told him. "We have to get tested. It's important."

"Jen, I'm so tired. I can't get out of bed. All I do is sleep."

"I know, me too. I sleep and cry and fight with Larry. This is my life now."

"I don't want to end up on the refrigerator truck."

"Or the Javits Center. Now there's a place I don't want to die."

That evening I materialized at the walk-in medical clinic. It was empty. A nurse saw me and brought me into an exam room immediately. She asked me the relevant questions.

"Have you been exposed to COVID?"

"Yeah, I'm an EMT. All my patients had it and so does my partner."

"I'm sure you have it. How long have you been sick?"

"This is day seven."

"What are your symptoms?"

"They roam. Headache. Sore throat. Dry cough. Chest pain. Accelerated pulse, my heart rate was a 104 two days ago. Fluey feeling. Body aches. Exhaustion. Shortness of breath. Rage."

"You have it," she said conclusively. "All of you first responders do. Let's swab you."

Has everyone been swabbed? Because that's a real treat, if you haven't. The nurse stuck a long Q-tip-like torture stick up my nose and reached so far back my eyes watered. It was deeply unpleasant. Then it was over.

"How long for results?" I asked, wiping my nose.

"You should see them online in forty-eight hours."

Four days later I got the results:

Negative.

How could that be possible?

"That's gotta be wrong," Robert said. "You have COVID. You have to."

Chief Suzy agreed. "That must've been a false negative. You had all the symptoms. Just think, you probably have the antibodies now. Woo-hoo!"

Woo-hoo.

15

CITY IN ARREST

The next week as COVID peaked I was still out sick. So were Nathan, Tommy, Lexi. All of us COVID Wave I first responders, it seemed. Fire Department data confirmed what EMS radios dispatched on the street:

EMTs and paramedics were responding to a surge in fatal or near-fatal out-of-hospital cardiac arrests suffered by New Yorkers whose true health issue was suspected to be COVID-19. From March 30 to April 5, 2019, there were an average of 69 cardiac calls a day, and 26 of those patients died. For the same period in 2020, there were 284 cardiac emergencies a day, and 72 percent resulted in death. One Sunday in April, out of 322 cardiac calls, 241 patients died, a death rate of 75 percent.

That April, first responders I hadn't heard from in months frantically got in touch. Our questions to each other were the same. Have you had it? What are your symptoms? Have you gotten tested? Are you back on the truck? What's it like out there right now? How are you holding up? Talk to me, talk to me, talk to me. First responders were not doing so hot.

Eyal, the walking-textbook paramedic instructor from my EMT school, told me he'd lost his brother to COVID. "I'm respecting this virus," he said. "It means business and touched very close to me." At Park Slope, one of our lieutenants lost both of his parents in the same week. Lexi's uncle died of COVID. In an effort to protect their families, EMTs and paramedics were sleeping in their cars, trying not to infect their loved ones.

We needed FEMA. I'd heard they were here. But even with extra units from out of town, there was no way New York City EMS could respond to the massive call volume when so many first responders were off the trucks, out sick, with everyone arresting in the street.

It wasn't just us.

A paramedic-firefighter from Paris sent me a message on Instagram one day, to see how it was going in New York. France was also getting decimated. I told him people were dropping dead, arresting in the street. "Same here," he said. "Everyone's going into cardiac arrest and dying at home."

Then things took an even darker turn in New York.

As COVID stretched ERs thin, New York state made a grim decision to change medical protocols due to the phenomenal number of cardiac arrests. One April night, Park Slope had an agency-wide Zoom meeting to update us on the shifting landscape. It seemed our protocols changed every time we blinked.

The pandemic changed the way time worked. Caused it to travel at warp speed and simultaneously decelerate and spin, a slow-motion whirling dervish of horror and cycles of catastrophic news mixed with long, lonely hours isolated at home, removed from friends and family. Every day was gargantuan, a thousand years long.

It was impossible to keep up with it all: the news, the deaths, the patients, the tests, the volume of calls, the PPE supply, the doctors' opinions about how the virus destroyed the body, the way I felt at any given moment about being on the ambulance, off the ambulance, at home, in the street, in New York City, which reporters kept calling a hot zone.

All of us EMTs at Park Slope gathered on our respective couches and logged onto Zoom one evening in April. Immediately, Lexi and Austin fell to pieces because I'd made my Zoom background a photograph of some firefighters who'd once come inside my apartment in search of a fire. (I didn't start it.)

"Girl, I'm dying over your background," Lexi said. We crowned each other with virus nicknames. Lexi was Saltyrona and I was Gingerona. Lexi also gave me a very powerful nickname years back, the Traffic Cone, since I was orange and so unmissable everyone stopped when they saw me on scene.

"Wifey," Austin texted. "Your background with suppression—it's beautiful."

Zoom life really threw me for a loop. The first thing I noticed was that my bottom tooth was much crookeder than I previously thought. All of a sudden, I felt like I needed dental work. That was weird. Equally weird was seeing people in virtual boxes, in their apartments and homes. Personally, I didn't need to see that. And I didn't want people in my house, either. Who invited you into my kitchen? Not me.

It was extremely strange, Zooming. Most of my crisis counsel took place over the phone. Huge group calls with twelve to fifteen people on them, CEOs and lawyers, grief counselors and crisis PR people, victims and sometimes law enforcement. I was a voice on the line. I wasn't a video or an in-person figure. I had clients I'd worked with for years who I'd never once seen or met in real life. Didn't mind that at all. I liked being a voice. In this way, I guessed in my day job I was similar to a 911 emergency operator. Seeing people on Zoom threw me off.

Back to Park Slope's meeting. Chiefs Beck and Hartford went over the new protocols. They were numerous.

PPE first. Now they wanted us to wear N95s on every call, for COVID and non-COVID patients. We were now to wear gowns and goggles any time we suspected a patient had COVID, or if the patient was confirmed to have COVID. Our agency policy was to use PPE more frequently than some other agencies, for our safety. That made me happy. Hooray Park Slope.

Moving forward, no more being dispatched internally. FDNY was activating all volunteer ambulance companies to work 911 tours to meet the surge in calls through its mutual-aid radio channel, MARS. Park Slope ambulances would now be dispatched by the Fire Department. I guessed I'd end up working for the FDNY after all. High-five, Pat.

On-scene changes: New York state was reducing the number of first responders on scene to try to limit our exposure to COVID. In practicality, that meant we might be canceled off a cardiac arrest, leaving ALS (paramedics) and CFRs (firefighters) on scene to handle the job. We were to follow the orders of dispatchers and conditions bosses.

Quarantine. In terms of those of us out sick and our return to work, due to the widespread transmission of COVID in New York, quarantine of asymptomatic healthcare providers was no longer recommended. We were essential, and the city needed us. Symptomatic EMTs and paramedics who were not hospitalized but had possible or confirmed COVID-19 were to isolate for seven days following the onset of illness; AND, seventy-two hours afebrile, without antipyretics; AND, with resolving symptoms—whichever was longest. In other words, we stayed off the bus for seven days then went back to work.

Lastly, compassionate CPR. Moving forward, if we were delivering compressions on a patient and no shock was advised by the AED, we were to stop CPR after twenty minutes. We then needed to call telemetry and ask for a pronouncement. If a shock was advised in the twenty minutes, we would transport to the hospital—even if no paramedics had arrived on scene. In this case, a firefighter could drive our ambulance to the hospital.

Whoa. Lexi and Austin and I texted each other shocked emojis. Did this mean what we thought it did?

While on Zoom, I Googled the new CPR protocols, which confirmed what our chiefs at Park Slope said. The Regional Emergency Medical Services Council of New York, REMSCO, issued a medical protocol advisory on March 31 tilted: "Temporary cardiac arrest standards for disaster response." REMSCO was responsible to the state of New York for coordinating medical services in all of New York City's five boroughs.

Effective immediately, no adult nontraumatic or blunt traumatic cardiac arrest patient was to be transported to a hospital with manual or mechanical compressions in progress without either return of spontaneous circulation (ROSC) or a direct order from a medical control physician unless there was imminent danger to the EMS provider on scene.

Effective immediately, in the event a resuscitation was terminated, and the body was in public view, the body could be left in the custody of NYPD.

Effective immediately, in the event NYPD response was delayed we were to call the following: Office of Chief Medical Examiner tour commander, or NYPD DOA removal.

In a normal world, we performed CPR and other lifesaving measures on scene even if there was no blood flow while en route to the hospital, and we took as long as it took to try to bring life back to arrested patients. Now, with few exceptions, that was no longer allowed. We were instructed to perform twenty minutes of CPR—"compassionate CPR," as they called it—then pronounce the patient dead on scene, then deal with the dead body.

News headlines were bleak. EMTS HAVE STOPPED TAKING PEOPLE IN CARDIAC ARREST TO CORONAVIRUS-STRAINED HOSPITALS. GRIM NEW RULES FOR NYC PARAMEDICS: DON'T BRING CARDIAC ARRESTS TO ER FOR REVIVAL. They called it compassionate CPR because it was a show, a performance of compassion for the families, a little dance to say, "We tried. For twenty minutes, we tried."

Many EMTs and medics felt this protocol change was bullshit. A death sentence for patients. Contrary to public perception, likely caused by inaccurate medical TV dramas, people believe CPR is a miracle cure. But statistically, cardiac arrest is an end-of-life emergency. The survival rate if a patient arrests outside of a hospital is only 12 percent. If CPR is performed, it can double or triple the chance of survival. Compassionate CPR was a performance of a save, not an actual save. It was a show for family members. It was about perception.

This sometimes happened on the street pre-COVID, too. I knew an EMT who responded to a train job where a guy got electrocuted on the track. The man was cooked. Liquidated. But there were bystanders watching, so a boss made him do CPR on the electrocuted patient. "Just put on a show," the boss told him, so people would think he was trying to save a life. When the EMT did compressions, he felt the patient squish when he pressed on his chest, like he was pushing on a waterbed.

These doomsday medical guidelines were unthinkable before COVID. That's how we referred to the old world now, as B.C. Compassionate CPR meant we'd leave patients to die in the field. If they died at home, untested, their deaths would go uncounted in the graphs and bar charts circulating in the news. The ones that boasted about hospitalizations being down.

When the Zoom meeting ended, Austin and I texted each other for an hour. We dove into the only oasis we had left, gallows humor and jokes about firefighters.

We were very sick, mentally. Our sense of humor was vile long before the Rona, but this meeting had made us sicker. It was the only way to survive, by breathing humor into it.

Firefighters had gotten some bad press as of late. The media informed the public of what we'd known for a while as EMTs and paramedics:

In March, FDNY had issued a temporary order that relieved firefighters of responding to the second-highest-priority jobs for patients presenting with fever, cough, difficulty breathing, and in some instances, patients who were unconscious—in other words, it pulled them off most of the COVID-19 jobs. The department was shielding firefighters from the virus, leaving its underpaid EMTs and paramedics to face the pandemic alone.

"We can't believe they would put out this order during one of the biggest citywide health crises," a paramedic told one news outlet. "The fact that they're abdicating all of this is just astounding. You're talking about people who call themselves the Bravest." FDNY was investigating three instances of firefighters responding to possible coronavirus calls who'd declined to engage with patients and left the job solely to EMS.

To some extent it made sense, that the department tried to protect firefighters from COVID. They lived together part-time, after all. If one of them got sick, they all went down. When an FDNY captain in Coney Island tested positive for the virus in March, thirty-three additional firefighters had to self-quarantine.

And while the rest of the world may have moved on from September 11, the Fire Department most certainly had not. FDNY continued to suffer enormous losses from that tragedy, with hundreds of its veteran ranks dying of WTC-related cancer from digging the pile, like Mike. It was understandable that in the pandemic, the department was trying to protect its veteran members. Even so, a woman firefighter friend who worked in Brooklyn reached out to me one afternoon and said she wanted to ride as a volunteer EMT with Park Slope. She wanted to help. Most first responders were wired to help. But that didn't stop me and Austin from cracking firefighter jokes.

"Why don't the firefighters stop clapping for nurses and help EMTs?" I texted her.

"Honestly!"

"Suppression. Eating their chicken and giving some claps."

"The world is ending, and their pay grade goes up each clap."

"The most powerful part of that meeting: a firefighter can drive our ambulance."

"There will be a docuseries on the lives of female EMTs when suppression hops on board to drive the ambulance to the hospital when they are there—or not there—for delivery."

"All female EMTs will be pregnant by summer. Married couples trapped at home will be divorced, and we will all be with child. Our babies will be born wearing goggles and N95s. We will name them Rona."

"When they do interviews of ladies for the EMS TV series, the first clips will be like, 'We responded to this eighty-eight-year-old man, a number of heart problems, he needed CPR, but all I could focus on was when the firefighters rolled up.'"

"I know we changed protocols to compassionate CPR, but I couldn't do it for twenty minutes because my arms were tired from hugging the firefighter driving my truck."

"My arms were tired and the only thing that made them feel better was to wrap them around a firefighter. While they drove us to the hospital. While they drove the DOA. To the hospital."

"I'm dead. Everyone on the street thanks to these protocols: also dead."

We were sick. But also strangely healthy. That's what people didn't understand about street humor. There was a sanity to it. It helped us survive.

For days after that grim Zoom meeting, I listened to the EMS radio from home. Most of us did. It was the only way to get the real story, the truth, the one the media and officials weren't telling, by listening to the street. The streets were talking.

On ambulances racing all over the city, paramedics were responding to back-to-back cardiac arrests for mandated sixteen-hour tours and losing the majority of patients. EMTs were sent to cardiac arrests alone, without medics to back them up, unable to do anything beyond twenty minutes of chest compressions and respirations before they pronounced.

Even in the best-case scenario, where paramedics were available and able to get a return of spontaneous circulation on a patient, or ROSC, within twenty minutes on scene, they transported patients to hospitals only to find no crash team ready to take over and revive. Instead, harrowed nurses advised there were no beds for the incoming patient, or the hospital had a bed but didn't have a ventilator. Supplies were gone.

Day after day, units radioed dispatch with nothing but fatal outcomes: "83R," "83D." Eighty-three was the ten-code for dead. R stood for attempt at resuscitation—now only a twenty-minute attempt followed by a pronouncement—while D stood for dead on arrival. DOA.

The poor medics. Poor patients. Poor everyone.

Listening to all the 83Rs and -Ds pouring over the frequencies, I worried for my first responder friends on the street. Like Eyal, who'd recently lost his brother.

"How are you holding up?" I asked him. "I'm thinking of you and sending love and light and prayers your way."

"I'm trying," he said. "I need all the support I can get. I'm feeling under the weather now but I'm at work upstate, teaching a paramedic class."

"Stay healthy. Be gentle. You're going through so much. I want to become a medic when this nightmare is over. I feel helpless. It's all intubations."

"I'll support you in every possible way. You're my rock now."

"We're in this together."

"I'm working, so I can keep my mind off things. But I'm not psychologically stable."

"No one in the field is sane right now. Deep breaths. One day, one patient at a time. You're not alone and we'll get through this. Let me know if you need anything. I'm here."

And Gabriel, in Queens. He was so young. In his early twenties. This was a lot for a new paramedic—for any first responder—to see. And while he was out on the street responding to the unimaginable, his mother was still hospitalized with cancer. By the end of April he'd worked north of fifty cardiac arrests. And thanks to the relentlessness of COVID, new protocols, and the bleak situation at hospitals, he was losing all of his patients.

"The inevitable has started to happen," he said. "People we RMA'd days or weeks ago are now dying. Five arrests for my unit today, all 83D except one who we transported to Elmhurst. Another ALS unit, same story, five cardiac arrests. Every other call being dispatched in Queens today was a cardiac arrest. If this is that peak that they keep talking about, I shudder to think of how bad this week will be."

The questions from family members were tearing him apart.

"I have to tell six or seven families a day, every day, that we did everything we could. And when you say that, you know you're lying to them because of these protocols. We do twenty minutes of CPR and if we don't get a shockable rhythm, we pronounce. I have family members saying, 'Why aren't you doing anything?' It's so fucked up."

Fire Department data confirmed Gabriel's words. First responders found 2,192 DOAs in two weeks in April. These at-home deaths lacked a lab diagnosis for COVID and took place outside of a hospital setting, so they weren't being tallied in the city's numbers and daily reports about infections, though the vast majority of patients who arrested at home were suspected to be COVID-related.

These were the uncounted dead.

The numbers of COVID-related deaths were much greater than what officials were reporting. The "hospitalizations are down, numbers of deaths are declining" press conferences of COVID were "the air is clean, keep digging" motto the city sold after 9/11.

First responders were dying from COVID, too. A lot of them. In April, the Fire Department lost EMT Richard Seaberry, a Black sixty-three-year-old EMS veteran who responded to recovery efforts at the World Trade Center and who'd worked the COVID pandemic, assigned to Station 53 at Fort Totten, in Queens. And Idris Bey, a Black, sixty-year-old FDNY EMT and beloved department veteran who also worked recovery efforts after 9/11 and taught for nearly two decades at the EMS Bureau of Training.

At home, unable to sleep and riddled with despair, I remained horizontal on the couch, feasting on unbroken hours of *Queer Eye* on TV. I wanted only to watch real-life stories about a group of diverse strangers who entered the lives of people who were suffering and tried to help them by making small changes that resulted in enormous positive upliftment.

Mainlining the news wasn't an option, relaxation-wise. The news was a hive of pain. Nurses at hospitals that lacked PPE were out in the streets, protesting. Healthcare workers were being fired or reprimanded for speaking to journalists, telling the public how bad things were on the street, how what first responders were seeing differed from what officials were reporting.

One day, the Fire Department appeared to have shut down a beloved Instagram account run by a Haz-Tac EMT instructor that featured stories about EMTs. Instead, the department showcased videos of turnout-geared firefighters clapping for healthcare workers—nurses. The clapping firefighters became another pain point in the EMS community, when paramedics and EMTs were drowning in DOAs and falling sick.

Outrage hit FDNY's social media accounts. Angry EMS workers lit up the comments section.

"Now can we clap for all those who actually performed life-saving procedures before the firefighters got to the hospital?" a paramedic said.

An FDNY EMT wrote, "This city is great man. Have them all gathered together, and instead of utilizing the firefighters while the city is on fire, have them being damn cheerleaders. Stop posting these, it's embarrassing to the FDNY."

Another medic said, "Shouldn't they be going on runs? Why is this a thing now? Limit their exposure?"

When the department started posting photographs of its EMTs and paramedics on social media, they got similar blowback.

"Maybe the city can thank them by paying them a livable wage?" one commenter said.

"Visiting EMS stations is nice. Making sure they get paid and get benefits like other 911 agencies is even better. This department has failed EMS for so long."

Engulfed in turmoil, the FDNY chief of department tried to contain the crisis, posting a statement reminding the public the FDNY is "the best Fire Department in the world"—a phrase they say constantly—adding, "We are all part of one department."

I mean, if you have to say something that basic, it's untrue. It's like when you go on a date with a guy and he keeps saying, "I'm a nice guy." If he has to say it, he's not a nice guy. It would be like me walking around saying, "I'm tall." You know why I don't say that?

I don't have to. It's obvious.

"It pisses me off," an ICU nurse who started her career in EMS said, "to see all the firefighters lined up clapping in front of the hospitals. Why don't you stop clapping and go help your EMTs and medics do CPR in the field? You like doing medical jobs when you're not needed, so why stop now? They're making themselves look like morons."

Speaking of morons, I was in another fight with Larry over the gentleman in the White House, due to Trump's suggestion that ingesting bleach and isopropyl alcohol helped kill COVID. People did it. They drank bleach! They listened to this guy!

WARNING DURING COVID-19 OUTBREAK: DO NOT DRINK BLEACH, the Upstate New York Poison Center said in a statement released that spring. Poison control centers in red states were exploding with calls about people ingesting lethal cleaning products. "New numbers show calls to Texas poison control centers have skyrocketed since the pandemic began: everything from kids licking hand sanitizer to adults asking how much bleach they should drink to kill the coronavirus," an article on News4 San Antonio reported. Health experts eventually stepped in to straighten the record: "It's very dangerous. You can get chemical burns inside your body from drinking Clorox or disinfectants," a spokesperson for the Commission on State Emergency Communications said.

I could not believe this was now a thing. Because the world was not surreal and dark enough before.

America, my people. Babies with guns. Take your cowboy hats off and put on your thinking caps. Come on, now. The world is laughing at us. We were in the fourth season of the silliest, most dangerous reality show running on the televised planet.

So I took my rage out on Larry. Screaming at cops was one of my specialties. I was a subject-matter expert in police-directed rage. Larry had pneumonia and had by this time tested positive for COVID antibodies, and I was still out sick with whatever I had or didn't have according to that sham-and-cheese swab test.

First, I played nice with Larry. You can't just go in swinging. You have to warm up, say hello. We talked about how hideous the virus was, how we both felt like shit. He said the NYPD was encouraging all of its sick members to get tested. Scarily, some cops were still testing positive as long as two weeks after being symptom-free. One cop racked up seven negative tests and was so short of breath he was on oxygen. The eighth test finally returned a positive result. We agreed the rushed-to-market tests, unregulated and unreliable, were a joke. We spoke about how young people were having COVID-triggered strokes, how they were fine, they were fine, then they dropped dead. Blood clot. Brain aneurysm. Larry said in Israel and South Korea, they were seeing people who'd recovered from COVID get reinfected.

"I'd like to thank the people of China for making this happen," he said.

That was all I needed to hear to put my gloves on. Let's fight!

I said, "Europeans brought it here. I'd like to thank our jackass president for telling people to ingest bleach."

"He was being sarcastic."

"You know he wasn't being sarcastic. He was being a fucking moron, as usual. And he walked his idiocy back. People literally drank bleach."

"People are fucking dumb."

"He is the king of the people. King dumb."

Mid-April, my rage stocks split after I saw videos of anti-maskers demonstrating in Colorado. Far-right groups took to the streets to bitch and balk about lockdowns established in the interest of preserving human life. Many of their signs featured Confederate flags.

I saw red. I thought it was a metaphor, but then I actually saw red. I thought of what Dr. Fauci said: "I don't know how to explain to you why you should care about other people."

One day on the phone with Mike, he said, "This virus is going to go away on its own. In the summer, when it gets hot, it just will go away."

No. It would not.

I didn't allow myself to empty my rage on Mike. I couldn't do it. But I did say, softly and firmly, "It's not going to disappear on its own, Turtle. COVID infects people in warm climates, too. Look at what's happening in Brazil and India. They're fucked. And those are hot-climate countries."

Then I called Nick and yelped into his earbud. I told him I thought alt-right domestic terror was going to become a problem in the pandemic. Mass shooters were bored. Quarantined at home. They had no groups to kill. No targets.

Mass shootings were down nationwide for the first time in years, thanks to COVID disallowing gatherings. However, hospitals had scores of sick people inside them, and terrorists loved crowds. Hospitals were soft targets. They didn't have the security infrastructure to protect patients. The seventy-five-year-old hospital security guard who just had a hip replacement and now manned the ER entrance was not going to stop an active-shooter event. I'd been inside hospitals when things turned violent. One patient walked right up to a nurse and punched him in the face. No one stopped him. Hospitals were a shooter's dream.

In the intelligence world, we looked at historical patterns to predict future crimes. Predictive intelligence, it was called. And I could not forget, as an extremist analyst or domestic terror specialist or whatever people wanted to call me, that after the San Bernardino mass shooting in 2015, when murderers were still on the loose and a manhunt was underway, hospitals in that area of California received this emergency alert:

MASS SHOOTING. THIS IS NOT A DRILL.

As ERs scrambled to triple their trauma-room capacity to triage and treat incoming gunshot-wound patients, Loma Linda Hospital faced a second emergency:

BOMB THREAT.

People forgot that. Civilians forgot—not intel analysts, and certainly not terrorists. Secondary threats were *always* part of mass-casualty incidents. That bomb was meant for healthcare workers and shooting victims. To blow them up.

This was America.

This was how MCIs worked.

And now, I saw, during COVID-19, the alt-right crowd was gearing up, taking to the streets. On the phone I told Nick it made sense to me, seeing that the NYPD had established a domestic terror unit last December, they speak publicly about the issue. Use the media. News was policing, too. Nick was the one who taught me that. Sometimes, if we saw a threat gaining traction online, the cops or feds called reporters. Let them know they were noticing an emerging threat pattern. Then journalists would write about it, and scared-off terrorists would go mute and scatter. It worked. I saw it work. I was part of it. The news could easily be used to make wannabe murderers aware they were being watched.

It was no secret that Internet surveillance was part of policing. Loads of cops took a swing at developing tech products when they retired. For the most part their software was garbage. Big Billie who never left Long Island or wrote a Boolean search string in his life and spent his time on the job tasing people was not talented enough to violate your civil rights. He just couldn't do it, even when he tried his hardest. The military could, and the CIA, surveillance products coming out of Israel sure had that capacity, tech companies like Palantir and Recorded Future, which cost millions to operate, those players could get some interesting data on you if they thought you might shoot up a hospital or school. People critiqued online surveillance as a policing strategy, but let me tell you something, OK?

If you think the cops and feds are watching you more pervasively than the CEOs of Google, Facebook, Twitter, and Amazon, who have more data on you and your online behavior than the intelligence and security communities will ever see in their careers, combined, worldwide, more data on you than I have in the galaxy of freckles on my face—personal identifying details like your birthday, favorite pet, book, drink, your address, and names of your family members and children—private information you give them, *for free*, to tech CEOs who don't even need a warrant or dollar to possess the keys to your life, you are flat-out wrong.

And none of the Silicon Valley billionaires are doing shit to curb mass violence or stop disinformation. "Not my job," they tell Congress. To the contrary, they openly allow falsehoods and hate. They sell it to you. It's their product. And you bought it.

So, circling back to that phone call with Nick, using the media as policing could help prevent violence. I'd seen it work well.

"I think it's a great idea," he said. "You should pitch it to the NYPD."

"You really think so? Maybe we could do a co-authored op-ed. They do that, occasionally."

"It's a good idea, Lioness. I think you're right. It's going to be a problem. You should reach out to them. They owe you a favor for all the free intel you give them. Use my name."

Loved it. Loved using his name. I crafted an e-mail to the relevant people at the NYPD and pitched the idea of an op-ed about alt-right extremism, domestic terror, and COVID-19. One of my contacts replied immediately. Great hearing from me, as always. Interesting idea. Said he'd approach the relevant chief.

I thanked him and waited. I waited a day. Two days. Two weeks. Never heard back. The relevant chief, I learned, was hospitalized with COVID.

As for the news, whenever I turned on the TV and listened to officials speak about the state of COVID, I felt physically sick to my stomach. I came from the "no clean politicians" school of thought. They all fatigued me. My wrath toward reigning officials was federal, state, and local. It was democratic in that way.

"Good news," the governor told the public in his press conference in mid-April, using bar charts to show that what we were doing in New York—social distancing, staying home—was working. "Hospitalizations and ICU admissions are dropping."

Sure were. Because guess what else was dropping? People were dropping dead in the street. What about the heartbreaking CPR protocols and the DOAs and uncounted dead who didn't get COVID tested, most of whom were poor and elderly, Black and brown? We were meant to take declining hospital rates and the allegedly flattening curve as an encouraging sign? How so?

All I could think of was that saying, "The first casualty of war is the truth." Listening to officials, you'd think things were going well on the street.

Things were not going well. It was worse than September 11. It wasn't a hot zone. It was a war zone.

Hospitalizations were down because people were dying in the field. It was all falling on the backs of medical first responders. On medics like Gabriel.

"I appreciate you reaching out," he told me one evening. "You're the EMS mother I never knew I needed. We first responders are our own grief counselors right now."

Grief counselors. Surrogate mothers. Freelance rescuers for friends and family. Doctors, too. We were doctors now.

In an effort avoid hospitals, many of us first responders in New York City gave up on the faltering healthcare system and took matters into our own hands, relying on one another for life-or-death guidance not only for ourselves, but for our loved ones. With the shortage of first responders and crushing influx of calls, everyone gave themselves a promotion in the medical field.

"Do you know anyone who could help me get a bag of fluids and IV gear?" Tommy asked me one April evening.

"What for? Are you a paramedic now?"

He said no, but he did give plenty of IVs when he was in the Army and went through the combat lifesaver course. His girlfriend's father, a sixty-five-year-old doctor, was sick with COVID and in bad shape. He hadn't eaten in days and his fever was high and unbroken.

"I got him an O2 tank and nasal canula," Tommy said, noting his oxygen saturation was at 91 percent. We agreed he merited hospitalization while knowing ERs were for worst-case scenarios only. Doctors were still releasing patients who were critically ill but weren't teetering on the brink of death. And even then, beds and ventilators were waning. I heard from Chad, who worked for a hospital and was now lending an extra hand in various ERs as an EMT, that one hospital in Manhattan ran out of walled oxygen inlets and was burning through small tanks.

A day or two later I sent Tommy a screenshot of the new EMS Viral Pandemic Triage Protocol for screening coronavirus patients, so he knew how to make decisions for the next person in his life who fell sick, and the next person, and the next after that. He thanked me and said his girlfriend's father was now in the hospital. He hadn't been able to break the fever. In addition to COVID, his chest X-ray showed pneumonia.

I worried for everyone. Lexi was still out sick, too.

"I'm feeling better from the Rona but now I'm having serious GI issues," she said. "I've been vomiting all day." She'd been out nearly two weeks with coronavirus, and her doctor had put her on antibiotics. "I think maybe it's the Z-Pak."

Zithromax (azithromycin), or Z-Pak, was an antibiotic used to treat bacterial infections.

I reached out to Mike in Vegas. Using him as my personal telemetry line, I asked Dr. Mike for advice. Aching to help, he was quick to deliver.

"She needs to eat something with the medication and take Zofran about half hour to an hour before taking it. Also clear liquid diet. Small frequent sips. Ice pops are great for this. Likely not related to Z-Pak, although azithromycin is an erythromycin base that does bother some people's stomachs."

I gave Lexi the news.

"Oh, shit," she said. "It's not related to Z-Pak? I just assumed. And yes, my doctor also gave me Zofran. Ice pops!"

"Ice pops!" I said. "Pop it, bitch!"

"Laughing my ass off. Hopefully it goes away."

"I hope so, ice-pop goddess."

"I love it," Lexi said. "Another nickname."

"We are the Rona queens."

Every mass-casualty incident, MCI, had its own unique anatomy. Because of my job, I was deeply acquainted with the structure of mass shootings. Disasters varied, but the arc stayed the same, more or less, with almost every mass-casualty incident. It was a five-part horror story. 1) Pre-attack; 2) attack; 3) secondary attack; 4) aftermath; 5) survivor and first responder suicides.

It was impossible for me to forget the fifth leg of every MCI. Sergeant Terrance Yeakey, who saved four people during the Oklahoma bombing, committed suicide after the event, at thirty years old. The officer who was with him and saved two women trapped on a ledge wound up with a drug conviction for felony-weight cocaine possession.

Paramedic Robert O'Donnell, who rescued baby Jessica from a well while all of America watched on TV, was given White House salutes and movie rights. Seven years later, he put a shotgun to his head and blew his heroic brains out. He was thirty-seven years old.

As for the COVID pandemic, in Europe suicides of healthcare workers had commenced. End of March, a thirty-four-year-old ICU nurse who worked in a hospital near Milan learned she'd been infected with COVID and committed suicide. In the UK, a nurse in her twenties who treated COVID patients at King's College Hospital in London took her own life.

In New York, COVID was already killing frontliners, with two suicides in April and more to come. John Mondello, a twenty-three-year-old new FDNY EMT based in the Bronx—which had one of the busiest 911 call volumes in the city—went straight from the FDNY academy to working the coronavirus pandemic. He killed himself after three months on the job. FDNY EMS Lieutenant Matthew Keene, who also worked in the Bronx, shot himself in the head in June. FDNY EMT Brandon Dorsa committed suicide in July. Doctors hurt, too. Dr. Lorna M. Breen, a forty-nine-year-old ER doctor who worked at New York-Presbyterian Allen Hospital, which got clobbered by COVID, also took her own life. "She tried to do her job, and it killed her," Dr. Breen's father said in an April 27, 2020, article in *The New York Times*.

She tried to do her job. And it killed her.

One day I reached out to the New York City Trauma Recovery Network, a local team of the EMDR Humanitarian Assistance Program that provided pro bono EMDR therapy to first responders and healthcare professionals who've experienced critical incidents. I didn't have high hopes that the social workers affiliated with the organization would respond in a timely manner, as I reached out at the height of the pandemic.

Contrarily, a woman named Linda replied immediately. "We are happy to help and have a team ready and waiting for all of you on the front line," she told me. "We served EMTs, FDNY, police, and other first responders after 9/11."

I sent Linda's e-mail to Chief Beck, to let him know we had help available. "This seems like a great resource," he said.

* * *

One April day, Nick's prediction that my crisis business would surge, that I'd become "a fucking funeral director," came true. A colleague looped me into a pandemic-related MCI. A nursing home with a massive double-digital loss of life.

COVID was fatal for the elderly. Across the country, officials had made some ghastly fumbles at the start of the pandemic, encouraging hospitals to release COVID patients back to nursing homes. Crisis contracts got signed fast. Immediately I engaged to help manage a nursing home with the aftermath. For a week I was on the phone with the embattled client, sometimes from bed, since I was still sick. It was a sad, difficult case, made more difficult by the fact that I'd been on the street and was still unwell. But it was money, and at this point all income was good income. I wanted only to listen and assist. The crisis case meant I could keep my beloved employee, which meant a lot to me.

My sweet nonessential friends were terrified for me now, their healthcare hero. Every time my phone chimed, I manufactured terrific amounts of fury at the assault by bottomless amounts of well-meaning worry. In the pandemic I developed a greater understanding of what my war veteran buddies meant when they talked about dying in the loneliness gap of the civilian/military divide. I wanted to speak only to first responders. I felt besieged and grew even more resentful. How was that possible?

Friends and strangers at various media outlets kept texting and calling day and night. News publications put notices online that they were looking for stories from "healthcare workers," "healthcare heroes," "first responders." We could talk to them in confidence, they said. We could go public if we wanted. Be featured. Have our names in the paper. Our pictures. Everyone working on the street was getting endless calls from journalists and civilian friends.

I bitched to Tommy.

"Do you get a lot of texts from your non-uniform friends constantly asking you about what's happening on the street?"

"Yes."

"I'm so tired of these questions. I'm not a frontline reporter. Read the fucking news."

"I marvel at the lack of understanding."

"You're so funny. I love you. Maybe one day I'll do a job in the Bronx, and you can clap for me. The clapping firefighter situation has to stop."

"I know," Tommy said.

At Park Slope everyone was personally touched by COVID, losing family members. I worried my mother was next. I couldn't sleep. I went days without rest. When I did manage to close my eyes for a nap, I had a nightmare that I walked into a store and saw my mom lying dead in the aisle.

Bakersfield was not yet greatly impacted by COVID, so my mom's behavior was somewhat loosey-goosy for my taste. She only left the house for essentials, she said. Then she admitted she ran errands to get birdseed, because she ran out, and said my stepfather was golfing. I thought my head was going to explode.

It was all I could think about when we got off the phone. My stepfather golfing, then coming home to my elderly mother. If he gave it to her and she died. . . . Where was her self-regard when it came to shielding herself from the virus? Where was his?

"They don't get it," I told my EMDR therapist one weepy session. "They're just going on with their lives as if people aren't dropping dead. I'm terrified my mom will get sick and wind up on a ventilator. I can't stop thinking about it."

"There's a name for the kind of grief you're experiencing," my therapist said. "Would it be helpful to know that?"

"Yes."

She sent me a March 23, 2020, article to read from the *Harvard Business Review* titled THAT DISCOMFORT YOU'RE FEELING IS GRIEF. I devoured the piece, which talked about "anticipatory grief," the feeling one gets when the future is uncertain. This type of grief sets in when someone gets a dire diagnosis, or the thought arises that you'll lose a parent one day—quite possibly soon. It helped to read that. To name what I was feeling.

What everyone was feeling.

"You're living on cortisol," Mike said one night. "The harsh, evil kind of stress I used to live on as an ER doctor." I cried and told him about the number of dead at the nursing home, and on the street. It felt so good to let it out.

"No one is in this crisis more than you are," Mike said. "Your EMT friends go and do the awful work of trying to save COVID patients on the trucks, and then they go home depressed and defeated because so few of their patients are surviving. You go home from all that you see on the street, and then you work a mass-casualty incident from COVID for your job. It's too much."

It was too much. I was afraid I wasn't going to survive.

One evening I rang Pat's friend Paul, also my friend, and asked him for advice about what to do with my in-constant-contact civilian friends.

"What did Pat do, when he was working a bad fire?" I asked him.

"Well, when Pat was alive, cell phones weren't a thing. So he didn't have to deal with what you're dealing with. We had landlines back then. You called him, and if he wasn't there, you left a message. But you're going through this with a cell phone, so people can reach you all the time."

"I don't want to be reached," I told Paul. "I don't know how to make it stop. I can't turn off my phone, because first responders are texting and calling me, too. And I need to talk to them and hear what's happening on the street, because it keeps changing. But this situation with my friends reaching out day and night isn't working for me. What would Pat do?"

"After the Watts Street fire," Paul told me, "when John Drennan got burned, Pat dropped off the face of the earth. No one heard from him for weeks. He didn't return calls and he didn't answer his phone. We all knew where he was, at John's bedside, up at Cornell's burn unit. So that's what Pat did, he dropped off the earth."

"I need to drop off the earth. I don't know how to do it with a cell phone."

"Your friends don't understand what you're going through, honey. You're at war, and they're bored at home. I felt the same way when I got home from Vietnam. People spit on me. Why don't you block the people who keep texting you? Just block them for now, and you can unblock them when you feel better."

"When will that be?"

I felt hugely relieved after speaking with Paul. He got it. He understood. I went through my contact list and blocked about fifty people. For the first time since the pandemic hit, my phone was quiet. At last, I could relax and watch *Queer Eye* in peace.

* * *

"Um, sis?" Felice said when she called a few days later.

"Yes?"

"I keep getting phone calls from our friends, saying they've been texting and calling you, and their messages aren't going through. Clara called. Natalie called. They're worried about you, so now they're calling me."

"I blocked everyone. This is perfect, that they're calling you now. This is wonderful."

"It is *not* wonderful," Felice said. "I think people are calling to talk to me, and they say hey, how's it going, then they're like, 'How's Jen? Is she OK? She's not returning my calls.'"

"You're my best friend," I said. "This is why you're my sister. You're also my emergency contact in the event of a disaster, by the way, so you're really doing your job right now."

"When will it end? I feel like your secretary."

"But you're not my secretary. You're the most important person in my life. Have I told you that lately? How much I love you?"

"Fine. I'll do it—for now. But I hope this ends soon."

Such a best friend.

After being home for two weeks, I was healthy enough to go back on the ambulance. So was Nathan. FDNY would be dispatching us on the 911 system now.

Can you believe it? I said to Pat one night in my prayers. *I didn't join FDNY. And yet I'll be working for your beloved Fire Department after all.*

16

LIFE ON MARS

Easter, Nathan and I decided. The day of Jesus's resurrection and greatest comeback. That's when we'd return to the ambulance. Seemed appropriate.

It was our first slated tour after being out sick with what we presumed was COVID. Nathan, untested, still couldn't smell or taste a thing. He had a lingering cough and exhaustion but was otherwise fine. I was still saddled with fatigue, not sleeping more than two or three hours a night thanks to my racing mind, but I was eager to get back on the ambulance.

Calls to the 911 system had reportedly plunged since we'd been off the street. On Easter, the Fire Department received 3,932 calls for people requesting ambulances, down from 6,527 calls on March 30, 2020. What did that mean? Why weren't people calling 911 anymore? Were they too afraid to go to the hospital, and get COVID? Or had all the people infected with the virus already died? I was confused.

COVID had scorched the city's poorest neighborhoods in the Bronx, Brooklyn, and Queens. Between March 1 and April 12, 2020, the Rockaways—where the poverty rate neared 20 percent, and 60 percent of the population identified as Black or Hispanic—reported 204 cardiac calls and 151 deaths. The year before, by comparison, the totals were 76 cardiac calls and 35 deaths. Brooklyn's East New York, where my EMT school was located, the poverty rate was around 25 percent, over 90 percent of the population identified as Black or Hispanic, and there were 168 cardiac calls and 114 deaths in 2020, compared to 79 cardiac calls and 34 deaths the year before.

What for some were just charts and numbers for us were human beings. Patients. People with stories. Families. Lives. And their lives were cut short not just by COVID, but also by the total failure of our healthcare system and underlying inequities. In the hospitals, ER nurses, doctors, and ICU nurses tasked with caring for vented patients got decimated.

"How's the ICU?" I asked a nurse friend who worked at one of the safety-net hospitals in Brooklyn. Safety-net hospitals served the city's most vulnerable patients, New Yorkers with low incomes, no insurance, or covered by Medicaid. These hospitals got pummeled during the COVID outbreak, which left them with scant resources and PPE.

"Nothing new," my friend said. "Everyone has COVID. Everyone is dying."

She described how fast the virus accelerated. How people went from talking to being intubated quickly. No agency nurses had been sent to her hospital to assist with the pandemic. The hospital had no temp nurses, nor had it received help from FEMA. It had the same ICU nursing staff, a third of them were out sick, and they opened twelve more ICU beds. Their solution was to put two nurses in charge of covering these dozen beds, which should have been covered by a minimum of six nurses. Like EMTs and paramedics, they received no hazard pay.

"All the ICUs are fucked," she said. "But my hospital is using this as a media opportunity. They're soliciting reporters. They brand themselves as a safety-net hospital that serves people coming out of the projects. But they provide shitty care. They're doing people a disservice. People could go to another hospital and get better care."

What's more, she said, medications and treatments for COVID patients changed constantly. It was all compassionate use, since no one knew what the virus was truly doing to people. "We just throw shit at the wall," she said. "No one is tracking outcomes, so we don't really know what works." Five of the safety-net hospital's staff members had died.

As for me and Nathan, our plan to ride Easter disintegrated the night before our scheduled shift. He called to say he had to leave town unexpectedly and was flying to California. The next morning he sent me a photo from the airport of the empty security line at JFK. He said he was wearing his grody N95 from our last tour and that everyone at the airport was on edge. He asked if I'd found a partner to replace him. I hadn't yet.

"Just take care of yourself. The Rona will be here when you get back, and I'm ready to ride with you as soon as you return."

"Yes, I'm looking forward to getting back on the bus."

"Same."

That week my apartment building got robbed—again. It wasn't a surprise. Management had fired Pedro, our "concierge." Packages got delivered and sat in the lobby for days. I ran into our super, Gilberto, and he told me Pedro was fine, he was managing.

"Do you remember him?" he then asked, getting his phone out and showing me a photograph of an older Hispanic guy.

"Yeah, I think so. Is that our old super?"

"Yes. He's a good friend of mine. He's dead."

COVID. These were half my conversations as of late. Nearly everyone in the city knew someone who'd died. All the chit-chat had trapdoors that dropped into basements stacked with corpses. Did I know so-and-so? Yes. Well, they're dead. Again and again, this was the ambient conversation in New York.

I was supposed to hang out with Ellery one afternoon and catch up, but we kept canceling on each other.

"Did you hear we got robbed again?" I asked him. "Someone came into the building and opened all the boxes in the lobby and took stuff. I don't think I had anything down there but if you have packages, get them quick."

Ellery said, "You clearly didn't see my Facebook post."

"I'm not on Facebook. What did you say?"

He sent me what he'd written: "Building theft. Woke up at 6 A.M. to a loud tearing sound coming from the lobby. Initially thought it might be the trash/recycle people, but the sound was too violent. I made it out of bed and opened the door to find someone in a mask and hoodie tearing through the uncollected delivery boxes. I yelled at them and they ran out the front door.

"Nearly every package is torn through, the contents taken out. He was ripping at the large box in the mail room when I opened the door. It's a mess! I sent a ticket but not sure what else to do. The building office is presently closed for holidays. The police are clearly overburdened right now, and this kind of theft is on the rise, so I doubt they will even come out.

"If you are away, there is no concierge, no one to collect your packages, so please don't continue ordering things unless you've made arrangements with someone in the building to collect and store them for you."

I sent Ellery three red hearts. "This is powerful. You're a Facebook activist!"

"It was scary as shit!"

"I bet! That sounds terrifying!"

We talked about crime being up on our block, every block. I told Ellery that I went to move my car one night then got an alert on Citizen, a location-based mobile app that monitored 911 communications and sent users alerts about nearby emergencies, that someone on our street was assaulting someone with a screwdriver, so I left my car and waited until morning. Two days prior to our conversation there was a man with a knife on our block. It was dicey.

Ellery replied with a frowny-faced, goateed, bespectacled emoji.

"By the way, do you think your COVID test was a false negative?" he asked me.

"Yes."

"I do too."

Since my test, I'd talked to a few nurses and EMTs and read one news report that posited 30 percent of swab tests were returning false negatives. But everyone on the street believed I had it. I wanted to get a serology test. None were available yet for first responders.

After a few days I scrounged together a few partners to ride on the ambulance with me. Driving to base, I was nervous to work. Even with lower 911 call volumes, I expected we'd be busy now that the Fire Department was dispatching us on MARS.

I worked one mid-April night with a personable EMT named Mark who preferred to drive the truck rather than tech. Fine by me. This EMT/sheriff has taken enough mirrors off cars.

The whole tour, four o'clock to midnight, we worked one job. And it was garbage. A frazzled lady called for an ambulance for an injury minor. When we arrived in her apartment, she had a loose flap of skin on her index finger. That was a bit too minor. We gave her a Band-Aid and said farewell.

Another Park Slope unit worked an eight-hour tour and responded to zero jobs. People were afraid to go to the hospital, it seemed. They'd seen the city's numbers. And those numbers were modest compared to the death toll we saw on the street.

It wasn't just us vollies who had dead tours. Rescuers on FDNY, hospital, and private ambulance trucks were doing one or two jobs a shift. Why was that? EMS dispatchers were sending the few jobs that came through to FEMA units.

We knew they were FEMA ambulances getting sent to jobs because they had three-digit unit numbers we'd never heard: 800 Nora, 800 Charlie, 830 David. Because they were from out of town, and didn't know the city, dispatchers had to spell out the street names when they were sent to job locations, which we locals found amusing.

"830 King you're going to Flatbush Avenue for the sick fever cough. F-L-A-T-B-U-S-H."

The thinking on the street was that since the government had called FEMA to save us, now that they were here—being dispatched from multiple staging units, including, as I mentioned, the Bronx Zoo—the city had to use them. At hospitals, ER bays were crammed with ambulances from out of town.

FEMA paid their rescuers better than New York City. Their EMTs and paramedics were compensated for 24/7 shifts at the rate of 1.25 their regular pay, plus overtime. They were supposed to be compensated for that, at least.

In June 2020, out-of-state EMTs and paramedics who worked the COVID peak in New York City sued FEMA subcontractor Ambulnz after the company paid its EMTs less than other FEMA first responders. When they weren't on the ambulance, these rescuers had to stay in their hotels and abstain from alcohol and sex, and were required to keep their emergency-responder radios with them at all times, which blared and kept them up all night. When the peak was over and they returned to their home states, Ambulnz asked them to sign release agreements relinquishing their right to recover unpaid wages.

So FEMA was still here for now, but they weren't exactly thriving in terms of how the government treated them, either.

But not all was bleak.

Soon, something special began to bubble from within the crisis. First responders from all over the world—paramedics in Paris, firefighters in

California—total strangers and people I barely knew, medical professionals of all types—began reaching out on social media, wanting to know what it was like on the streets in New York City, voicing their support and alliance, asking if there was anything they could do, wanting to know how we were holding up in the hot zone.

By now I was so slaphappy from lack of sleep and death that every time I heard that phrase, "hot zone," I fell over laughing. It sounded like a poorly written sentence in a romance novel. "Come closer, darling. Step into my hot zone."

Across the world we all said the same thing, give or take. People died en masse. In the street. Everyone arrested. DOA. Every government failed. In some COVID-ransacked European countries—Italy, France—things were now getting quieter on the street. But first responders across the globe were bracing for another flare-up when lockdowns lifted. Another wave of COVID patients in winter, when flu season began. On Instagram, I had a little chat with a firefighter named Christopher who worked in Paris.

"In France, it's calmed down a bit," he said. "For a long time we've been confined, since March. When the city opens in May, it's going to be a disaster."

"Disaster," I agreed.

One April night I worked another MARS tour with Friedland, a blond-haired, glasses-wearing EMT, the one who was a two-donut-at-a-time Sweets in the Street customer. He was in paramedic school at night. On the ambulance, he passed time reading books on his Kindle. At one point, he managed to find a radio station that played only Led Zeppelin, which was all we listened to for hours.

"Why do you think it's so slow out here?" I asked him.

He turned to me and said, with deadpan frankness, "The 911 call volume is low because the virus has finally accomplished what FDNY and EMS has been trying to communicate to people for years: Don't call fucking 911 unless you're dying."

Made sense.

Around five o'clock, the CAD number for jobs was at 2,150—a slow night. Half of what New York City usually fielded by way of 911 calls pre-COVID. I'd never seen the street this quiet.

We were in what the Fire Department called a "multi-year low." At some point, Friedland called MARS to do a radio check. Checking to see that a dispatcher could hear us was his sly way of making sure the dispatcher remembered we existed, and hadn't forgotten us, which happened sometimes.

"93 King radio check," he said.

"93 King five by five, loud and clear."

Bored, a few of us local EMTs from various departments shared videos with one another of FEMA ambulances crashing and rolling over. Apparently, several out-of-town units had crashed since they'd arrived in the Big Apple. One Brooklyn first responder's theory was that they didn't know how to drive the trucks in New York City. Some of them blew through red lights and busy intersections as if they were in Nebraska.

New York City was not Nebraska. Drivers here didn't care if you were in an ambulance on the way to save a life. They didn't yield or stop. And bikers—don't get me started on bikers. I could write a paper about vigilante-attituded bikers' disobedience of basic driving rules that resulted in seeing them get squished like bugs on windshields by cars. Helmets only did so much.

As jobless hours on MARS passed, some duty officers at Park Slope felt sorry for us, sitting on the ambulance for eight hours, rotting. It was an awful feeling, since the public was lauding us as healthcare heroes. One night a guy walked by the ambulance and saluted us.

I felt ridiculous. I didn't deserve a salute. I wasn't doing anything to help, not right now. I talked to military friends who said what people really didn't understand about war was how fucking boring it was. I guessed the same was true for first responders at this time.

There we were, Friedland and I, sitting on the ambulance, bored out of our minds with FEMA running in circles around us. Just when I'd gotten used to things calming down on the street, with fewer people calling 911 for COVID-related complaints, I got my first gunshot-wound patient.

If cardiac arrests were the meat and potatoes of a first responder's life, shootings were the caviar.

Pre-COVID, very few shootings came over in our coverage area. Tonight was different. Out of the blue, Friedland and I got dispatched to an emergency in the projects.

Friedland put his Kindle away and drove toward the job. That's when PD came flying past us, lights-and-sirens, RMP after RMP blazing to the same place we were heading, apparently. My heart started racing.

We arrived on scene with a flock of cops. Friedland hopped off the ambulance and said, "What happened?"

"Guy got shot," one of the cops said.

My first shooting! So exciting!

I grabbed the tech bag and Friedland, the stair chair. The stair chair? I thought. For a shooting? Why he didn't grab the stretcher I had no idea, except to say that everything was happening fast, it was an active crime scene, and we were so full of adrenaline we made the best decisions we could. One time, I accidentally grabbed the stair chair instead of the stretcher for an arrest that turned out to be a DOA. "Nice stair chair for the arrest," an EMT said. I thanked her and asked her if she wanted a ride, since the DOA had better options.

Tonight, Friedland and I trotted to onto scene and found a lean, Black, teenaged boy sitting on the steps. He was hunched over, his white T-shirt pinked by blood. A bullet had pierced his upper right arm, which had a tourniquet just below his shoulder.

"Who put the tourniquet on?" I asked the bald white housing cop standing beside him.

"I did," he said.

"Time?"

He gave me the time and I jotted it down on the little fluid-proof notepad I kept in my leg pocket. In EMT school they told us to stick a piece of tape on the patient's forehead and write the time he or she was tourniqueted, but I couldn't bring myself to stick tape on the patient's forehead. With bleeding controlled, there wasn't much for us to do for the shooting victim aside from load and go and give him some oxygen en route to the hospital.

As we packaged him up in a sheet a rowdy crowd gathered and swarmed the scene. Kids, mainly. "Who shot you?" they wanted to know. "Hey, man, who shot you, just tell us and we'll take care of it." The patient's mother stood by her son, crying, grabbing at the sheet. We had to tell her she couldn't come with us to the hospital because of COVID, since no visitors were allowed, which made a wail come flaming out of her mouth. I felt so sorry for her. This was my first experience managing a bereaved family member during COVID. But not my last.

It took several cops to control the crowd. They struggled to clear a path for us to get to the ambulance. The thought crossed my mind that seeing that no one knew who or where the shooter was, I could easily be shot dead. It wasn't a lingering fear, just a passing thought. I could probably get shot right now.

As for the crowd, no one was wearing masks or social distancing, that's for fucking sure. Bystanders had taken out their phones and were recording videos of us, as usual. I knew I would wind up on Citizen. It wouldn't be my first rodeo. On the street, sometimes Citizen alerts beat our dispatchers. The people had phones, after all. And when people recorded us, those videos wound up on Citizen. By this point, I'd been a shining star on the app many times. I considered myself somewhat of a Citizen starlet.

Finally, we got through the crowd and loaded the patient onto our bus. The bald housing cop rode along with us. This was his shooting victim before he became our GSW. Gunshot wound.

On the ambulance, Friedland took vitals and cut off the patient's shirt in search of an exit wound, then called a note to the nearest trauma-receiving ER to tell them we were coming through. Friedland worked fast. I blinked, and he had the patient's vitals. EMTs who'd been on the street for a long time were mind-blowingly speedy. I was impressed.

I was also underwhelmed by the medical trauma. The gunshot wound was elegant. A pierced dark hole with a little spurt of blood. Nothing compared to that uncontrolled bleeder Lexi and I'd had. The patient complained of thirst. He kept asking me for water, which was a bad sign. It meant he'd lost a lot of fluid volume. The least I could do was give him a hit of O2.

I reached in the tech bag to get out the oxygen tank, but it was stuck to the Velcro sleeve we kept it in so it wouldn't fly loose. When I rode with Nina, she always made sure to take the tank out of the Velcro sleeve or at least unbuckle the straps when it was resting in the bag. I thought it was a quaint little thing she did when she prepped the tech bag. But no.

I realized how crucial her minuscule gesture was when I struggled to get the oxygen free of the Velcro. It made no sense to unfasten the oxygen from the Velcro tank that secured it to the tech bag from a safety perspective, since it could easily become a missile. But it made equally no sense, I realized on the truck, to have the oxygen secured so stickily that it was an epic struggle to wrest it free when a patient was critical and time, let's just say, was of the essence. Our back doors were open, and the crowd was closing in. Everyone was watching me go to battle with the oxygen. I felt dumb. What else was new? Just another night in clown town. Finally, Friedland saved me and ripped it out of the bag in one strongman gesture, bless his soul.

The housing cop kept trying to get information from the patient about who shot him. But the guy didn't want to talk. He didn't want to be a rat. No one wanted to be a rat.

Transport to the hospital was butter. The patient didn't enjoy it much, but he was stable. He complained of thirst the whole time and called me a bitch for not giving him water. I didn't have any water to offer. And, like I said, he wasn't thirsty, he was bleeding internally, possibly bleeding to death, which I didn't feel was appropriate to point out.

Friedland hadn't found an exit wound, and as he drove fast and smoothly to the ER, I wondered if our patient would survive. Fifty percent chance, I guessed. That tourniquet had been applied fast, so that was good. But gunshot wounds to upper arms or thighs were often fatal, since they were near important arteries. Brachial and femoral.

If a bullet graced one of those gushers, the patient would bleed out within minutes. When bullets entered the body, they whizzed around and caused lacerations and crushing wounds, puncturing tissue and bone, often creating cavities that could be up to thirty times wider than their track. Cavitation damaged tissue, organs, and bones from shock waves. If bone greeted the bullet, it often stopped it in its path. So it was impossible to see from the outside how bad the damage actually was.

When we got to the ER and pulled out the stretcher, the housing cop complimented Friedland on his graceful driving. He was right. Nathan should take a driving lesson from Friedland—as should I. We rushed the patient inside and Friedland bounded into the trauma room and shouted out the information the professionals needed to proceed. "We have a 19-year-old male, gunshot wound to the upper right arm, tourniquet applied at 22:31, no exit wound found, pulse 78, BP 110/78, respirations 18 per minute."

I didn't know what else he said. I wasn't paying that much attention. "Words, words, words," as Hamlet said.

Doctors and nurses took over, transferring the patient onto an exam table, stripping him, and getting up to whatever they got up to with gunshot victims. They found the exit wound below his elbow, which the bullet had shattered. That must hurt. We rolled the stretcher into the hallway, and Friedland peeled off the bloody sheets and went searching for a fresh set.

A cloud of languor hung over me.

The ER nurses seemed by the bounce in their steps, grateful to have received our medical present. Something other than a sick, dying COVID patient who needed a vent. One of them came up to me and said, "Thanks for bringing this one in."

I went up to the housing cop standing outside the trauma room with his back against the wall. For crimes, cops had to stay at the hospital for hours, sometimes all night. He had to find out who shot the guy. That was his task, and one I didn't envy.

"Good job with the tourniquet. You saved that guy's life."

"Do you really think so?"

"Yeah, definitely. He would have bled out on scene."

"Thank you for telling me that."

It seemed like he'd never received a compliment in his life.

"When this is all over," I said, "and they have Rona Medal Day, you're going to get medal for that save."

He took me seriously. "Will there really be a medal day?"

"No, sweetheart. There won't be any medals at the end of this, if any of us are still alive."

When I got home that night I showered and climbed in bed and saw that our job had indeed wound up on Citizen. There we were, on video at the shooting. One Citizen user noted the huge crowd and wrote, "Ya'll are supposed to be social distancing."

I was awake all night, elated I'd saved a life. Well, Friedland and the housing cop did most (all) of the saving. But at least I hadn't gotten in their way or created a problem for them. I'd been mildly helpful. I gave myself a B–.

The next day everyone at Park Slope sent me congratulatory texts and messages. It was the best night on the street I'd had since the pandemic kicked off. Larry texted that afternoon and told me places were now doing serology tests.

"Get one," he said. "They're more accurate than the swab."

I doubted that. But I told him I would. It felt good, to know he was out there, looking after me. Trying to help.

But of course the good feeling didn't last. That appetizer of despair I'd tasted before, over the shooting victim's mother not being able to come to the hospital with us—that was about to become a five-course meal.

A week later, on MARS, Friedland and I got dispatched to a sick patient, a Russian man in his eighties who lived with his son at home. When we got inside the apartment and found the patient lying in bed, he was contracted and shivering, so short of breath he could barely speak. A sour odor rose from his bed. While I took his vitals his son explained that his father had pneumonia. He was also a smoker. And had diabetes. And a history of heart disease.

"He hasn't been outside at all," the son said. "I don't want him to catch COVID because of his medical history and age, so I've been really careful. I only go outside for groceries, and I always change my clothes and wash my hands when I come home."

The patient was warm to the touch, and his blood sugar level was worrisome, over two hundred. Sugar that high could damage to the body, cause blindness and strokes, kidney failure and heart attacks. When Friedland saw the patient's glucose level, he told the son we had to take his father to the hospital and explained why.

The son's face drained of color. He had a tormented look in his eyes and seemed afraid and near tears. I could tell he was trying to understand what to do and reckoning with the fact that he had no choices. I could almost feel his anguish in my chest, a pressurized heartache that said, "Imagine yourself in my shoes."

When he spoke his voice broke. "I understand. If he needs to go, then I need you to take him. He's been coughing like crazy for days. Our thermometer says he doesn't have a fever but I'm not sure it's working right."

This was the worst part of the virus I'd experienced by far, standing with this man in the throes of loss. Being the one to strain him further, taking away his father, the person he'd broken his back to protect. That was the thing about being a first responder during COVID. We had to break the families' hearts. Go into their homes and brutalize them by removing their loved ones.

Friedland and I walked to the bed, sat the patient up gently, and collected his belongings. We helped him into his robe and got some socks and slippers on his pale, hairless feet. He was so underweight Friedland

and I lifted him onto the stretcher as if he were a pillowcase of bones. We bundled him up in a blanket; his teeth were clattering, and his son set a phone in his father's lap.

"Let's get his cell phone charger, too," I said.

A day or two before, Robert reminded me to have patients take their chargers with them to the hospital. Across the country, COVID patients sent to ERs alone were losing communication with their families because their phone batteries died in the hospital, and ICUs lacked chargers, which were now a life-sustaining piece of equipment in terms of saying final words.

Robert's uncle, a Navy veteran and pediatrician, had been on a ventilator for two weeks in isolation and not even his wife could visit, but hearing familiar voices from his family telling him to keep fighting kept him alive. Robert was so moved by his uncle's situation that he and his family made it their mission to try to make sure patients in ICUs didn't die alone, cut off from their families, because of something as small as a cell phone charger. They organized a GoFundMe campaign that raised over $41,000 to purchase chargers for isolated COVID patients.

When the son returned to the room with the charger, he started to put on his coat, and looked around the room for his shoes. He was standing there in the bedroom with his eyes darting all around, living in some world we no longer inhabited, where he got to accompany his father to the ER. This just about killed me.

"I'm so sorry, sir," I said. "But you can't come to the hospital with us. They won't allow any visitors right now."

The son looked at me with a pained expression, and I saw the world's sorrow slash his face. "I knew that," he said. "Right, I heard that. I guess I just. I didn't fully understand until. I really can't come with him? He's my dad."

I almost lost it.

What a crown of despair this was when I had to tell families their worst nightmare was coming true, we were taking their parents to the hospital without them, almost certainly to die.

"I'm so sorry. I wish we could bring you with us, but we can't."

He nodded. Then he led us outside the apartment and came with us into the elevator. We descended and went outside. The air was cool and fresh, the building surrounded by lush flowering plants. The air smelled so good. We loaded the patient into the ambulance and the son squeezed his father's foot.

"I love you, Dad," he said. "You'll be home soon, OK?"

The patient smiled. Friedland closed the ambulance doors.

I stood in the grass with the patient's son. He rubbed his temples, took his face in his hands, and convulsively wept. The virus did that. Made hard men weep. I knew this. I'd seen it. COVID taught me this lesson with each patient and family member, a dozen nightmarish variations on the same theme.

"This is so sad," he said. "He's my father. He lives with me so I could take care of him. This is it? This might be the last time I get to see him? This is unbearable."

Unbearable.

"I know it is. It's so awful. I promise you we won't leave him alone for one second. We'll be right there with him the whole time. And when we get to the hospital the nurses will take good care of him, I promise. We'll be his family tonight. We can do that. He won't be alone, I promise you."

"I don't know how to thank you. All of you, for doing this. I don't know how I can ever repay you for taking such good care of my dad. Thank you. You're angels. God bless you."

"It's our pleasure. It's an honor."

And it was. It was an honor and a sacred privilege for me, for all of us EMTs to help people feel a little less frightened and alone. But it was also shattering.

When we got to the hospital, the patient had a fever, 102. The triage nurse told us to go to the back and put him in an isolation room.

Room was the wrong word. The back section of the hospital had been transformed into an assembly of makeshift stalls divided with flimsy partitions. The doors had plastic windows cut out of them. They were horrible, the isolation rooms. They were sadness constructed. Before we said goodbye to our fevered patient, he told me he had to urinate. I found him a container from the hospital restock cabinet and a handful of paper towels. I handed it to him, then closed the wobbly door and left him alone in his room.

Then I stood outside and stared at him through the plastic window. I knew a nurse would check on him in a few minutes but leaving him there—even for an instant—brought tears to my eyes. It damaged me in profound, delicate ways. I felt watermarked with sorrow. There was no washing it off.

I couldn't get the sight of this man out of my head for weeks; he followed me everywhere, and every time he came floating across my field of vision my eyes glassed and I felt like a traitor who'd broken her promise not to leave him alone.

First responder or everyday person, no one got to skip this part of the pandemic. The part where feeling registered, when suffering landed. You could try to Netflix it away or ward off pangs of grief with news and numbers, bar charts and politics. But it would find you, sorrow. At least it always found me.

Over the next week I grew more worried about everyone I loved. I thought often of Kentaro, my beloved street husband, my frequent flier, and wondered how he was faring in the pandemic. No EMT I was in touch with had transported him since COVID flared up. Was he drunk? Sick? Dead? I thought about Mike, in Vegas, and how COVID intercepted our marriage with Ylfa, annihilating his cancer treatment in New York, his plan to move here.

I missed Mike. My mom. My friends.

Tears helped. And prayers. Phone calls to Ylfa and Mike and Felice. One night I baked chocolate chip banana bread and cookies. I ramped up my meditation practice and sat for twenty minutes each morning.

Everything helped. I couldn't say it worked and I wasn't coming unraveled. But it gave me a chance to inhale and exhale in the city where no one could catch their breath.

One Saturday morning I awoke with an urgent desire to buy more plants and turn my apartment into a greenhouse. I was halfway there already, pre-pandemic. "You know there is such a thing as too many plants," Nick said the first time he walked into my living room.

I disagreed. That April, the virus pushed me over the green edge. I was turning into a full-blown Plant Lady. We were even sicker than Cat Ladies, I thought. We were way worse off in terms of strangeness.

"Is it Plant Lady Saturday?" Mike asked these weekends when he called. It sure was. My husband knew me so well. I was at Home Depot. I came home with a dozen new leafy children. Begonias. Monsteras. Gardenias, with their rich waxy blossoms. I slept with them near my bed, and they perfumed what little sleep I got with their strong, sweet smell. They made me feel as if I were in another world—a better one.

I wasn't the only one rewilding. Jeremy came into the hallway in his forest-green robe one day—every time I saw him now, he was in his robe—and when I peeked inside his apartment, I saw an explosion of plants.

"Wow. When did you get all those plants? Look at your hydrangeas. They're thriving! You're such a good plant father."

"Right? I'm buying so many plants right now. What do you think?"

"It looks amazing. I just bought more plants myself."

One unremembered day of the week I made a telemedicine appointment with my GP, so I could get a referral for a serology test for COVID. The blood tests were more accurate than the swab, everyone said. In the afternoon I logged onto my computer and my doctor's face filled the screen.

"You're alive," I said.

He laughed. "Yes."

We discussed the virus. He said he'd been out sick with a fever two weeks ago, but his bloodwork came back negative for COVID. That sounded suspicious. I told him all my patients had it, they were dying of it, and my partner had it, too.

"I'm sure you have it," he said after I described my symptoms. "Hopefully you have the antibodies."

He wrote me a requisition and said he'd leave it at the front door of his office. He suggested I make an appointment early in the morning to get my blood drawn at LabCorp. The line was long, he said, and they were careful about who they let in. The next day I drove into Manhattan. It was a ghost town. The streets were eerily empty. No people, no cars. A few busses floated by with nobody on them. Homeless people wandered around with their palms cupped, begging for money.

I picked up the referral from my doctor's office and walked up the block to LabCorp. A nurse in sky-blue scrubs asked if I'd been exposed to COVID and experienced symptoms, and I gave her the story.

"I'm sure you have it," she said, drawing my blood.

The test results came back pretty fast, three days later.

Negative, negative.

No active COVID infection, no antibodies.

"Jen, that can't be right. You had it," Nathan said when he came back from California.

"Are you ever going to get a test?" I asked him.

He said he would. A week or so later he waltzed into a medical clinic in his EMT uniform, to expedite the process and cut the line. It worked. Nathan's COVID antibody test came back the following day.

Positive.

"These tests are bullshit!" I told him when I saw him on the ambulance for our next tour. "How's it possible that all of our patients have it, you have it, I rode with you while you had it, we both got sick at the same time with the same symptoms, and you have antibodies, and I don't."

"I'm sorry," Nathan said. But his laughter indicated he was not sorry, he was amused.

"When they hand out the Rona Medals," I told him, "you're not getting one."

17

MAY DAYS

As the weather warmed in May I wanted only to be outside, like most New Yorkers who'd been compliantly cooped up all spring.

One bright afternoon I drove to Prospect Park to stroll around the gravel paths. I needed to be surrounded by my beloved friends—trees and plants. Get some fresh air and decompress after witnessing so much suffering. Let nature do its healing work on my shot nervous system.

I strolled into the park and stopped fifteen feet in, stunned to see it packed with people. Families playing with their unmasked kids. Teenagers kicking soccer balls around. Happy, laughing couples sitting side by side on blankets. My vision blurred. I saw only a smudge of green speckled with dead people. I couldn't understand what I was seeing.

Thousands of people had died on the city streets. Many more than reported in cheerful, declining numbers circulated by officials. It would take a decade, maybe longer, to get an accurate body count. It would take a governing body established in the aftermath of COVID, which was still ongoing, to review the disaster and points of failure. Something like the 9/11 Commission, which deconstructed the emergency response to the terrorist attacks and tried to understand and patch up the places where overlapping systems collapsed and failed.

For now, there was no end to the virus in sight. All the talk in the news was about the possibility of a second wave. I thought of all the patients we'd lost. I saw them now, in the park. Sarah. Margarite. I'd held her fevered hand. Listened as she coughed, gasped, suffocated to death, rushed into a room to be intubated and vented, then probably loaded onto a refrigerator truck. I saw the first responders who'd committed suicide across the world. And Mike in Vegas, whose cancer was advancing faster than we'd anticipated, who was now in and out of the ER, vulnerable to catching COVID and dying of it due to his compromised immune system. The chirping birdsong in the park suddenly sounded like it was coming from an Alfred Hitchcock film. I turned around and walked out. Ran. I couldn't get out of there fast enough.

When I got back in my car, I felt nauseous. I put my head on the steering wheel. So much for nature.

I wasn't the only first responder alarmed by the crowds. One afternoon, Chad texted me a photograph of a sunny field in Central Park, the grass littered with sunbathing New Yorkers on blankets. "Here's your next round of patients," he said.

Driving home, I wished for a different country. But nearly every nation-state was raging against their government for botching the pandemic. Raging at each other for not taking COVID seriously enough. I wished New Yorkers would take COVID as seriously as we first responders had been forced to take it. It was impossible to communicate the devastation were seeing up close. The news was bad. But the street was worse.

At the same time, I identified with people who wanted the unmasked world back. The world of sunny days in the park and splashes in the sea at Riis Beach. The days of hugs and kisses hello and goodbye. COVID was turning into a mental health crisis due to people being isolated and trapped indoors. Not everyone was safe inside, stuck at home with their families.

If this pandemic had happened at a different point in my life—when I lived in Bakersfield, or was a young drunk woman, or newly diagnosed with cancer, or reeling after 9/11—I didn't know if I would have survived it. The isolation gutted people. You know what happens to newborn babies who don't get touched. Babies who don't get human contact in the first few days and weeks of life suffer long-term health problems related to deprivation.

In the pandemic, the same sad math seemed to be coming true for adults. On the ambulance in May, the calls coming over the radio were hideous and tragic. Drug overdose. Drown. Someone shot in the face. Stabbed in the train station. Female with lacerations to her wrist, unresponsive. Cardiac arrest. Jumper up. Jumper down.

I had to get away. Get out of the city for a few days. Drive upstate. Escape New York. But first, I had to age.

On my birthday that May, loads of friends sent me loving messages and cards and texts. My friend Steve from my writers group texted and asked how I was.

"I've been better," I said. "My friend with cancer has been in the ER. I'm working a nursing home mass-casualty incident. Still loads of sick COVID patients on the ambulance. But today is my birthday. So I'm watching *90 Day Fiancé*. How are you?"

"Happy birthday! I'm fine, what can I complain about in this context? How are you taking care of yourself?"

"Turning my phone off was my biggest act of self-care. And I'm eating homemade banana bread. And I talk to Felice every day. And take walks. And I bought a new vibrator. Is that enough?"

"You decide if it's enough, but I'm glad you're doing all these things. I say buy ALL the vibrators."

In March, as 8.6 million New Yorkers were locked down at home, the city's health department released a two-page document discouraging residents from having in-person dates, casual sex, or sex with anyone they didn't live with, since COVID-19 could be transmitted through the saliva exchange involved in kissing. "You are your safest sex partner," health experts said. The document encouraged residents to use "pleasure devices" and have video dates. "Sexting or chat rooms may be options for you." Loads of media, from *Vogue* to *The Wall Street Journal*, published articles about sexting and how-to guides on making love, sweet virtual love, in COVID isolation.

I texted Tommy. "City is selling sexting to the people. We were ahead of our time."

"Way ahead."

"If we co-taught a pandemic sexting class, we'd be millionaires."

"Billionaires. There is a need we could fill."

"An essential need, and we are essential workers. We created this art form. We broke this art form."

"Worldwide."

"It's true. People struggle with this. We have PhDs in it."

"Our sexting was some of my best work. In life."

"Trust me, I know. I also feel I performed at a top level."

"The best. Ever."

Mike called. I said farewell to Tommy and talked to him for a while. My husband said happy birthday and asked if I'd checked my mail. I had not. Did I have a present? I loved presents! I ran downstairs and looked. In my mailbox, surprise! A birthday present from my husband. I ran upstairs and tore it open.

Card first. Mike had written me a beautiful note telling me how much he loved me, and what I meant to him. He said he wanted me to have this. Janet had given it to him, his late wife. What was it? I opened a little folded packet. My eyes bulged when I saw what I unwrapped.

In my hands I held the most beautiful necklace. A thick gold chain with a caduceus, the symbol of medicine, its staff entwined by two snakes and a pair of wings. Much greater and more powerful than the EMT symbol patched on my uniform, the Rod of Asclepius with its single snake.

I put the necklace on and looked in the mirror and cried. Then I called and thanked Mike. It was one of the nicest things anyone had ever given me. From now on when I worked on the ambulance, I could wear Pat around my wrist and Mike around my neck, to protect me. We weren't allowed to wear jewelry on the street, since patients could strangle us with necklaces. But I wore mine anyway, tucked beneath my shirt.

It was the happiest birthday. It was gold.

A few days later I hopped in my car and sped upstate, to a little Airbnb in Kingston I rented for a few days.

Perfection.

Except there was no toilet paper. Apparently, a lot of hoarders lived upstate. Thanks, hoarders. I would have brought toilet paper from Brooklyn, had I known. But it was otherwise lovely to get out of the city. For days I went on walks. Sat in the sun. Read for hours. Napped. My God, I loved being alone. No one understood that about me. Well. No one except writers.

"Tell me something," Mike said one night when he called. "Did you go upstate with Tommy?"

"What? No, silly. Tommy isn't in my real life. He's only on my phone. I came up here by myself, to relax and read and write."

"You can tell me the truth."

"Turtle, I am telling you the truth. Why would I lie? You sound like a jealous husband. Remember, our marriage is fake."

"It is *not* fake," Mike said.

One morning I went on a walk along a trail and forgot my mask in the car. I figured it was OK to keep walking, since I was outside, and it was early, and there weren't many people around. The few joggers I saw weren't wearing masks, and I was fine with that. It was somewhat unhealthy to work out in a mask. Hard to breathe. As I was walking, I got attacked! This hippie-looking older white lady saw me and laid into me for not wearing a mask.

"This virus is very serious!" she screamed at me. "You have to take this seriously! It's fatal! People are dying!"

I raised my hands in surrender. "I know it's fatal, I'm a healthcare worker. I forgot my mask in my car."

Exasperated, she stormed off.

Bitch. Get control of yourself, I thought. Contain your hippie rage. She probably hogged all the toilet paper. Who did she think I was, some rich neoliberal hipster who lived in Williamsburg and sat around all day watching CNN, vaping weed and posting Instagram stories? I was healthcare hero! #FirstResponder.

I tried to keep walking with my shirt over my mouth, but now I was too ragey from being screamed at to enjoy myself. After ten minutes I turned around and stomped back to my car, kicking rocks. Along the way, I saw the screaming lady lying on her back on a slab of rock, sunbathing.

Are you kidding me? That rock was public property. It was nasty. It was probably dripping with COVID. I'd never sit on that rock in the pandemic, let alone lay on it. You and your terrible attitude are probably getting COVID right now, I thought.

But did I say that?

No, I did not. Because I was not a bitch.

In May, news broke about a new COVID condition.

Children were no longer thought to be invulnerable to the virus, as previously believed. Medical journals and media outlets reported kids were showing symptoms of COVID-19 inflammatory syndrome, with clinical features that resembled Kawasaki disease. These children reportedly presented with fevers for more than five days, rashes, conjunctival injection, and swollen lips. Some had extremity swelling and desquamation of the fingers, peeling skin. Always something new on the street these days.

One tour, MARS dispatched Nathan and I to a job for an "unknown." The location was three blocks from where we were posted, on streets with numerals. When Nathan asked me to GPS the job for him, I understood he was fried.

"Drive straight four blocks," I said. "Count the numbers."

When we got to the building on a quiet treelined street and went inside, a blonde-haired woman came running downstairs in a mask and stuck out her arms as if to stop us. She looked afraid.

"Stop, stop! You don't have to come upstairs."

We asked her what happened. She told us her daughter had an unusual event. She was sleeping soundly, then half an hour later she came out of her bedroom waving her arms and screaming like a zombie. The woman and her husband couldn't tell if their daughter was crying or laughing. They couldn't get her to speak or respond to them for five minutes. Panicked, having read the news about children coming down with COVID, they called 911. But then then their daughter returned to normal. She started speaking again then went back to sleep. They tried to cancel the 911 call. The woman didn't need us.

"How old is your daughter, ma'am?" I asked.

When the woman said "Three," I felt the ground open up beneath me.

With pediatric patients, they couldn't verbally express what was happening to them, medically, so we couldn't just clear the scene without examining the patient. Nathan and I asked the upset mother if we could come upstairs and check their daughter out, just to be sure she was safe. At the foot of the stairs, the mother agreed, saying again she'd overreacted and didn't need EMS. She said her daughter had no rash, swelling, fever, or nausea. She was perfectly fine.

"That's good," I said, walking up the stairs behind her now. "Since we're here, we'll just take a look."

We went into the child's dark bedroom and switched on the light. Lying on her back in a crib, a little rosy-cheeked girl with a rash above her upper lip roused from her slumber. Seeing us, her eyes widened with fear. Nathan and I were in uniform, wearing N95 masks. Imagine being a little kid and waking up to find two uniformed, masked aliens in your bedroom, looming over your crib, staring down at you. The poor girl couldn't unfasten her gaze from us. Her eyes were wide. She looked at us like we were from Mars. Which we were—FDNY MARS.

She appeared to be fine, just as the mother said. No swollen limbs. No strange marks on her skin aside from the rash above her lip, which we would ask the parents about.

"Does your tummy hurt, sweetie?" I asked her. Head shake to indicate No. "Does anything hurt, anywhere?" Again, a shake of the head to say No. "Would you like for us to leave you alone now so you can go back to sleep?" Strong nod to say yes.

In the living room, Nathan and I chatted with the rattled parents. I asked if the rash above their daughter's lip was there before. Her mother confirmed that it had been; she'd had that rash on and off for a year from licking her lip.

"Have you had COVID?"

The husband said, "We've both been sick. But we haven't been tested so we're not sure."

"Have you seen kids dying of it?" the mother asked, stepping closer. "We've been reading the news. Do you know anything about what's happening to kids who get COVID?"

"We haven't seen it personally, no. But your daughter has no symptoms. It's possible she had a nightmare or night terrors. We'd be happy to take her to the hospital if you'd like."

"No," the mother said. "That's what we think, too. We think she had a nightmare. This has never happened before, so we panicked and called 911."

"This is really scary for kids. It's normal to have nightmares at this point. For all of us."

After that call, Nathan drove to a deli and bought us ice cream. At seven o'clock we heard a ruckus and circled the block. What was all the noise? I couldn't tell where it was coming from. Then I saw people standing outside in the street, holding signs for healthcare heroes, clapping as we drove by in the ambulance, dinging cow bells. *Wow.* One man flagged us down at a stoplight. He ran up to our truck and handed us two homemade masks sewn out of blue-and-black *Star Wars* fabric.

"My wife made these," he said. "We want you to have them. You guys are heroes, being out here. We're so grateful for you. Thank you for your service. My wife will be so happy to know I gave you her masks."

Nathan and I were happy, too. We put on the homemade masks and our goggles, then took pictures of each other.

"*Return of the Jedi*," I said. "I love it."

"Jen, these people think we're heroes," Nathan said.

"They really do."

The clapping was nice, actually. I'd been such a bitch about the clapping firefighters and now that I was the recipient of applause, I was retrospectively glad the hose-draggers had been standing outside hospitals, clapping for nurses. The nurses deserved it. We all did. Firefighters, too. And cops. They'd been buried in a rubble of corpses.

This was exactly why social media would never be my medium. Because I ran my mouth, and then two months later, I disagreed with myself. My friends knew this about me. "You remind me of something I just read in one of Henry James' letters," my writer friend Josh said. "An Englishwoman took James to task for summing up certain English manners through characters in one of his stories. James replied: 'Nothing is my last word on anything.'"

In May there was a sweetness in the air, cowbells and applause for firefighters and cops, EMTs and paramedics, nurses and doctors, all of us on the front lines, a rising-from-the-ashes feeling of unity among first responders on the streets, in the hospitals, ERs, and ICUs, EMTs and paramedics throwing their arms around each other, embracing in tears. A feeling that we'd made it, we survived, that the peak of the virus was behind us.

We did it. We were alive.

I remembered that feeling after 9/11. Pure love. It started on 9/12, and I never wanted it to end. The coronavirus pandemic brought that feeling back in May. I finally felt it. That sense of unity and love and unspeakable tenderness.

And who, in my virus-besieged city, my home, which for the second time since I'd lived here endured catastrophic disaster, my city scattered with white tents and refrigerator trucks, hospitals deluged with bodies, blowing up with infected patients, running out of PPE and ventilators, COVID spreading at breakneck speed, so rapidly the release of daily numbers came as a crushing shock to the system all spring, who had spoken from the heart of COVID?

Governor Cuomo.

Listen:

"Bring down that anxiety, bring down that fear, bring down that paranoia," he said in a March press conference I was only now getting around to listening to, as the street quieted down. His voice was so low and soothing, seared with emotion, it became my mantra the rest of the summer. I often listened to the audio recording before I rode on the ambulance. You listen, too:

"We're going to get through it," he said, "because we are New York, and because we've dealt with a lot of things. And because we are smart. You have to be smart to make it in New York. And because we are united. And when you are united, there is nothing you can't do. And because we are New York tough. We *are* tough. You have to be tough. This place makes you tough. But it makes you tough in a good way.

"We're going to make it, because I love New York. And I love New York because New York loves you. New York loves all of you."

Beautiful. A perfect crisis communication. I wondered who wrote it.

MARS sent us on no jobs the rest of the night. It was exhausting to sit on the ambulance for hours and do nothing. Physically and psychically. Just being in uniform drained me, even when we were just sitting there, available for jobs. After a while my neck hurt. My back. My head. My rotator cuff, which I'd injured ages back, who knows how, and I'd already blown through two cortisol shots and my doctor said, "No more." Maybe I'd hurt it on the ambulance. Maybe working out. Maybe just being forty-five. At my age, sometimes I hurt myself just getting out of bed. As hours passed, I felt dirty, lonely, tired.

Driving back to Bed-Stuy around one o'clock in the morning, I could barely keep my eyes open on the road. When I got home I stripped, bagged my uniform, took a hot shower and two Aleve, and crashed. I couldn't use the words "fell asleep" these days. I just passed out like I used to, when I was a drinker. The next morning I woke up with the chemical taste of my N95 mask in my mouth and an e-mail from my mom.

Bad news.

My favorite uncle, the sheriff, had had a heart attack. He'd been medevacked out of Sequim, Washington, and rushed to a hospital in Seattle for emergency surgery. *Oh no.* I sent my mom and aunt e-mails and told them I loved them. Then Mike called.

More bad news.

* * *

Mike found out he might not get into a clinical study to do radiation and chemo at once. He was crushed. And in pain. His ribs hurt, and his back and legs. He'd put all his hope into this plan. On the phone, we had a long talk about plans, and what he could control. How he couldn't keep giving all of his power away to doctors, hanging his hat on a magic-bullet solution.

"Every time you go to the doctor you have a plan for what you want, Turtle. You've made your mind up. Then the doctor tells you the plan won't work, and you spiral and start burying yourself. Quit burying yourself. Next time when you go to the doctor, you can have your plan. But let's leave some room for another plan to emerge, so you don't keep tanking when your idea doesn't pan out."

"You're so smart," Mike said. "How can I ever thank you?"

"I'm not as smart as you or Duck. And you can thank me by staying alive."

"OK," Mike said. "I'll try to do that."

Onto lighter subjects, to laugh away our sorrows. I told Mike I felt ridiculous for never working an arrest, the meat-and-potatoes emergency of the street. I felt like a fake first responder. He listened then disagreed that working an arrest meant anything in terms of my capabilities as an EMT.

"Speaking of meat and potatoes," he said, "did I ever tell you about the time I pulled a potato out of a patient's ass?"

"No, Turtle. I believe I would have remembered that."

"I won't go into detail. But let me just say if you're looking for anal stimulation, don't use a potato. It expands when it mixes with the liquids in the anal cavity."

That's what it was like being one of Mike's wives.

Pat, I asked that night in my prayers. *Can you let Mike stick around? We really love him. And he's sober now, like you always wanted. It's like having you around again. I get to have a brother. He helps me so much. And I really need him. Can he stay?*

Even with the lighter call volume on the street, by mid-May I felt done. Cooked. Salty. My previous dreams of becoming a paramedic fled. I didn't know what I would do next, EMT-wise. Or if I'd even stay on the ambulance. I was wearing down.

Tommy felt the same.

"I'm roasted," I told him one afternoon.

"We all are," he said.

He'd just come off a twenty-four in the Bronx and went on run after run all night. He had a raging headache from carbon monoxide poisoning. Like me, Tommy was struggling to empathize with regular people these days. Even his girlfriend, who was bereft after her doorman died of COVID. She was upset, but all Tommy could muster on the feeling front was "meh."

"I can turn on the switch and go cold and emotionless at times like this. It's a very well-trained survival mechanism of mine."

"Oh boy, that must be fun for your girlfriend."

"It's like a dude just got smoked by a train, let's scrape his body off the tracks and go back to the firehouse and watch a movie. It's just too hard to take it all in. I've seen too much. So when her doorman died, I didn't know what to say beyond, 'Yeah, it sucks. It's awful?' You know the deal."

"Yeah. I have friends texting me about how they're having a hard time staying home and they're bored and don't know what to do with their time, and I'm like, 'OK, well, I'm loading Grandma into the refrigerator truck right now, so let's talk later.'"

"Exactly!"

"My humor has gotten very dark."

"Dark humor is the best."

"It's all we have left."

Most of our patients had COVID in May, even the ones who called 911 for other complaints. The lead singer in the emergency band might have been an injury or a motorcycle accident, but COVID was always the backup singer.

We usually found out too late that we were assisting a suspected COVID patient to put on goggles and gowns. One tour, Nathan and I took an intoxicated woman to the hospital and the triage nurse said, "Oh, her again? She was here yesterday for the same thing. By the way, she's positive."

Good to know.

Here's a stunning fact that became laughable during COVID, when one of the primary symptoms of the virus was a fever: EMTs in New York City don't carry thermometers on ambulances. There's no way for us to take our patients' temperatures. We find out patients have fevers later, too late for us to put on PPE, when we triage them in the ER.

Another night we went on a call for a "sick" patient, but the sick turned out to be secondary to a universe of other problems. We parked on a dark, empty, industrial block to find an emaciated white woman screaming at a large Black man to give her money after what appeared to be a sexual transaction. The man ran off and the patient screamed at us to follow him.

"Get him!" she said.

Um, no.

We offered to call the police, but the woman didn't want that. She wanted us to chase whoever that man was down the block on foot. Do I look like a cop? Do I have wrap-around sunglasses on? Do you see me going on a hot-action foot pursuit? People watched too much TV.

"We're not cops," I said. I found myself saying this constantly on the street. It bears repeating: We're EMTs. We're not cops.

Finally, we got the livid patient onto the ambulance, where she said she had a fever, cough, and was a self-described junkie. She had track marks railroaded across her arms and legs, open sores, and head and body lice.

The second she said "lice," Nathan quickly and politely escorted her off the truck. Then he threw a sheet over her and wrapped her up like Yoda. Outraged at being cocooned, she shucked off the sheets and cursed Nathan. I couldn't blame her. She looked ridiculous. She looked like two-dollar ghost. Then she took off down the street. Bolted.

Once she was out of sight, Nathan had some sort of OCD-like reaction. He was pacing all around, taking his hat on and off, itching his scalp. He was clearly shaken up. I'd never seen him so freaked out. I guessed he was afraid of bugs. Never knew that until now. He made me pitch everything the woman touched into a dumpster on the street. He spent the rest of the night slathering himself with squirts of hand sanitizer. He even slapped some on his face. Most hospitals had no disinfectant wipes sitting around anymore. What they did have they kept for themselves, hidden in ER nooks and crannies. We cleaned the ambulance after each run with our own dwindling supplies.

The depressing show kept rolling. The most depressing show on earth. Everywhere we turned we brushed up against tragedy.

One night as Nathan and I walked into the ER, a nurse walked past us, pushing a bed bearing a sheeted corpse.

Later, while we were standing in the hospital triage line, a note came over the PA, but we didn't catch what it was for. Three or four minutes later a fleet of paramedics rushed in with a sheeted woman face down and rear up on the stretcher. One of the medics had his hand deep inside her vagina while his partner tried to cover the woman's face and shield her from COVID. The medics blew past nurses and doctors and bolted to the elevator bank.

"Jen, did you see that?" Nathan asked me.

"I did. What the fuck."

Breech birth, we later found out.

That poor woman.

That night when I got home, I stayed up late reading about breeches, and what to do if you respond to a complicated childbirth in the field. I read for hours. I learned that it depended on how the baby was breeched. If the infant's head was stuck in the vagina, you were supposed to insert a gloved hand into the patient to create an airway for the baby, so the infant didn't suffocate. The thought of just having seen, in a matter of minutes, a corpse on a stretcher chased by a potentially suffocating baby stuck inside a mother whose face was smothered in a sheet due to COVID with a medic's hand shoved inside her—it was too much to process. I'd never get these images out of my head.

Enough was enough already. It was May. Call volumes were down. When was this COVID situation wrapping up? I didn't know how much more slow-rolling tragedy I could take. I didn't know it yet, but there was no end in sight. Au contraire, the city was about to erupt in protests.

18

APRIL SHOWERS BRING MAY PROTESTS

Last week of May, just when I started to get my sea legs for the pandemic, started feeling like maybe COVID Wave I was behind us, and I'd narrowly escaped drowning in a cauldron of despair, a white police officer in Minneapolis heinously murdered George Floyd, a forty-six-year-old Black man, during an arrest for allegedly using a counterfeit twenty-dollar bill. Pinned to the ground, the cop kept his knee on George's neck for over eight minutes—even after he lost consciousness, and after paramedics arrived on scene.

Eight minutes. Eight minutes and forty-six seconds.

Immediately the video of the killing went viral. Protests commenced in Minneapolis. The city was set on fire. Three days later, on Thursday, May 28, demonstrations commenced in New York City. First, with a peaceful assembly of protestors in Manhattan.

The next night, Lexi and I picked up a tour on the ambulance in Brooklyn.

If we'd been out sick and missed the peak of COVID, we now had front-row seats to the protests about to erupt across Brooklyn.

Out of the gate, joy. FDNY dispatched us to a job for an "unknown." Lexi hit the lights and sirens and gunned it to street corner where a group of bystanders gathered around a downed man on the sidewalk.

"Did you call this in?" I asked the crowd when I slid off the truck. They nodded. Step aside, step aside. On the sidewalk, a man was lying recumbent against a wall. He propped himself up and was halfway into a seated position when I recognized him.

"Kentaro!" I screamed. "It's me, Jennifer! It's your wife! I'm so happy to see you, my love! I've been so worried about you."

Baffled, the bystanders wandered away, looking back over their shoulders at the scene.

Lexi stood back, giggling as Kentaro looked up at me in fuzzy recognition, squinting one eye. Then he smiled, reached inside his duffle bag, and pulled out a stuffed yellow lamb. He handed me the gift.

"Jennifer, this is for you," he said several times.

I loved my present. My husband was bombed. He'd drank two bottles of vodka—minimum. An empty beer can rolled into the gutter when he adjusted his dirty coat.

Clutching the lamb, I turned to Lexi, who was standing back a few feet, letting me enjoy this intimate moment with my husband. "He gave me a lamb," I said.

Lexi gave me a frowny-face. "You can't keep it."

"Really?"

"No, girl. It's all he has."

Oh, damn it. She was right.

With sadness, I handed the lamb back. It was ratty with worn-down, nubby fur. I still loved it. I would have kept it, if Lexi had let me. Fifteen or so minutes later, at the hospital, everyone in the ER screamed with delight upon seeing Kentaro. He was a gift to us all. Several nurses came over and shook his hand.

When Lexi and I put him on a bed, I went to get fresh sheets and heard one nurse say to another, "It's his third visit this week."

Then, as I passed by him, a doctor came to Kentaro's bed and said, "Tell me what's going on. And I'm not going to kiss you."

Aw. They knew my husband. They knew he didn't want to go to rehab or detox. He just wanted some kisses. Such a love. I was so glad he was healthy—healthy-ish.

Hours passed without another run. Then night fell, and in the new darkness, the radio exploded with jobs.

10-13! 10-13! Police vehicle on fire! People destroying property at Barclay's Center. Large crowd approaching Prospect Park. 10-13! 10-13! PD requesting backup. 10-13! We got airmail coming over on Atlantic Avenue. I need a bus forthwith! Put a rush on the bus! 10-13!

By quarter to ten that night, we'd heard six 10-13s, assist police officer, come over the air. In four years at Park Slope, I'd heard one.

With the dispatcher's voice dripping from our ears, Lexi and I sat on the bus in stunned silence, our gaze fixed out the window. "What the fuck" we whispered to one another as we listened to the echo chamber of incoming requests for help.

Police were receiving "airmail" in the form of thrown bottles, bricks, and other projectiles flying at them through the nighttime air. More than five hundred protestors surrounded the Eight-Eight precinct in nearby Fort Greene, a ten-minute drive away from where we were sitting. We opened our phones. Saw videos. Someone had tossed a Molotov cocktail into an NYPD van that was now on fire, burning in the street. We looked at each other.

Ruh-roh.

My phone buzzed. Nick. "Please be careful, dear Jennifer. Bad times. Head's up and safe always. I love you very much."

"Love you, too."

"Look at rooftops. Be tactical where you go and how you enter and leave."

"10-4."

My friend Peter, a retired paramedic from California, sent me a message. "Hey, checking on you. Hope you're safe and not on duty, and if you are be safe!"

"On duty. Shit just got crazy."

"BE SAFE!"

"10-13! 10-13!" the dispatcher said. There were so many 10-13s coming over, each radioed request like a round of ammunition, members of service requesting ambulances.

Alert from MARS dispatch: "Be advised stay safe. Please be careful. It's madness out there. I'm here if you need me."

We'd never gotten a message like that from a dispatcher. The golden rule in the world of first response was stay calm. Let calmness flow out of your eyes, your mouth, your hands in the face of the unimaginable. Otherwise your panic saturates the scene and ramps up everyone's blood pressure when you need to function and perform. After the young FDNY EMT killed himself during the peak of COVID, dispatchers had started sending us texts for mental health services and counseling available to us. Tonight, it seemed their worry for our wellbeing thickened.

Soon, we heard dispatch rush an ambulance to a stat ep, short for status epilepticus, or seizure, reporting over the radio that a cop had pushed a female protestor to the ground, she hit her head on the sidewalk, and she was now having a seizure.

"Oh, wonderful," I said to Lexi. "The cops pushed a protestor at a protest against police brutality. That's going to go over well. They can't even keep their shit together for ten seconds."

The MARS dispatcher came over the air and told all units to stay away from the protests unless we were sent to a job. Then Park Slope's dispatcher radioed the same thing. All EMS units were instructed to avoid the protests unless dispatched to an emergency at one. Someone told us the Fire Department pulled all of their units off the street, ordered them back to base after it was reported that bottles and other objects were also being hurled at EMTs and paramedics, shattering ambulance windows.

Lexi and I stayed on the street.

We sat on the truck in tense silence and listened to the radio firing off 10-13s, waiting for our unit number to be called. Around ten o'clock, we got assigned to an injury in Fort Greene then canceled en route, preempted for the higher, meaning higher-priority, job.

"You're going to a PD-13," dispatch said. "93 King, I need you for a 10-13 at Prospect Park."

Here we go.

"I don't like this," Lexi said as she switched on the lights and sirens and sped toward the park.

For better or worse, as EMTs and medics, we were smack in the middle of the chaos, responding to clashes between police and protestors that resulted in injuries. As EMTs we treated all patients, always, on all sides. Rape victims and rapists. Assaulters and assaulted. Hate crime victims and their attackers. Drug addicts and dealers. Tonight, dispatchers sent EMTs and medics across New York City to assist police officers requesting backup, the now-constant call for 10-13s, and also sent ambulances to protestors injured by police officers. If the patient had a heartbeat, that was our patient.

"We don't have bulletproof vests," Lexi said as she drove. I looked at her. She was green.

"We'll be OK, girl."

"I don't like this," she repeated.

When we got to the dark street edging the park, hundreds of protestors, swarms of people, thick lines of riot-geared police filled the blocks. The scene was jarring. It was so loud and crowded and swaying I could barely hear anything but screaming. There was too much going on, so many people, demonstrators shouting, waving signs, some of them throwing bottles, glass breaking on concrete, everyone shoving each other, shoving police, cops pushing people, forcing their way through the crowd. After seeing so much death it was a burst of aliveness like I hadn't seen in months, years, ever, not in real life, high-velocity rage, images flying at me, so many people, I couldn't not look, take it all in, feel responsible for what I saw.

"I don't want to get out," Lexi said now that we were parked. "We don't have hardhats."

We did have hardhats. But they were in an outside compartment.

"I'll get out. Let me go talk to the cops and see what the deal is."

I was feeling strangely fearless. Maybe it was the adrenaline. I'd been much more terrified responding to COVID jobs than protests. What was there to be afraid of, getting shot? That seemed unlikely. And if I got shot, Lexi was there, and very good at CPR. I didn't have any fear someone would kill me at all. Although, I really didn't want to get a bottle or brick thrown at my head. I'd seen enough concussed patients to know I didn't want to become one myself.

I slid off the ambulance and walked up to a short brown cop. Protestors threw shit at us. Glass bottles broke by my boots while others crashed and broke open near the ambulance. There were objects of all kinds flying our way. Airmail. I couldn't hear anything anyone was saying. So much shouting. Pure rage.

"You guys need an ambulance?" I screamed at the cop over the noise. "We got a 10-13!"

"Nah, no one's hurt! They just called for a bus for backup just in case!"

"10-4! We'll be in the truck!"

I climbed back on the ambulance. Now Lexi's face was white, her eyes open and pupils pinned, tiny as gnats. She said nothing. Most people prefer to think of their first responders as robotically brave and emotionless, unhuman, rather than traumatically stressed, toxically overdosed on death and violence to the point of psychosis.

"I don't want to stay here," Lexi said. "It's violent. They're throwing things at us."

I gave no shit. I was buried alive, I guessed.

"We'll be OK," I told Lexi.

"I hate this. I'm scared."

"You're OK, girl."

We radioed dispatch and told them there was no job. Just protestors and cops, no injuries so far. They told us to hang out for a minute. Standby. Standby meant stay. Standby meant be ready to act.

Lexi opened her mouth to speak.

"I know," I said before she got a word out. "You don't like this. It's OK, honey, we're good. Relax. We're on the truck."

I was being a bitch. I didn't have any emotional blood left. Not even fear, the cheapest emotion in town. COVID had drained me of inner resources. The kind I needed to be compassionate to my partner, who was rightly afraid. That was the healthy response. The city was getting torched in front of our eyes. We, too, were receiving airmail. The sound was incredible, so loud it was like a plane was taking off inside the ambulance, inside my eardrums, we could barely hear a word we said to each other, surround-sound chaos and pain, everyone in front of us moving and sloshing around, the crowds, the cops, as if we were on a stormy sea, about to be pitched under.

After some time, we checked in with dispatch and said there was no patient or injured MOS, and dispatch cleared us from the job. Cops lifted a barricade so we could get out without a problem. Lexi came back to life, her cheeks flushed with color.

"I'm sorry," I said to her. "For being a bitch."

Not long after we became available, we got sent to a women's shelter for an intoxicated patient who'd fallen off a chair. Much tamer landscape. In the shelter, a short Black woman cop asked us how it was out there. We said violent. She shook her head. "A month from now cops are going to start committing suicide."

"Yeah," I said. "We all are."

We took our fallen patient to the ER. While we were there, we saw two riled-up skinny white dudes with shaved heads and neck tattoos who had scratches all over their arms. They looked like they'd been wrestling with a tumbleweed. I wondered if they were protestors. They seemed happy, fired up, excited to be in the hospital. They were smiling and looking all around like something important had happened to them. I wasn't sure what.

I hated them.

Back at base at the end of our tour, around midnight, I apologized to Lexi again for being a heartless bitch. There was a look of crestfallenness on her face, a look of incurred injury. I left marks on her, and I felt horrible for it. She forgave me and said it was OK, but I still felt awful. I loved Lexi. Who had I become? What had the street done to me? What had being an EMT?

An hour or so later, when I got home, I tried to key into my building and my fob didn't work. It was two o'clock in the morning. I wasn't sure where I was. So much had changed. The world, the country, the city, the street, my building. More than half the tenants had moved out. Left New York. My super, Gilberto, said the building was 80 percent empty now. Most people weren't paying rent. I still had my friends here, thank God.

I called Jeremy. No answer. Called Ellery. He picked up in a soft voice, and minutes later shuffled groggily into the lobby and let me in. "I'm so sorry," I whispered, as if he were still asleep. He was moving soon. Out to a little seaside community near the Rockaways.

Maybe I should move, too. These days there were moving trucks double-parked on the blocks nearly every day. Mass exodus. But I didn't have the energy make any major changes. I barely had the energy to wash my hair.

Inside at last, back in my apartment, before I showered, I caught a glimpse of my reflection in the bathroom mirror. I didn't recognize the woman staring back at me. My forehead and cheeks were red and dented, carved with mask marks, the skin at the bridge of my nose chapped and bleeding from where the metal bar of my N95 clasped, my hair was matted and stuck to my face, plastered with sweat to my forehead, my face gaunt and colorless. I looked like I just got back from Afghanistan.

"You did just get back from Afghanistan," Nick said when he texted to see if I'd made it home safe.

My first responder friends were worried about me. Firefighters and cops and EMTs and paramedics. Them only. Everyone else had moved on to the new crisis unfolding on the streets across the city. The country was on fire. The applause that had come our way last spring, after COVID, stopped. The show was over. No one cared about EMTs or paramedics anymore.

I didn't care about us anymore, either.

* * *

That night, I worried for my friends. All of them. On all sides. Protestors. Cops. Felice, Natalie, Jeremy, Ellery, Ylfa. Mike, sick in Vegas. Everyone I loved. The list of suffering was exhausting, a CVS receipt of heartbreak unfurled in my chest. I crashed like never before. Slept a deep, morphine-like sleep until late Saturday afternoon. I wasn't sure what day it was when I woke up.

I called Felice. She was weeping. Natalie, the same. All of my Black friends were destroyed. So much sorrow, all I could do was listen. Let my quietness catch their tears. I said nothing about my night. Felice always quoted Audre Lorde, who said "There is no hierarchy of oppression." But I felt there was. Felice and Natalie's pain as Black women soared above mine.

We all suffered, as women. Felice and I once talked about how, when we walked down the street at night, we both looked around in imagined fear that we could be dragged into the bushes, murdered or raped by some dude. If the dude was a white man, I felt afraid. If it was a Black man, I felt more afraid. No matter how many Black people I loved or antiracism books I'd read, I'm sure if you strapped a heart rate monitor to my chest, my heart rate would be higher for a Black man than a white one. Racism was in me, in my nervous system, of course it was, that stuff was embodied, for me at least, it was an undeniable fact.

And if in that same imagined scenario of being a white woman in danger, a narrative pounded into my head since birth, taught to me in a thousand ways, learned, I saw a cop appear on the nighttime street, I immediately felt better, safer, like everything would be OK. Not for one second would I think the cop might kill me. That was where the hierarchy of oppression came in. Because in that same scenario of a woman walking alone at night on a dark street, with a man appearing behind her, then a cop, at the sight of the cop, Felice would feel even more afraid. She said, "Then I'd think 'Oh, no. Now I'm going to get shot in the street and turned into a meme.'"

Never once had I thought that. Feared I'd be shot by a cop in the street. Or in my own house, like Breonna Taylor. Not all EMTs were alike. There was a hierarchy of oppression. Just being Black in this country was a life-threat, a 10-13.

One of the worst sounds available to me on this planet was the sound of my sister weeping.

* * *

Later that same day, I checked my e-mail. A long, agency-wide update from Chief Beck and a correction request from a duty officer for one of my charts from the night before. I'd forgotten to write down the job number and needed to call MARS to get it.

The e-mail from Chief Beck said there were large protests with riot-like behavior that occurred at Barclays Center and police precincts directly adjacent to our coverage area as a result of controversial law enforcement events across the country. There was credible evidence some folks in these events were intending to create mayhem with violent behavior exhibited not only toward law enforcement but also the greater public-safety community including EMS, fire, and hospital emergency departments.

Beck reminded us that our safety was the priority. He told us to remain vigilant on the scene of assignments, and also while posted waiting for calls and traveling around the community. We were not to wear our uniform to or from our shifts. To remove ourselves from scenes that were unsafe. Be calm, professional, and patient with members of the public. If operating at the protests, to wear full PPE, including goggles and helmets. To stay with our partners at all times. He thanked us for everything we were doing.

After I digested the information, I rang MARS and spoke to an EMS dispatcher and told him I needed one of our job numbers from the night before. He asked for my unit number and I gave it to him.

"Oh, hi," he said. "I was your dispatcher last night. I was so worried for you guys. You had so many 10-13s coming over."

"It was crazy."

"You were so nice on the radio."

"That was my partner Lexi you spoke with. She's really nice." *I was a bitch.*

He gave me the job number I needed and told me to stay safe.

Protests flowed through the city that Saturday. There was no room in the news for the public to hold stories about EMS workers and fire trucks attacked at various protests. But the street told the story nonetheless.

Demonstrators threw projectiles at FDNY ambulances and broke their windows, reportedly attacking two crews. "Just know I have been and will be at every 10-13 for my people," a Latinx paramedic wrote on

Instagram. My people, in this instance, appeared to be his fellow members of service—cops.

I stopped looking at social media.

That afternoon Ylfa and I called Mike. He was suffering so much. In pain, the cancer worsening, treatments failing. We still spoke to him day and night and texted each other constantly. Reality was failing us, so we turned to fantasy for hope.

Duck and I reminded our Turtle he needed to stick around, since he had two wives. And he needed to make us legitimate, we had to get married. We decided to hold our wedding at Pat's tree, just the three of us and our minister, Michael Daly. And Paul could come. And Bobby. And James. We could time it for 9/11 and be together for the anniversary this year. Mike loved the idea.

He was still sober. And we reminded him that it was a miracle. "It's a fucking miracle," I said, and he laughed. Stage four cancer, agonizingly sick in a pandemic, and the man was sober. Heroic. He'd have six months in June.

"We're so proud of you, Turtle," Ylfa told him.

"And Pat is proud of you," I said.

"Pat's been waiting for this for a long time," Ylfa said. "You answered his prayers."

"I feel closer to Pat than I ever have," Mike said. "And I was so happy walking around in New York with you guys, going to shows and I don't know, just being around you. You guys gave me a whole new life."

"We didn't do it," I said. "It was all Pat."

"It was all Pat," Ylfa agreed. "It was divine intervention."

"And no one has saved more money than you by getting sober," I said. "Most people save some cash. You saved thousands of dollars since you stopped giving out personal loans."

Mike laughed and laughed. "You guys really saved my life. I never would have lived this long if it weren't for you. I probably wouldn't have even gotten treated. I'd just be sitting at the bar by myself, drinking and depressed. I'd be burying myself. And instead I got to have a life. We had so much fun together in New York. I want to come home."

"We want you to come home, too," Ylfa said.

"Yes," I said, "and we need to get a dog. You're not Fifty-Percent Mike anymore, since you're taking all your medicine, so we can't name the dog

Fifty. We can name him after Ernest Shackleton, the arctic explorer in Ylfa's play."

"Yes!" Mike said. "We'll get a dog and name him Shackleton!"

Ylfa's play about the explorer soon went up on Zoom, and Mike and I went to it. We loved seeing our talented wife shine on screen. Even if the screen was Zoom.

"Duck is so beautiful," Mike said, watching Ylfa perform.

"Yes, she is. Inside and out. She's a goddess."

"One day we're all going for a trip in my RV."

"Oh, Turtle," I said. "I love you so much. And I'm never getting in that fucking RV."

With 911 calls down, the Fire Department was soon releasing all mutual aid units. The next day was Park Slope's final tour on MARS before we returned to normal, serving the community and being dispatched internally. But normal?

Normal was very, very far away.

Sunday afternoon, before I headed to base, May 31, Beck sent around another e-mail. He told us to don bunker jackets and helmets now if we got dispatched to a protest. To practice wearing the gear before we left base if we hadn't worn it recently.

"Make sure the helmet ratchets are secure to your head."

Well, I guessed this was what they called wartime.

Beck reminded us to stay away from protests unless we were called to an emergency at one. "Please don't forget there is still a pandemic," he said. "Make sure you're wearing your N95 masks at all times."

He thanked us for our hard work and said that making sure we got home safe to our families was the utmost priority.

What family? I thought.

It took me an hour and a half to drive from my house to base, rather than the usual twenty minutes. I didn't mind. It was inspiring to see throngs of people filling the streets, most of them peaceful and masked. Aliveness combined with care for others. One of my favorite pairings in humanity.

At the same time, I feared the huge gatherings would cause COVID to spike. While New York City had finally quieted down on the virus front, thirty-three states were seeing upticks in cases. Florida. Texas. Nevada.

California. So much for those theories that COVID would just go away on its own or die out in warm weather. When I parked near base and walked inside the garage, I grew nervous for what the night would hold, if this night would be anything like the last few.

Wow, was my sense of impending doom accurate.

If Lexi had been frightened to get off the ambulance with airmail flying last Friday night, and I'd been irrationally relaxed, this Sunday evening Nathan was overeager to be part of the action.

Leaving base, he said he hoped we got dispatched to jobs at the protests. Gone were the slow days on the street. The second we logged onto MARS, we got sent to an "unknown" at a brownstone on Sixth Avenue. No EMS was needed, the job description said. It was a lift assist. Someone needed help getting off the floor.

The run turned out to be Nathan's dream job, helping his cherished people—the elderly.

We descended a set of mold-thick stairs and crept inside a basement apartment where an Italian woman in her eighties told us her husband had fallen down. She wasn't strong enough to lift him. She led us to her husband, an Italian man in his late eighties who was laid out on the floor. Helicoptering above him, we asked if he was hurt; if he'd lost consciousness; hit his head. No, no, no. He wanted only to be picked up.

Nathan and I laced our arms under his armpits and eased him onto his feet, then walked him to the kitchen and sat him down at a long table. We took his vitals and assessed him for trauma just in case. He was fine. At this juncture, our work was finished.

But not for Nathan. For Nathan, the party had just started.

While I packed up our equipment, by myself, Nathan sat beside the couple and did a deep dive into their lives.

The things I learned: They'd been married for sixty-five years. The wife complained her husband wet the bed every night and refused to wear Depends. "I'm not wearing diapers!" he shouted. She had to clean up after him every night. He was unsteady on his feet and refused to use his walker. "I don't need a walker!" he screamed. Instead, to make sure he didn't injure himself, he started wearing a hardhat around the house. "That way if I hit my head, I don't get hurt," he explained to me.

Made sense.

The husband was furious his wife had called 911, and couldn't understand why she didn't call their neighbor, a cop who lived across the street. "Every time I fall, we just call our neighbor, and he comes over and picks me up. He doesn't mind. He's a good guy," the man said.

The wife grew frustrated. "I tried calling him, Victor! I tried and he wasn't home!"

"Nonsense," the husband said. "You didn't try."

Then he turned to Nathan and said, "She lies all the time, my wife. Sixty-five years I've been dealing with this. Lies."

I said, "Well, sir, to your wife's credit, the cops are a little bit busy at the moment."

"No, she didn't call him," the patient said. "He would've come. He comes over every time I fall."

I gave Nathan a look that said, *OK, buddy. Time to go.*

But no. Nathan wanted to stay longer in geriatric heaven and talk more with his new friends.

I picked up our equipment, by myself, and lugged it back upstairs and outside, by myself, and sat alone on the ambulance. Ten minutes. Fifteen. Twenty. Unbelievable. No time with the elderly was enough time for Nathan. Ten more minutes passed. *Are you kidding?* I thought. *Wrap it up, Nathan. Land the plane.*

Finally, he came bounding out of the apartment after God knows how long on scene, beaming with joy and stories.

"Jen!" he said, climbing into the driver's seat. "They got married in Italy, and they fucking *hate* each other!"

"Cool story," I said.

As Nathan drove away at last, he told me all about their lives, their entire lives on earth, eighty years of stories, while I rubbed my forehead and listened to him go on and on, longer than *Anna Karenina*. Nathan had not only heard their whole life story, he'd also tested the wife's Life Alert bracelet to make sure it was working, in case she wanted to use that to alert 911 for her husband next time, instead of calling 911.

"Unbelievable," I said.

Almost immediately we got sent to another job near Prospect Park, standby for a possible explosive.

Yikes. I guessed now we might get blown up? That would suck. On the way to the run, it struck me that I'd been scared all spring of dying of COVID, but now it was summer, people were protesting, and I hadn't once considered the possibility that I might get blown up at an explosives job.

At least we had hardhats and hazmat gear on the truck. That would probably help. I hoped if something exploded and we got hit, I kept all my limbs, especially my hands and fingers, so I could still write and take care of my plants.

On the way to the job we got canceled. FDNY sent one of their ambulances instead of us to work the explosive standby. I didn't care either way. I still had the emotional life of a rock. But Nathan was disappointed.

"Damn," he said. "I wanted that one."

Everything I treasured about being a first responder was contained in our next emergency. Twenty or so minutes later Nathan and I got dispatched to our third job, a CVA-C, cerebrovascular accident critical, medical speak for acute stroke. Time-sensitive, this job.

Nathan sped lights-and-sirens toward the Gowanus housing projects with the windows cracked to let in rushes of fresh air while I gloved up and put on my N95. Now we were there.

Inside a small, well-kept apartment we found a frail elderly Black woman lying in bed. She was whimpering and crying to her daughter on a phone sitting on her pillow. In the bedroom, the woman's son told us why he'd called 911. His mother had stage four lung cancer, hypertension, and HIV. Fifteen minutes earlier, he'd come into her room and found her staring blankly at the wall, unresponsive. He'd suspected a stroke.

I looked at the patient. She was so tiny. She looked around eighty years old, but she was only sixty-three. In bed she was crying into the phone, telling her daughter she couldn't breathe.

Hearing her words—I can't breathe—was like hearing fingernails drag across a chalkboard. I felt sick. With COVID patients that was the gasped complaint—I can't breathe. At protests over countless Black people murdered by police—I can't breathe. And five months later, Mike, the cancer infesting his lungs—I'm having a hard time breathing.

What did we have as human beings except for our heartbeats and breath? Nothing. That's all we were, medically, and maybe spiritually, too.

That's what made a sentient life. But difficulty breathing was not a symptom commonly associated with strokes.

"Give me a big smile," I told our patient. Her lips moved evenly and bilaterally as she showed me her teeth. "Perfect. Now close your eyes and hold your arms out with your palms facing up and keep them there until I tell you to relax." She nailed it. Neither arm drifted down. "Now squeeze my hands," I said. Normal grip strength. "Beautiful. Now repeat after me, 'You can't teach an old dog new tricks.'" The patient's speech contained no slurs, errors, or missing words.

"Negative for stroke," I told Nathan as he talked with the patient's son. That was good news. But now we had to figure out what was really going on.

Our patient was screaming in pain, still saying she couldn't breathe. Snot bubbled from her nose. I asked her to tell me what hurt most. She shrieked and said her neck and chest, then repeated that she couldn't breathe. Her vitals were normal aside from a speedy heart rate, to be expected from a woman riddled with cancer who had a history of hypertension. Every time I had a patient with cancer my mind flew to Vegas, to Mike, and stabbed me with pain and prerecognized death.

Her sugar was normal, too. And the pulse oximeter we'd slipped on her finger told us her oxygen saturation, SpO2, was in a normal range. Sometimes knowing this detail calmed patients down.

"You're getting enough oxygen, sweetie," I said when she cried out again that she couldn't breathe. "Do you think maybe it's hard to breathe because you're in so much pain, and it's really upsetting?"

"Yes," she said softly.

"There we go. That makes so much sense. Pain is so stressful."

We spoke with her son, who said this was his mother's baseline. She was always in this much pain. Can you imagine? Just moving in bed or sitting up sent her into fits of agony. Three months from now Mike was in this state. His bones so gnawed away by cancer that when he rolled over in bed, his rib broke.

Tonight, we needed to take this woman to the hospital, but were mindful that moving her would cause even more distress. We took our time. The patient's son hugged her so he could ease her into a seated position. She stopped crying when we sat her up. She blinked, as if in wonder, and looked relieved.

"You look like you feel a lot better sitting up," I said.

"Do you feel better now?" Nathan asked her.

She nodded, and smiling said, "Yes."

She kept telling her son to go get her something. "Get me that thing for my nose!" she said. I had no idea what she was talking about. Her son giggled and left the room.

"She's asking for a surgical mask," he said when he returned, handing it to her.

We helped her son dress her. We put on her slippers. Got her phone and charger, ID and insurance card. Slowly we scooched her onto the stair chair and bundled her up in a sheet. Finally, we were ready to go.

Nathan wheeled her out of the apartment and into the street. Outside, the sky was black, the air cool, and our patient was no longer wailing in pain. A small victory. I ran ahead to the ambulance to pull out the stretcher. Nathan and the patient were chatting, getting to know each other. No one did more talking on scene than Nathan—no one. He won the race toward talking.

I threw our equipment on the truck and pulled out the stretcher. Now we just needed to transfer our cute patient from the chair onto it and load her inside the ambulance. Her pain level remained manageable, but she was frightened and whimpering.

"I don't want to die," she said. "I'm scared."

Then something unprecedented happened.

While we were in the street transferring our bundled-up, scared cancer patient from the stair chair to the stretcher, working as tenderly and slowly as we could, trying not to hurt her or exacerbate her pain, a car pulled up beside us.

Oh? What was this? A white woman driving, round-faced and blonde, the kind of woman who looked like she shopped at Whole Foods. She rolled down her window and leaning over, said something I couldn't hear. My attention was where it should have been, on our patient.

Nathan looked at the driver and said, "I don't know."

Then our patient said, "Turn around, then turn left at the corner, then, I can't remember where you go after that."

Nathan said, "Jen, can you give her directions to the Brooklyn Bridge?"

I turned, and I glared at this white lady's face, and my white lady face said it all. My face said, *Really? You're asking us for directions right now?*

In the middle of an emergency? With a sick patient in pain out in the street? While we're trying to get her inside the ambulance without hurting her?

"No," I said disgustedly. "I don't know how to get there. And this isn't a really good time for this."

The woman paused. Then she looked at me and screamed, "I have a right to ask you for directions! You are a public *servant*!" She said it like a slur, then peeled off.

"Mmm," the patient said. "She has an attitude."

In the street all three of us laughed. It felt so good to laugh. I loved this emergency. It just kept delivering.

We loaded our patient into the truck without a hitch, and before Nathan closed the doors and went to the front to drive, he said, "Jen, she makes hats. Ask her to tell you about the hats."

On our way to the hospital the patient and I had a nice, relaxing chat. We did not talk about cancer or dying. We did not talk about police brutality or COVID-19. We talked about hats.

She made hats. All kinds. Not the easy ones, either. Complicated hats. Brims and feathers. When we got to the hospital, she was cheerful and in much less pain. We triaged her and discovered she had a fever, 101 degrees. Suspected COVID-19. We had no gowns or goggles on, as usual, since we hadn't known. The nurse pointed us toward an isolation room.

Ugh.

We rolled the stretcher to the back of the hospital. Next, we needed to transfer our patient one last time, from the stretcher onto the bed. She got upset again and cried. I slid my hand under her armpit, but she didn't like that—not one bit. She wanted to put her arms around my neck. She raised her arms as if to hug me.

Nathan shook his head and said, warningly, "Jen."

I ignored him.

The patient threw her arms around my neck and pulled my face close to hers, so our foreheads were almost touching.

"This is how my son moves me," she said, her fevered breath rushing across my face. "He hugs me."

We didn't hug patients when we moved them. And with COVID patients, we weren't supposed to get close or touch them without goggles and gowns.

But what was I going to do? Tell this dying woman with stage four cancer, hypertension, and a low-grade fever that qualified her for COVID isolation, who was in ten-out-of-ten pain as her baseline and was now totally alone in the hospital, which she would likely never leave, that she couldn't hug me? Put her arms around my neck and touch my forehead to hers?

No. I couldn't do it. I let her hug me all she wanted. Nathan sighed and looked away.

After a moment, I peeled her clasped hands off my neck and said, "In order to slide you over without hurting you, we have to put our arms under your armpits and move you like that, but it's going to be fast and smooth."

"Can I scream?" she asked. Her voice trembled and tears journeyed down her cheeks.

"You can scream so loud. You can scream as loud as you want. But we're not going to hurt you, I promise."

We counted to three and slid her over. She didn't make a peep. She paused for a few seconds, then looked up at me, and beaming with gratitude, said, "You should teach my son how to move me like that. That was better than the way he does it."

I loved her. I loved every minute of this call. It was wonderous. Maybe that was why they called being a first responder a calling. Because the sacred started with a call.

After we cleared the hospital, Nathan taunted me with that white lady's phrase. "Jen, you're a public servant. Tie my shoes! Clean my boots! Give me directions! You're a *servant*!"

Yes, I was. And there was nothing I would have rather been.

The rest of that night on the street was a bit tense.

We drove past Barclays Center to get to an EDP and had trouble reaching the job location because of the protests. Robert texted us to avoid Barclays. Police had requested a level 3 mobilization, sending all units to Brooklyn, which was a problem because Manhattan had also called for a level 3 mobilization for extra units, for violence in progress. Fires, and stores being broken into and trashed.

A hospital paramedic who also volunteered at Park Slope texted us and said to avoid turning down Fourth Avenue because cops were receiving airmail. Objects were flying. Once again, ambulances were also reportedly getting struck. Nathan avoided that street and drove to get us milkshakes at Häagen-Dazs.

Making decisions was not Nathan's strong suit. Inside, I ordered a cookies-and-cream milkshake while he stared at the menu and deliberated. As soon as the woman behind the counter finished making my shake, Nathan decided he wanted the exact same thing.

Typical. Signature Nathan move.

Before I could finish my shake, we got sent to another job, this one at a men's shelter on Atlantic Avenue.

Again we had trouble getting to the shelter because half the streets were barricaded or filled with riot-geared police and protestors. When we got to the shelter it turned out to be a 93 Refuse All. A man had been punched in the face by another guy, but he didn't want to go to the hospital because he had asthma and COPD, and he was afraid of contracting COVID.

When we cleared the job and got back on the ambulance Chief Beck texted.

"Massive riot with explosives outside the hospital. Please do not transport patients to Brooklyn Hospital."

I relayed the message to Nathan, who rarely checked his texts. About the violence against first responders, he said, "They clap for us at 7:00 and throw bottles at us at 7:01."

Driving back to our area, we accidentally ran smack into the protests outside Barclays Center, because the other streets we tried to turn down were barricaded. I didn't see any violence in progress. Mainly bored-looking cops standing around in riot gear and throngs of peaceful masked protestors in the street.

Nathan saw his favorite pair of redheaded hospital paramedics standing outside their parked ambulance on Atlantic Avenue. They were working standby at the protests, wearing hardhats, goggles, and masks. They looked hilarious geared up to the eyeballs, like combat medics at war.

Nathan stopped at a green light to talk to them. He was famous for stopping at green lights. The medics had been standing there for hours. So far, their night had been eventless.

"There's so many PD-13s coming over," I said to them.

One of them said, "Yeah, but they're all bullshit."

* * *

Our last run of the night was a street job, and a very sad one.

It came over as a sick patient. But when we got on scene, we found a twenty-six-year-old homeless, Black, pregnant woman who said she felt nauseous. On the ambulance we talked with her for a long time. She didn't know how far into the pregnancy she was. She worried she had HIV. She said what made her sick was that earlier that night, she'd snorted heroin.

Nathan said, gently, "You know that's bad for the baby."

I said, "Nathan. Let's go."

He nodded and went up front.

On the back of the bus, the patient was notably high. She had a five-year-old daughter in foster care. She lived in and out of shelters, but lately she was living on the street, sleeping in a friend's car. She was thinking of becoming a vegetarian, so she would stop doing dope.

I remembered that logic from my drinking days: Maybe if I move to New York City, I'll stop drinking. If I just drink beer, instead of vodka, that means I don't have a problem. If I can stop for thirty days, that means I'm fine. Maybe if I just cut back. If I only drink on weekends. As long as I don't drink during the day, or at home, then I'm cool. Then I'm definitely not an alcoholic—I'm normal.

At one point I, too, became a vegetarian. Now this may come as a real shock, but it turns out vegetarianism doesn't stop alcoholism or drug addiction.

On the bus, the patient was nauseous. I handed her an emesis bag and she quietly puked while Nathan drove us bumpily to a hospital that didn't have explosives outside it.

In the hospital, I made Nathan hunt down a fresh emesis bag, which he did. When we triaged the patient, the nurse asked her why she was in the hospital.

"I feel sick," the patient said.

I gave the nurse a little more information. "She's pregnant, she doesn't know how many weeks along she is, she snorted heroin this evening, then she felt sick; she was actively vomiting on the bus. This is her second pregnancy. No medications, no allergies. She lives in and out of shelters and she's currently sleeping on the street."

The nurse said, "Ah."

It's difficult to tell the full story—it's hideous, at times. But you have to tell it, unedited. Otherwise, no one can help you.

On the way back to base, Nathan avoided protesting Atlantic Avenue and managed to find an open street that led to Eastern Parkway. I told him he shouldn't have said that thing to the patient about heroin being bad for the baby. That drug addiction wasn't a moral issue, it was a disease, a sickness. He didn't know I was sober. No one on the street did. My partners just knew I didn't drink.

I guess they know now.

"OK," Nathan said. "I get that, you're right. But Jen," he said, glancing sidelong at me. "Remember, you're a public servant. Give me directions!" he said, cracking himself up. "Answer my questions! I can ask you whatever I want—you're a SERVANT!"

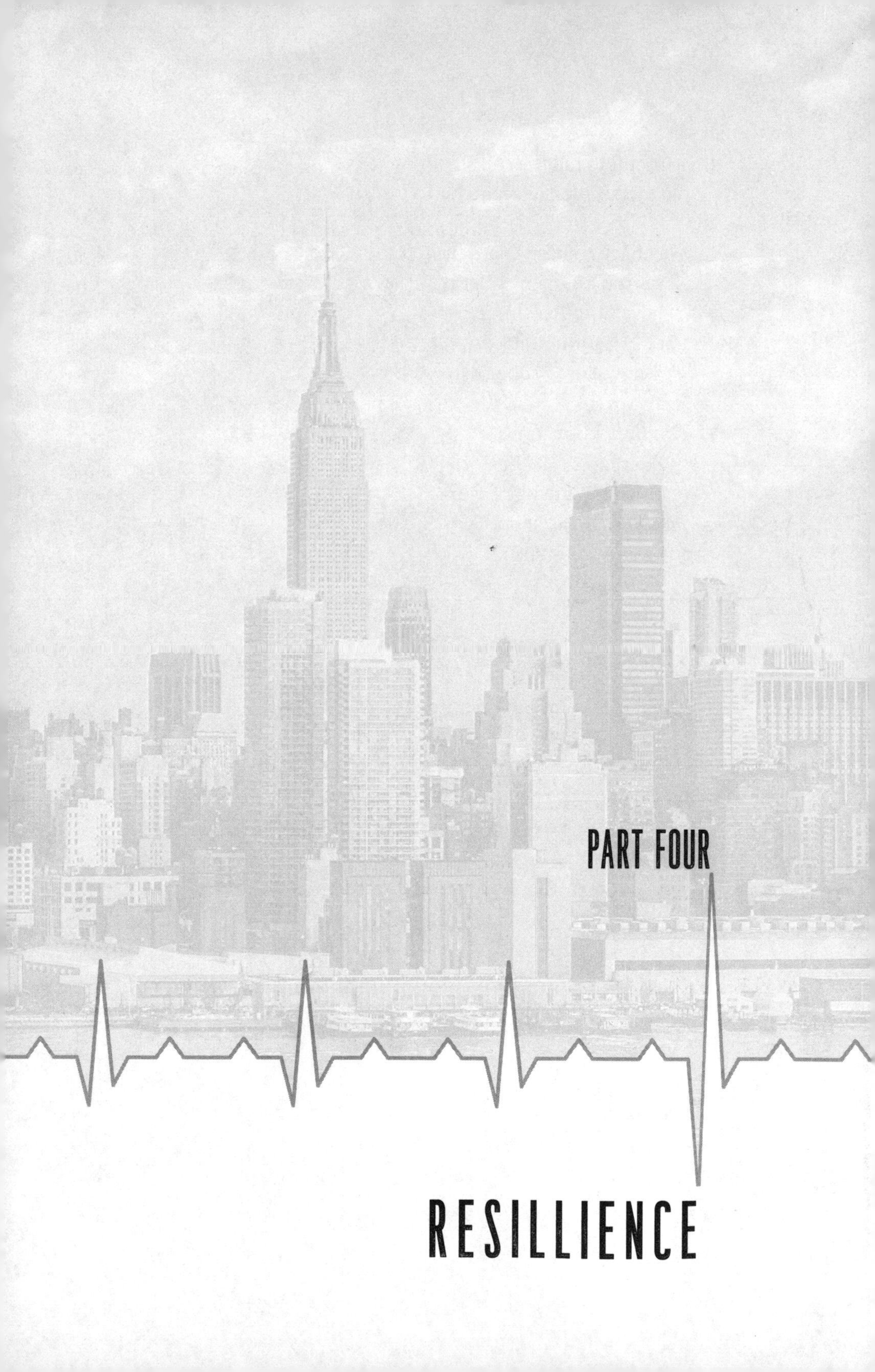

PART FOUR

RESILLIENCE

19

PANDEMIC BIRTHDAY

If COVID had been the street's main dish in springtime, by June the virus was plated with a generous helping of protests, many of which grew violent at nightfall. I'll leave it to medical anthropologists to write books about the connection between pandemics and mass demonstrations throughout history.

But briefly. As for the anatomy of the disaster, as far as coronavirus and protests went, around the world, tens of thousands of people took to the streets, seeking justice. From what? In America, systemic racism and police violence. In France, systemic racism and police violence. In Ireland, Italy, Spain, Hungary, the UK, systemic racism and police violence.

Variations on a theme. In Brazil, systemic racism, police violence, and the government's response, or lack of response, to the COVID outbreak. In far east Russia, falling living standards and the dismantlement of social safety nets. India, anti-Muslim government laws.

Iran saw protests the following month, in July, against the regime's ongoing human rights violations. In August, anti-Kremlin protestors flooded the streets in Russia. Chilean protestors had been in the streets back in May over food insecurity during the country's COVID lockdown. Ecuadorians had also protested in May, against economic inequality and government corruption, when the country became South America's worst-hit nation per capita with over 3,200 COVID deaths.

Here, those numbers were child's play. By the first of June, 98,536 people had died from COVID in the United States since the pandemic began—not including non-hospital deaths. Even mortality data that started including at-home suspected COVID deaths was thought to be grossly underestimated, as it failed to account for DOAs found by first responders.

Meanwhile, the media released stories, images, and videos capturing eruptions of civil unrest between protestors and police.

Violence against other first responders went underreported.

As EMTs and paramedics who were still working coronavirus, and now protests, many of us returned to our baseline state of invisibility. Gone were the days of applause and cowbells. These were nights of cop and protestor clashes. On the street, we were pitched into the middle of these events, and performed our duty to treat people injured on all sides of the line. At times, EMTs, paramedics, and firefighters were attacked for being of service. For wearing a uniform.

In the Bronx, people threw bricks at Ladder 37, shattering the rig's windows while firefighters were responding to a blaze. Crowds in Atlanta broke the windows of a fire apparatus while firefighters were extinguishing a restaurant fire. Ladder 23 in Cleveland was struck by projectiles on the way to a fire and went out of service due to a shattered window.

People threw rocks at Charlotte firefighters while they were attempting to perform a confined-space rescue to treat an injured protestor who'd fallen through a sidewalk grate. In Austin, crowds set fires, then tossed firecrackers under firetrucks while rescuers attempted to extinguish the blazes. A firefighter was attacked in Rochester when he approached a fire scene. Heartland Fire & Rescue's vehicles were set on fire in La Mesa, California. In Grand Rapids, crowds threw a firecracker or similar explosive toward a firefighter responding to a dumpster fire; the firefighter was knocked to the ground and was seen clutching his ears.

EMS work was indeed different at demonstrations. It was at times more dangerous than the work of other first responders, since the majority of EMTs and paramedics worked unarmed and unprotected. With few exceptions—rescuers trained in rapid care and extraction for terrorist attacks, mass shootings, et cetera—most EMTs and paramedics did not receive or wear ballistics vests, even though in urban environments we constantly responded to emergencies where patients carried firearms and other weapons. In New York City, lots of knives.

EMTs and paramedics were also attacked and targeted these punishing nights. At a demonstration in New York City, people threw bricks at an FDNY ambulance and dented the back. Denver Health's paramedic division reported numerous instances of attacks on ambulances, EMTs, and paramedics attempting to treat injured protestors during demonstrations. In Cleveland a crowd surrounded an EMS vehicle, striking it with multiple objects as one person jumped on top of it while an EMS supervisor was trying to reach a patient.

Violence flowed both ways.

Police officers nationwide inflicted bodily harm on street medics—a loose term for a medical professional with an unknown level of training operating on the street, or simply a layperson trained in first aid. A Marine veteran who worked the COVID outbreak at Kings County, Brooklyn, piling hundreds of dead bodies into refrigerated morgue trucks, was beaten and kicked by NYPD officers one Saturday night while wearing his hospital ID. In another instance, a white male NYPD boss pinned down a white male street medic wearing the red cross insignia on his helmet at a protest, holding him down with a knee on his back and threatening to drown him in the milk he carried to treat tear-gassed protestors. "I'm a medic! I'm a medic!" he screamed during the recorded attack.

The mayor's line that the cops were "overwhelmingly acting appropriately" fell on deaf ears. The same could be said of the protestors being "overwhelmingly peaceful."

Because we co-responded to emergencies on the street as one interconnected, emotionally distressed family—fire, medical, and police—many front-line personnel expressed unity during protests while others called out the cops for being a bolt of racist lightning.

Emotions ran high.

White male firefighter on social media: "Thank you to our brothers [*and sisters, beep beep*] in blue for protecting us the entire night."

Black EMT: "They can't stop killing us, man. When's it going to stop?"

Puerto Rican firefighter, posting a photograph of Black Lives Matter painted in bold yellow letters across a Brooklyn street with a quote by Martin Luther King: "The time is always right to do what's right."

Snoop Dogg posted a meme that said, NO ONE EVER MADE A SONG CALLED "FUCK THE FIRE DEPARTMENT,"which I thought was pretty funny.

And also pretty uninformed (sorry, Snoop, I love your music). Black firefighters had to litigate their way into the FDNY, which, unlike the NYPD and EMS, both agencies stunningly diverse, was still a big fat bowl of macho-man milk.

The firefighting side of the FDNY was the least diverse civil service department in New York, wildly out of synch with the city's demographics. Fire was cited in media outlets as 70 percent white, 8 percent Black. Diversity in the FDNY came from its terribly paid, devalued EMTs and paramedics, who were largely women and people of color. Many male EMS workers joined the department through EMS so they could advance to becoming firefighters, creating a constant shortage of EMS workers.

Several associations within the FDNY that represent Black, brown, Asian, and women firefighters actively participated in BLM protests. "Over the past 50 years, Black men and women firefighters and paramedics have endured and fought against institutionalized government systems that perpetrate racism, discrimination, harassment, hostile work environments, or retaliation in fire departments throughout this country," Gary Tinney, northeast regional director for the International Association of Black Professional Firefighters, said in a June 7, 2020, *Daily News* piece. "Our work continues."

White supremacy was alive and well in the FDNY, and if you don't believe me, just ask a Black New York City firefighter—if you can find one.

We're all in this together?

After several violent, fire-filled nights here in "looted" New York City—*looter* according to who, James Baldwin would ask, pointing out that America had been looting Black people of cash, jobs, dignity, respect, and humanity for centuries—the mayor announced a citywide curfew to try to curb civil unrest.

In early June, state politicians steered protesting, otherwise locked-down New York City toward cautiously reopening, calling it a "triumphant" moment and congratulating New Yorkers for flattening the COVID curve and being "smart."

On the street, I did not feel triumphant.

One night, when Austin and I were on the bus, a pickup truck roared by with two huge Confederate flags billowing in the wind. I'd never seen Confederate flags in over twenty years of living in New York City. Were these people locals? That June I saw an awful lot of out-of-town plates—Georgia, North and South Carolina—on cars speeding around the city during the protests. My sense was that it was both: New Yorkers mixed with white alt-right folks who came here to co-opt the BLM movement and start what the kids called "drama."

As for New Yorkers being smart, that was not my first observation in June.

One evening, Austin and I worked standby at an event in Queens. The son of a volunteer EMS chief was graduating from middle school, and the chief wanted a procession of ambulances to whoop and beep around the block. As EMTs, we did these sorts of events for other agencies and for the community often. Funerals. Graduations. Fundraisers. Touch-a-truck events, where we showed little kids around the ambulance and introduced them to medical equipment, so in the event of an emergency they wouldn't be frightened. The chief's son was apparently having a tough year and needed cheering up.

"You know who else is having a tough year?" Austin said as she drove us to Queens on expressways jammed with traffic.

"Everyone," I said. "Everyone is having a tough year."

When we got to Queens, we parked alongside six or seven other ambulances in front of the school. We greeted the EMS chief, a big, chipper white guy in his fifties, I'd guess, with a very strong handshake. He thanked us profusely for coming all the way from Brooklyn.

We told him we were happy to help out. Anything for the kiddos. I felt awful for children who'd been locked inside for long, touchless months, and even more awful for their trapped parents.

While we waited to partake in the fanfare, I pulled a pair of scissors out of my backpack and handed them to Austin. I asked her to check the back of my hair, to make sure it was straight. I'd cut it myself, like many quarantined New Yorkers. It wasn't my best idea, but compared to being on the street, it wasn't my worst one, either.

"Wifey, it looks even!" Austin said, clipping a strand. "You did a great job!"

I wouldn't go that far, but it wasn't horrible. Also, who cared what my hair looked like? I hadn't been on a date in nine months. Austin told me she liked the T-shirt I was wearing under my uniform, which said STOP SCREAMING, I'M SCARED TOO!

Half an hour later we hit the lights and brought up the rear of the parade of ambulances that circled the school. The leafy blocks had pretty, fenced-in houses. Queens. I never understood Queens, personally. Queens eluded me. I couldn't imagine living in a house in New York City.

To my surprise, families came outside and whistled and clapped for us. I was shocked by how uplifted I felt to see and hear people's appreciation. I was so moved. Austin was, too. It occurred to me that we'd been through a hell of a lot these last few months, and due to the trashed state of the world, it had really sucked to be so quickly forgotten and cast aside. The fact that these people, families in Queens, came out of their homes just to wave to us and cheer—it moved me in a way I found impossible to communicate. I was speechless in a good way, the best way. I was unraveled with gratitude.

Now I understood, retrospectively, why that housing cop I'd told did a great job applying a tourniquet to our shooting victim had been so profoundly grateful when I told him he'd saved that guy's life. No one ever did that. No one said something as simple and kind as *Thank you.*

Helping the middle school kid who was having a hard time wound up helping me. I beeped the air horn and Austin laughed.

"Wifey, you love the air horn."

Wifey did. I was in this for the air horn.

But soon this "triumphant," "New York smart" situation ended.

Listen to this.

Back in Brooklyn sometime later, when Austin and I rounded the corner to return to base, we saw our block was crammed with double-parked cars, many of them luxury vehicles. Well-heeled white couples in business formal, women in below-the-knee skirts and blazered men, were headed toward a corner building where the top-story windows were bathed in purple light and smoke from what appeared to be a smoke machine wafted outside, with disco music thrumming.

Oh? What was this? A party? During lockdown? Indoors? Please tell me this was not happening.

In front of our garage, we were unpleasantly surprised to find a car parked beneath a sign that said NO PARKING. AMBULANCES ONLY. This happened constantly. Reportedly, our landlord wouldn't let us paint the garage or sidewalk red to make it clear this was an active driveway.

Usually when this happened, we waited around for a while, hoping whoever had parked illegally would appear. We canvassed the block, asking whoever was in sight if the car belonged to them. If that failed, we called one of the precincts in our area or texted cops we knew and asked them to send someone over to write a ticket, which had to get done in order for us to advance to the next step, call a tow truck. Often, this rigmarole took hours. Now, with the cops tied up at the protests, it could take half the night.

It wasn't just any car blocking our garage. It was a BMW with no license plates. No license plates typically meant the driver was up to no good.

I walked over to the restaurant on the corner and asked the owners sitting inside if they or any of their patrons had perhaps accidentally blocked our garage? The owners were a couple. They said they had the same problem tonight, that there was a party going on at the other end of the block.

A party. At a "triumphant" moment in time. When New York City was still on lockdown, and gatherings of ten or more people were forbidden. New York smart, alright.

Back at the garage I relayed the message to Austin, and together we lumbered down the block, toward the disco music and fake smoke. We just wanted to go home.

As we approached the corner a goateed white guy sitting on the stoop of his building looked at us and said, "Oh, thank God!"

"We're not cops," I said dismally.

From the front people often mistook us for police, which these troubled days was more hazardous than usual. We walked up to a muscular security guard manning the door.

I said, "Hi, sir. Is there a party going on here?"

He shrugged. "I don't know anything about any party."

"Interesting. Because it sure looks like there's a party."

"I don't know anything about it," he said, grinning. He gripped a tiny flashlight, the kind you shine on driver's licenses to check a person's age. He was cute, the security guard. He had a playful, boyish demeanor, and his cheeks were dimpled. I wanted to slap him. More couples strolled toward the building where the party wasn't happening.

"Here's the thing," I said to the guard. "A BMW with no license plates is blocking our garage so we can't park our ambulance, so we're going to have it towed. And my guess is that whoever owns this nice, unmarked luxury vehicle may be upstairs at this party you don't know anything about, so we just wanted to give you a chance to tell them to come down and move their car before we have it towed."

Just then, a second security guard poked his bald head outside and began transmitting a message over a handheld radio. "I think it belongs to someone upstairs."

"That would be our guess as well. They have ten minutes to move it," I said, and now I felt like a cop. I was acting like one.

As we walked away, the goateed guy on the stoop said, "Is this even legal, what they're doing? Having a party right now?"

Still walking, I said, "No."

"Man, this is bullshit! I'm going to call the cops!"

"You can call the cops," I said, "but they're a little busy at the moment."

"I don't care! I'm calling 911 right now!"

I didn't care, either. I was exhausted and miserable. Outside the garage, Austin and I stood on the sidewalk, shaking our heads at the situation, thinking of our dead patients and the unmasked, unlocked states upticking with COVID, waiting for the partygoer who owned the BMW to appear and move his car, so we could park and go home.

After ten or so minutes a short, slender white man came dashing down street, wearing a crisp blue dress shirt and slacks.

"Sorry, sorry!" he said, scrambling through his pockets.

I stepped toward the vehicle. "Is this your BMW? With no license plates?"

He pulled keys out of his pockets and jangled them in the air. "No, it's not mine. I don't know whose it is, but I have the keys to it."

How convenient. New Yorkers. So tough and smart. So cooperative. What a triumphant moment.

After he sped off, Austin looked up at me and said, "This is the kind of thing that makes you hate people."

"Yeah," I said, kicking the curb. "We're all going to die."

Two days later, after seventy-eight days of stay-at-home orders and a higher death toll than all but six countries, New York City was slated to enter Phase One of reopening. Just a few more tortured days of isolation until we could gather outside in small, masked, socially distanced numbers. COVID deaths were down, they said.

But were they? Who counted?

Off the ambulance, life wasn't exactly a day at Riis Beach. Every time I talked to Felice or Natalie, to any of my friends, Black, brown, or white, queer or straight, they told me they'd been sobbing, heartbroken by the state of the world and plagued with a feeling that they weren't doing enough to help, that this pandemic of COVID dovetailing with the pandemic of racism was relentless, endless. I felt that way, too. I felt gutted.

June was Felice's and Natalie's birthday month, those tricky Geminis. I offered to bake them birthday cakes. Sweets in the Streets was out of service. My beloved cofounder and partner, Nina, was still stuck at home, miserable. But I could bake. Birthday cakes to fight racism, that's what I offered. No idea why more people didn't think of this as a solution for systemic change.

Felice didn't want my homemade cake. "But I'd love an ice-cream cake from Carvel," she said. "The one with vanilla on top and chocolate on the bottom and a cookie crust layer."

"Done."

"Really, sis? You'll get me my favorite cake?"

"Are you kidding? For my sister's birthday? In a pandemic? When everyone is dying of COVID and a cop just strangled a Black man to death for eight minutes? Yes. I'm buying your cheap, store-bought cake. And I'll deliver it to your door."

Felice wept, then said, "Sister, I'm so excited. I love that cake. And we'll get to see each other. I haven't seen you in months. I don't know how I'd get through this without you. You're my fire escape."

I thanked her and told her she was my fire escape, too. Felice and I had recently listened to a beautiful podcast by one of our favorite writers, a poet and novelist named Ocean Vuong. In it, he talked about how the question "How are you?" had become meaningless, because people didn't tell you how they really felt. What suffering people needed was an emotional fire escape. Someone they could talk to openly, who could listen and pull them out of the wreckage.

I didn't know how I'd get through this, through anything, without Felice. Or Ylfa. Ylfa carried me through the pandemic, the summer, 9/11. She carried Mike, too. He was struggling.

Natalie didn't want my homemade cake, either. She wanted my salty honey pie. That was quite popular in my circle of friends. Lexi nicknamed herself after it, calling herself Salty Honey. I told Natalie I'd bake that pie for her and drive it to her house, after I dropped off Felice's cake. I hadn't seen any of my non-uniformed friends in months, and I missed them terribly.

Scores of my Black friends were now struggling with the same thing I'd dealt with during COVID: their phones were blowing up. Suddenly every white person they'd ever glanced at, now forced into awareness that Black people had been suffering relentlessly for four hundred years, started calling them constantly, to check on them, saying things like "I see you."

I felt bad for them. I told them blocking people had helped me a lot when healthcare heroes were trending and everyone discovered EMS workers existed. I was concerned white America would forget and abandon them and their pain and move on to another disaster quickly. The presidential election was coming up.

Around this time I watched comedian Dave Chappelle's *8:46*, in which he discussed, among other things, the killing of George Floyd. He ended the show with the aside that white women should shut the fuck up. So I did that, too.

I called Felice and said, "I'm going to take Dave Chappelle's suggestion and shut the fuck up."

She said, "I think that's a solid position."

As far as what the cops were thinking went, which people kept calling and asking me about like I was some sort of cop whisperer, on the street police officers switched to twelve-hour shifts.

That June I wasn't on good terms with Larry or Nick, who went into what I could only describe as "cop mode."

Police officers were on a lot of e-mail lists, Nick included. He took this opportunity to blast out many e-mails. Most of them contained articles he knew flew in the face of everything I believed. He gave no shit. COVID was over, as far as the historical moment was concerned. Policing took the wheel.

One of his e-mails included a link to a *Wall Street Journal* op-ed titled THE MYTH OF SYSTEMIC POLICE RACISM. So that's where he stood. It was penned by a secular conservative commentator, a white woman who, during the pandemic, publicly articulated her position that the coronavirus was no deadlier than the flu, calling shelter-in-place policies "unbridled panic."

Having seen dying COVID patients close up, gasping for air, and having heard my Black friends' stories and tears for twenty years, Nick's e-mails made me feel angry and hopeless. I couldn't even look at his messages in my inbox. Deleted. Marked as spam.

Larry's lungs still hadn't recovered from COVID, so he was on restricted duty inside the precinct. When he texted, he mostly sent links to various police-reform Senate bills he wanted me to reject. "Vote Nay and pass it on!" He didn't think all cops should be punished for "the sickening actions of the asshole cop in Minnesota."

After receiving half a dozen Senate-related texts, I told him to stop sending me police-reform bills. I reminded him Mike was sick, people I loved were decimated, the world was on fire, and I was exhausted. Then I asked how he felt.

In a crisis, thoughts were like ribs inside an arrested patient. You had to break them to get to the heart.

"Don't tell me what you think," I told Larry. "Tell me how you feel."

"I'm not sleeping at all," he said, "and my anxiety levels are through the roof. I haven't seen my family in two weeks because we're on mandated twelve-hour shifts. I see them briefly in the morning when I get home and before I collapse in bed at night before coming back to this hell. I'm sorry I haven't checked on you. I know you're on the front lines, too. And I know we disagree about politics. But please know that I love you and I worry about you. I think about you all the time and know we've all been through hell these last few months on the street. And I'm not the most emotionally available person on the planet, but I'm working on it. I'm sorry to hear about Mike. Poor guy has been struggling for a long time with this unfair disease. My prayers are with him. My prayers are with you, for strength and resilience."

Resilience. I loved that word.

One June afternoon, out of the blue, I heard from Rafael, the detective I'd dated several years back. The pandemic did that. Brought all the exes back, a marching band of sad trombones.

"Well, well, well," I said when he called. "The last ex to straggle back."

He laughed and said, "That's not why I'm calling."

Oh?

Rafael had a personal matter he wanted to talk through. He also wanted to know how it had been on the street, as he'd been injured and off duty for over six months. How strange, that he'd been the one who'd helped me get onto the street, back when I was a regular person. And now I was on the street, and he was at home. I gave him the long, sad story.

"One of my coworkers said it was worse than 9/11," he said.

"Yeah, it was. Cops got stuck with all the DOAs. Thousands of dead bodies. They're all having nightmares. They'll retire."

We talked and squabbled for a long time. About racism and policing. Rafael never denied racism, or racist policing. He knew both existed, he'd experienced it personally.

"You think people at Ralph Lauren don't look at me funny when I walk in a store?" he said. He grew up in a Hispanic neighborhood with mostly white cops. "You think the cops didn't stop me and jiggle my balls and search me for drugs when I was a kid?"

The phrase "jiggle my balls" really stayed with me.

At the same time, Raphael said, he believed the BLM movement was the biggest scam in town, that it filled the pockets of white politicians, Democrats, and did nothing to help Black people, especially poor Black people. He also believed the reason he became a detective and didn't wind up on drugs like other people he grew up with was because of his family. His family taught him to respect the police, so that's what he did.

I disagreed with both of his arguments, and we went back and forth for a bit. I railed against him about Trump, and what it felt like to work a mass-casualty incident he minimized and sold as a hoax, and to have had cancer and been unable to get health insurance because of my "preexisting condition," and how I didn't come from a bang-up family like he did, and that respect argument he used was dangerous, the same logic used against rape victims that went, "If you hadn't worn that short skirt, you wouldn't have been attacked." It freighted victims with blame.

Then we came to some agreements that surprised me.

Universal healthcare, for one. We both agreed it was humane and necessary. And that higher education should be free, and people shouldn't graduate college with $80,000 of debt for an English degree. That cops shouldn't be wasting their time harassing young Black kids for stupid shit like jumping turnstiles and smoking weed and riding their bikes on the sidewalk. That you couldn't pretend brutal cops didn't exist, or that it was just a few bad apples. We both knew it was a bad-apple orchard, and no one did anything about it. No one wanted to be a rat. And no one was surprised when the guys who snapped and murdered someone broke headlines.

"*Eight. Minutes*," Rafael said with disgust.

I loved him, Rafael. I don't remember if we said that when we hung up, or ever, but that's how I felt. We never fell in love when we dated. I found his politics dangerous and repulsive, and he found mine equally idiotic and noxious. But we respected and valued and trusted one another, and in that way, as first responders, people who worked on the street, I loved him for sure.

All through June, Ylfa and I were in touch with Mike every day. His mouth was now riddled with sores from chemo, and tumors had infested his spine, sending him into agony and compromising his ability to sleep and walk. He was in enough pain to warrant a trip to the hospital, but there was no way he was checking himself in. "If I go to the ER it's going to be palliative care from then on," he told us one night on Zoom. "I'm not there yet."

What a roller coaster we were on, trying to support him from afar, unable to accompany him to doctor's appointments or give him a hug. Hearing him in so much pain soured my days.

It was hard to sleep, as fireworks burst through the night. For hours I trolled Zillow, looking at faraway houses I couldn't afford, dreaming of places I might move. Vermont? New Hampshire? Maine? I didn't know anyone in those states.

Felice was on Zillow, too. We considered leaving New York. Felice rejected the aforementioned geographic suggestions. "I'm not trying to be the only Black person in town," she said. Should she move south, to New Orleans? Nashville? Somewhere musical and warm? Abroad, to a Black island? St. Lucia? Martinique? We still had our jobs, thank God, unlike so many people. We toyed with the idea of taking a *Thelma & Louise* exploratory road trip to examine our options in real life, except in the end we probably wouldn't drive our car off a cliff.

The news that summer was hideous. Social media, too. I couldn't take it. Tommy, either.

"I don't have all the answers," he said. "Not by a long shot. I'm genuinely trying to understand. But at least I know there's more to the story than what the news shows. Fox News: all cops are perfect heroes. CNN: all cops are racist, white killers. OAN: global warming is a Chinese hoax. MSNBC: capitalism is worse than communism. It goes on and on. It's a goddamn menu. What would you like tonight? Anger or fear? Anger? Here's CNN. Bon appétit. I blame the media for inciting fear and hate."

"I hate the media right now."

"Hate."

"Social media is worse."

"I just take it off my phone."

Same.

Sleepless, firework-filled nights, I took shelter in a meaningless—meaningless—reality TV show called *Love Island*. Felice watched it, too. It had no plot. People sat around in bikinis and dated one another then abandoned each other for a hotter person who walked onscreen in a bikini. That was the show. I enjoyed it immensely. It was like having people over. I bought four bathing suits during the pandemic, probably triggered by all the time I spent on *Love Island*. That's what I said to Felice whenever she called: "I'm in Australia. I'm on *Love Island*."

"I'm also on *Love Island*," she said. "I'm in the UK."

"I can't understand anything they're saying with those accents."

"I watch it with subtitles."

I looked for *Love Island* on the street, too. Not the reality TV show. But I looked for moments of humanity, unity, love. I looked for things I'd never seen before or hadn't seen enough. And one night, I found some hope.

The next Sunday, mid-June, Nathan and I worked a Tour 3 together. On the way to base I drove past a gargantuan protest for Black Trans Lives outside the Brooklyn Museum. Holy shit, the crowd was impressive, and important. That year at least twenty-two transgender people had been killed just for being themselves, and their healthcare protections had been repealed *during Pride Month*. So despite the fact that it took me over an hour to get to base, I thought it was worth it.

When I walked into the crew room, I ran into Soo. She'd transported Kentaro to the hospital and he'd asked her about me. "Do you know Jennifer?" he'd said.

My husband! He remembered me! I loved being remembered! Being forgotten and left behind was my greatest fear. Half the time when I signed off on texts to first responders I loved, Tommy and Larry and Nick, that was my closer: "Don't forget me." "Never," they swore. The world had already forgotten us EMTs and paramedics. But Kentaro hadn't.

When Nathan came to base, he grabbed Barry, one of the young and relatively new EMTs. He dragged him outside and said they needed to talk. About what, I had no idea.

"Jen, come over here," Nathan said, wiggling his fingers.

Outside, Nathan gave Barry a fatherly lecture because he'd apparently transported a shooting victim to the ER without calling a note, and the nurse's eyes had practically popped out of her head when she asked Barry what was wrong with the patient and he'd said, "gunshot wound."

"You have to stop riding with new people," Nathan told him. "And you have to stop doing stupid shit if you want Jennifer to like you. I can only help you so much."

I said, "I like you, Barry. And who cares if I like you or not?"

Nathan said, "Jen. He cares. Right Barry? Don't you want Jennifer to like you?"

"Yeah," Barry said, staring at his boots.

"I like everyone," I said, then realizing that was blatantly untrue, I said, "Almost everyone. Why would I not like you?"

Barry looked up and said, timidly, in an injured voice, "You called me an asshole on speakerphone."

I sucked my teeth. Whoops. Now that he mentioned it, I faintly recalled that. Sounded very familiar. Barry had responded to one of our jobs a month or so back, an MVA, which was dumb of him. We were on the same team. We hadn't called for another unit.

"You did an asshole thing," I said. "But you are not an asshole."

I liked Barry. He was young and loved to work on the truck and learn. What more do you want in an EMT? Nathan squeezed Barry's shoulders and we parted and started our tour. When I called dispatch, they advised us that one of the hospitals in our area was on diversion.

"For what?" I asked. Sometimes one or two hospitals went on diversion for a particular call type. Almost always, 99 percent of the time, hospitals diverted EDPs or pediatric EDPs, the patients who, as I mentioned, ERs didn't have the capacity to handle and, frankly, didn't want. That evening the dispatcher said one hospital wasn't taking *any* patients because of protestors surrounding it. It was a safety-net hospital. It treated the poorest, Blackest, brownest, oldest New Yorkers devoured by COVID. And now these sick people couldn't get treated there because of the protests. This disturbed me.

Hours into our tour, I noticed Nathan hadn't said much. He seemed down. I asked if everything was alright, and he said he was fine. Just tired. And he wanted a serious run.

I didn't care what kind of job we went on. I just wanted to work. I was restless. And I was driving. For once, Nathan let me drive.

At one point, his paramedic pals sent him a video he showed me, of protestors throwing trash cans and bottles at a police vehicle, breaking its windows. The cops backed up and fled. The scene looked chaotic and violent. It did not look "mostly peaceful." There were plenty of videos circulating on social media showcasing the reverse, police attacking protestors.

Later that night, things dramatically improved on the truck. More than improved. I struck EMT gold.

At twenty-two hundred hours, a confirmed arrest flew over the air. Before the dispatcher finished sending the full address, Nathan was on the radio, saying we were 63, headed to the job.

"Here we go, here we go, here we go!" he said. "Jen! Time for your first arrest!"

At last! Happy birthday to me! I was a Taurus, my birthday wasn't in June, but tonight was my night!

The arrest was in the projects in Red Hook. I battered Nathan with questions as I drove. "Do you want me to do compressions or bag? Should I grab the scoop and the stretcher? How many other units will be there?"

"Jen, relax. And stop asking me so many questions, just drive. And go faster. You're decelerating. You're driving like five miles an hour."

Was I? I stopped talking and drove. That was hard. I was a nervous talker. I got anxious and I talked. My heart pounded, but in the good way. It was excitement rather than fear. I was ready! Eager to be real. Three fucking years without an arrest!

We got to the projects and parked next to two hospital ambulances, an FDNY SUV, and a fire rig. Last responders. Womp womp.

I hopped off the ambulance and grabbed the tech bag. Just as I closed and locked the door, I realized I'd forgotten to grab goggles and gowns. I'd completely forgotten about COVID. What's that? Never heard of it.

"Do you have PPE?" I shouted at Nathan as he trotted away.

"No! Grab some for me!"

Grab some for me. I was his secretary. I was his mother. If I missed this arrest because Nathan forgot PPE and treated me like his bag boy, he'd never hear the end of it.

After I grabbed our stuff and looked around for my partner—darkness. Nathan was in the wind. Hey, where'd did he go? I swiveled around and saw no sign of him at all.

Bastard! Some kids looked at me like the lost, emaciated white lady I was. Did my partner just abandon me on scene? I didn't think to walk up to the parked fire engine and ask the chauffer rotting behind the wheel to point me in the right direction. I just wandered around the projects lost and alone, saying hello to people until I stumbled upon some housing cops standing outside a building, yucking it up. I asked them if this was the arrest, and they nodded and led me inside and upstairs, to an apartment on the second floor.

Door was open. I stepped inside and set the bulging, green tech bag on a table by the entryway, where an FDNY lieutenant with silver hair nodded approvingly at me.

Loved that. Loved feeling like I belonged. *Hero's here everyone, hello, good evening, here to save a life.*

I glanced in the living room. A fleet of gowned, masked, gloved first responders was hard at work. They hovered over a bare-chested man lying dead on the floor. A sweating EMT knelt beside him, doing chest compressions, while a woman EMT bagged the patient, and Nathan's pals, the ginger-haired paramedics, prepared to intubate. Nathan stood among the rescuers with his hands on his hips looking down at the patient. Glancing at the scene in progress in the living room took a millisecond, but it felt like an hour-long movie.

In the entryway, I opened the sealed PPE bag. The FDNY lieutenant said to me, in the tone of a man asking a woman to dance at a ball, "Do you need help with your gown?"

"Why, yes," I said, slipping my arms in the paper sleeves.

"I never met a Murphy I didn't like."

"I was *designed* to work in this field."

He snickered and stood behind me, tying my gown at the waist and neck. I adored him for helping me. So loving. Looking over my shoulder at him as he finished tying my gown, I said, under my breath, “This is every woman’s dream.”

He snorted, laughing.

Soon I was in the sweltering living room, standing beside Nathan. Ready! I could feel my uniform filling with sweat. The mask and goggles—it was like having a wet cat on my face. The rescuer on the floor had switched out. Now a firefighter was sweating out compressions. Not terribly well, I might add. He wasn’t pushing hard or fast enough on the patient’s chest to the beat of “Staying Alive,” which they taught us in EMT school. Plus, his elbows were bent. I may have never done CPR myself, but I’d practiced on an awful lot of dummies, so I felt justified making a mental note of his mistakes.

Looking around at my colleagues, I noticed one EMT, a young girl with frizzy brown hair, staring blankly at the patient. I knew that look, that face. Those eyes like blown tires. She was in shock. This was her first arrest for sure. Possibly her first day on the job. She was a frozen ice pop. I used to be her once.

That’s when Nathan did it. He stepped forward, tapped the firefighter doing CPR on the shoulder, and made a terribly loud announcement in the otherwise silent room.

“Hey, buddy, let my partner switch in and do compressions next, when you get tired—she could use the experience.”

My eyelids came down. *She could use the experience.* Thanks for the public service announcement. I vowed to scream at him later.

Soon the heaving firefighter rose to his feet, and I knelt. My turn to pray.

My first round of compressions went OK, I guessed. It took some getting used to, the feeling of the patient’s ribs snapping beneath my hands, because of my hands.

You have to break the ribs to get to the heart.

“Jen, press harder,” Nathan said. He was my professor—of humiliation.

I did two or so minutes of CPR then another EMT switched in and I bagged the now-intubated patient. The medics administered another shot of epi. So far, no luck. The patient wasn’t coming back. The room was hushed and quiet. All you could hear was the sound of medics rustling open packets of medicine, and the whoosh of us breathing beneath our masks.

That's what I always found most touching about serious emergencies. The silence. How the noise of the world fell away, and everyone worked sacredly, silently, and together, breathing and moving and working as if we were all one.

At one point, someone asked the patient's age. Nathan walked over to an unopened birthday cake sitting on a table and said, sixty-five.

Oh, no. Did the patient just have a birthday?

I'd seen the cake when I first walked in but hadn't thought anything of it. Sixty-five was so young. I wanted our guy to come back to life.

After another ten or so minutes, I switched back in to do compressions. Nathan stood across from me, holding an IV bag, squeezing it so the medicine would flow through, into the patient's veins. My second round was much better.

"Good CPR! Good CPR!" the medics said, looking at their EKG machine.

"Thank you!"

I didn't expect to receive compliments at my first arrest. I loved compliments. Give me a compliment and I thrived. The lieutenant and firefighters left. There were two medics and two EMTs and an FDNY conditions boss on scene, so she let them go. Because 911 call volumes were now lower, ERs were calmer, and paramedics were available, the medics took as much time as they needed to on scene to try to revive arrested patients. Low CPR survival rates and statistics don't matter to first responders. What matters is that we get to try as hard as we humanly can, for as long as we can, to save lives.

Tonight more time passed, and I lost hope. The paramedics called the medical director. After forty-five minutes or so, they pronounced and wrote down the time.

All of us stood in sweat-drenched silence, breathing heavily, around the body we couldn't bring back to life. The shattered-looking EMT stared at the floor. She was traumatized for sure, but I was feeling steady, considering. Arrested patients were dead, as everyone reminded me, so no emotional connection between me and the patient, the patient and anyone, had been established.

Four of us lifted the body onto the couch. Then we covered it with a sheet, carefully and slowly, to make sure the patient looked dignified.

I lowered my head and said a little prayer for our patient, wherever his spirit had gone.

Quietly, saying nothing, we packed up our things. And quietly, with heads bowed, we stumbled outside. The cops came inside as we left, to stand guard over the body.

Outdoors, the nighttime air was cool and magnificent. All of us ripped off our masks and goggles and trashed our gowns and gloves in a big red bag. I rubbed my eyes, which were stinging from sweat.

One of the medics said to Nathan, "Thanks for coming. Who's your partner who's never had an arrest?"

"That's me!" I said. "The one you said did good CPR!"

"Oh, that's you?"

What was I, forgettable? Get it together, guy. The medic had just seen me recently at an anaphylactic shock, where Nathan had announced that I'd never worked an arrest. No one in EMS remembered anything. It was too much to process. The patients, first responders, COVID, protests, peace, violence, life and death, and death, and death. It seemed never-ending.

"Hey," I said to them. "Was that other woman new?"

"Yeah, she doesn't work 911," the medic said. "I think she works transport."

"She looked traumatized."

"That was definitely her first arrest. Probably her first dead body, too."

Rough. No happy birthday for her. Or for the patient.

I went back to the ambulance and sat beneath the overhead light, typing up the patient's chart for a long time while Nathan stood around and fraternized with the conditions boss and the medics. He returned to me twenty or so minutes later and started the truck.

"Jen, congratulations," he said, pulling into the street, heading back to base. "You had your first arrest."

"Yes," I said. "We did good. Thanks for helping me. And thank you for telling the entire fucking room I could *use the experience*."

Nathan balked. "Jen! I'm telling you, no one cares."

"Next time, why don't you get on a megaphone and stand on the couch. And thanks for abandoning me on the way to the job while I got all our PPE, since you forgot it."

"Oh, yeah. I forgot mine. I just grabbed some from the medics."

"I was walking around like a missing child."

"I'm sorry!"

"Abandonment is an actual crime, you know. It's illegal."

An hour or so later, before we left base, Nathan apologized for being in a strange mood that night. He told me his close friend's father who'd been sick with COVID had been taken off a ventilator and died earlier that day. Nathan knew the guy well. That's why he was quiet that night. And the arrest didn't help. Losing the patient.

I felt awful.

"Why didn't you tell me that earlier? I was so hard on you tonight. I would have been so much nicer. I'm so sorry, honey."

Nathan took off his hat. "It's OK. It's sad, but it's OK."

Driving home later, I felt horrible for roughhousing with Nathan. All those hours on the truck, teasing him for this or that thing, and that whole time he'd been grieving. What a time we were living in. Everyone registering so much sorrow. Near constant, the feeling of loss.

When I got home, I was glad to have worked my first arrest, satisfied as a first responder, even though we'd lost the patient. But I was disappointed in myself, too. I regretted not being kinder to Nathan. He was such a sweet guy. And he didn't need me needling him all night.

I tried to hold that in my heart moving forward, through all the rage and hate exploding in the world. The fact that you never really knew what people were going through at any given moment, what they were carrying inside them. You only knew that life in 2020 was brutal, precious, and very short.

I knew I wouldn't stew or maybe even remember that particular patient in the better years of the future. But I'd remember his age. Sixty-five. Written in frosting on his uneaten birthday cake. And I'd remember how rough I'd been with Nathan at a time when he needed tenderness.

A few days later, it was Felice's birthday. I needed to see and celebrate my sister.

I showed up at her door in a mask with America's favorite cake in my hands the following Tuesday. She came downstairs naked-faced and threw her arms around me.

"No!" I said, inching my head away from hers. "Sis, you can't hug me, I'm a dirty healthcare worker! I'm with COVID patients every tour!"

"I know but I can't not hug you," Felice said, stepping away. "I forgot my mask upstairs."

Then I stepped six or eight or ten feet back and we stood on the sidewalk for a long time and talked about everything, everything.

I missed my sister. I was tired of not seeing my friends. I don't remember how long we stood there. A while. Driving away, to Natalie's house with her salty honey pie, seeing Felice grow smaller in my rearview mirror, my eyes glazed with tears.

Twenty minutes later, on a different Brooklyn street, Natalie appeared. She was masked. We didn't hug.

I handed her the bagged pie. "Happy birthday, my beautiful friend."

She thanked me, then we stood in the street for a while and talked. Natalie had been crying for days. Her cousin tried to talk to her father, a cop, about what was going on in the world as it concerned policing and Black America, but he couldn't hear it.

"They can't listen right now," I said.

Natalie didn't know what to do. "This is so bad. It's so bad, and it keeps getting worse."

"This is all we have," I said, waving my hands between her and myself, then fanning my arms out at the street, the pie, the sun shining above us. "This moment. This is it. You and me and a salty honey pie and a moment of sunshine together on the street in Brooklyn, and both of us healthy and alive. This is it."

"This is it."

"And it's a lot. I love you so much, and I'm so sorry for what you're going through."

Natalie's uncle had had a stroke, and he'd been hospitalized. Thankfully, he was stable and tested negative for COVID. But her aunt, the person Natalie was closest to in her life, the woman who raised her, and was like a mother, had stage four cancer and wasn't doing well. In August, a month and a half from this day, her uncle would get discharged and return home from the hospital. Her aunt would die at home, with Natalie at her side the entire time. When she passed away, Natalie bellowed out in agony and fell to the floor, and lay heaped there, sobbing. Her husband, Pete, scraped her off the floor and carried her to bed, then stayed with her. I loved him for that. Taking care of my girl.

This world.

I wasn't sure how much more we could take.

Then another Black man would be shot seven times in the back by police. Felice would lose a friend to cancer. I would deliver another Carvel cake to her door that said HAPPY BIRTHDAY on top, the smallest gesture to try to soften her grief. It just kept coming, tragedy on top of tragedy, a thousand-layer cake of pain for everyone on earth.

"Thank you so much for the pie," Natalie said that day on the street. "I'm going to eat the whole thing."

"It's the least I can do—literally."

Natalie laughed in my face. "Jen. You're on the ambulance in a pandemic. While your friend is dying of cancer. You're out in the streets saving lives. You could die, too. I'm so worried about you. I think about you every day. I think, 'Jen could die.'"

"Nah," I said, shaking off the suggestion.

"Jen," Natalie said. She was a lawyer, so she liked to win arguments.

"Alright, alright. But right now, today, both of us are alive."

"Yes. This is true."

"And this is all we have. A moment together. And a pic."

"This is all we have."

"And it's a lot. It's more than most people have right now."

"It's a lot."

20

IF THE WORLD WAS ENDING

In July I tapped out on fireworks. Snap, crackle, pop, all day and night. I got no sleep.

Auditorily terrorized New Yorkers who hadn't fled the city back in spring, when COVID blew up, now flooded 911 with noise complaints, creating a strain on the emergency call system.

In June, firework-related complaints increased 4,000 percent from the previous year. By the end of that month, fed-up Brooklyn borough president Eric Adams, a Black politician and former cop, urged people to stop calling 911 for "nonviolent acts" like noise complaints. Adams suggested people handle urban unpleasantries like noise neighbor to neighbor. Stop over-relying on the police, was his view. If you don't want cops, stop calling them. Take petty matters into your own hands. Manage your own life and neighborhood. Community policing.

In July, one woman followed Adam's advice. She walked over to some kids setting off illegal fireworks in her neighborhood and asked them to knock it off. They shot her eight times, so she was dead. After her murder, Adams spoke in the press and said her killers should be brought to justice.

But where was justice taking place? Courts weren't holding in-person sessions during COVID. Bail reform laws enacted in 2020 stopped jails from holding people on bail and probation. And jails and prisons released people because of coronavirus. So brought to justice where? What did justice even mean in the overlapping pandemics? What did anything?

Police did well financially after the protests in New York City. Overtime payments to cops quadrupled in the two weeks following civil unrest after the killing of George Floyd, with the city paying $115 million in police overtime.

Hundreds of cops handed in their papers over the summer. Some believed demoralized officers were quitting out of frustration. Others believed they quit in 2020 because they were financially incentivized to do so after working so much overtime. Their pensions were more valuable now, based on their "final average salary." The protests may have simply sped up the inevitable retirements of veteran cops who were a year or two away from leaving anyway. Regardless of why they quit, between June 29 and July 6, police retirement filings increased 411 percent from the same period in 2019. There were so many officers filing papers that pension fund appointments got backed up. The NYPD couldn't process the paperwork fast enough.

The last time cops quit in this big a wave was in the aftermath of 9/11, when they were treated, as one media article phrased it, as "unimpeachable national heroes."

Over the summer, murder in the city also increased.

Pandemic or no pandemic, crime always rose in the summertime.

In July, citywide shootings were up 177 percent from the previous year. Media sources like *The New York Times*, *Wall Street Journal*, and CNN ran dramatic headlines. 64 SHOT, 10 DEAD: SPIKE IN GUN VIOLENCE ALARMS AN ON-EDGE NYC. NEW YORK POLICE DEPARTMENT BRACES FOR SUMMER UPTICK IN CRIME. 1-YEAR-OLD KILLED, 3 INJURED IN SHOOTING NEAR NYC PLAYGROUND. Same thing across the nation. Homicide and violent crime were up in big cities run by Democrat and Republican mayors. Every time I opened Citizen in Brooklyn these days, it alerted me to nearby violent crimes. Two people shot dead. Three people killed. Man brandishing firearm 300 feet away from you. Would you like to record?

Why no, I would not.

Despite the rise in shootings, violent crime was still lower than peak levels seen in New York City in the eighties and nineties. As was true with understanding COVID, it would take criminologists years to analyze attributing factors to recent surges in crime. But that didn't stop the media from running a storm of headlines about murder or discourage politicians from offering theories on crime patterns that warranted years of analysis. Consider the source for these news articles. Data used in crime reporting was typically drawn from police departments.

Theories about spikes in homicide and violent crime circulated in the news varied: bad economy and poverty; notable increase in gun purchases in 2020; social displacement and people going stir-crazy from COVID lockdowns; protests over the police killings of George Floyd and others, with some suggesting cops were pulling back from their duties; bail reform laws; and increased community distrust of the police, among other opinions.

So that was New York in July. That was many major cities in July.

Regardless of political leanings, New York City was certainly experiencing a reversal in terms of poverty and crime from recent years. These problems never left New York City, of course. Politicians just swept them under the rug. "Cleaned up the city" so people who paid $15,000 in rent and shopped at Neiman Marcus didn't have to see overdosed heroin addicts and homeless people crumpled on the subway steps.

But first responders? Cops, firefighters, EMTs, and paramedics? We never had a rug. We saw those people every hour of every week of every tour every year. This wasn't a new world to us. Everyone who worked on the street faced violence and poverty in New York City nonstop. It was the rich who didn't have to deal with these "unpleasantries" anymore—not us.

So in a weird way, for me, it was refreshing to see everything laid out on the table. When things were on the table, we could look at them together, as a nation, rather than pretend they weren't there and dump them all on first responders.

Like cancer, death, terrorism, white supremacy, gun violence, wildfires, like every crisis, the COVID pandemic was a bullshit eliminator. People paying $15K in rent and spending ten bucks on grande soy lattes while half the city was sick and dying on the street without health insurance was bullshit. Many of those people left New York City. They fled. They ran for their fucking lives. And I didn't miss them. I hoped they enjoyed Vermont.

As for me, even at the height of my exasperation with fireworks and shootings, I was glad to be surrounded by my people, the reason I moved to New York City in the first place—New Yorkers. Immigrants and families and artists and weirdos and servicepeople. I was Irish. My family immigrated here from County Cork, Ireland, one of the original "shithole countries." That was how my Black neighbors referred to me whenever they saw me. Not as the white woman, which I was, but as "the Irish lady."

Everyone please call me that from now on. I'd love an Irish passport.

Felice often reminded me that when the COVID pandemic first kicked off, I said something along the lines of *Everyone is more themselves in the pandemic.*

It was true. The lonely were lonelier, the angry were angrier, and the cheaters were cheatier. The corpses of everyone's character defects floated to the surface of their personalities.

The same held true for the city, I thought. New York, New York, big city of dreams. Big city, big shadow. So also big city of shitty healthcare. And racist policing. And a homelessness problem. And a mental health crisis. Every person, city, and country has a shadow. The pandemic introduced us to our shadows.

I appreciated that.

But due to the fireworks and shootings, it was still way too loud for me to relax around here in July. I was tired and jumpy. I had to get out.

It was time for that *Thelma & Louise* road trip.

In early July, Felice and I discussed leaving town and agreed to pack up, hop in my car, and drive far, far away. We agreed on dates, we thought. Fourth of July—a firework nightmare. But then we realized our work schedules conflicted and we couldn't escape New York at the same time. I had to get out, with or without her.

"I'm coming to see you," I told my friend Rafa, who lived in Providence, Rhode Island.

I packed my things and loaded my car.

"What time are you leaving?" Jeremy asked me. "Have you eaten? Want to grab lunch?"

We grabbed lunch. The ramen spot we liked was open again, so we went there and sat masked and outside, in a quiet, pebbled garden. We slurped ramen and caught up.

Jeremy told me he grew up in a poor Black neighborhood he described as "basically, an open-air drug market." He felt he was biased against the police, because growing up, the only cops in his neighborhood, who were mostly white, were brutal. Whatever happened to someone between getting arrested and arriving at the precinct jail was off the books. Cops were known by name and by the ways in which they tuned people up before arriving at the precinct. So it was hard for him, he explained, to take in alternate narratives, like the one I mentioned, about people not realizing how much cops did for us as EMTs and paramedics. They protected us from patient violence.

"But they don't protect me!" Ellery had cried when we talked about this on a separate summer day, and sitting now with Jeremy, I could still hear the outraged despair in Ellery's voice ringing in my ears. "I know," I'd said to him. "I know."

What did we *do* about all this? Stop having police altogether? Even Bernie Sanders didn't go that far. Jeremy, either—at first.

"I respect detectives," he said. "If someone walked in here and shot you right now? Some of those blue people would come, but then they'd have to call detectives."

"That is correct."

"Basically, we need a bunch more people like you. I want you to be online making sure people don't shoot up schools."

"Yeah, because I track white dudes. Mass shooters are mostly white men. But the people I send intel to track everyone. After 9/11, that became the world."

"Fuck it, then," Jeremy said. "Burn it down. It gonna be rough for a while, but we've been there before. We've done that. We know how to do that."

My dentist said the same thing one day, when I went to get my teeth cleaned.

"Jen!" she said. "I'm so glad to see you. I've been so worried about you. I'm so glad you're OK. How're things on the street?"

"I've been worried about you, too. I'm so glad you're open again. I was afraid to come see you because I didn't want to infect you or your patients, but I haven't been sick or symptomatic for ages, and my teeth are dirty. The street is fucking crazy. The cops are done. They're cooked."

"They gotta change, Jen. It's going to be rough for a while, but we can do it. I grew up in Brooklyn when bullets were flying. I ran for my life. We can do it again. We know that life. We can go back to that if we need to. But they've got to change."

"They've got to change," I agreed.

My escape-the-pandemic trip to Rhode Island didn't go so hot.

First, I got stuck in ungodly traffic, since I left late in the afternoon on July 4 weekend. The three-hour drive from New York City to Providence took me over five hours. The sky opened up and gushed rain. Sheets of rain that slid down the windshield and made it impossible to see and stressful to be on the highway. In the fast lane I sat like a squatter, jammed bumper-to-bumper with what appeared to be half the vehicular world.

At least three times on my drive, a sad song came on the radio, "If the World Was Ending." The song answered the musical question with the refrain "You'd come over, right?" It was the quintessential 2020 pandemic song, playing all the time. In the car when it came on, I wept and thought about Mike. I tried to memorize the lyrics, so one day I could sing it to him.

When I got to Providence, I checked into my hotel room. It had a window that looked out on a parking lot. When I'd booked my hotel—which gave no discounts to first responders; I asked, then I hung up on the guy when he said no—I was told my room had a "river view."

It had a river, alright. A blue thread of river hiding behind a giant parking lot.

For three days, Rafa and I spent hours walking around outside in the sun, talking about everything. Rafa was one of the smartest, funniest people I knew, and we teased each other mercilessly, which was fun. At one point he tried to shame me for not knowing the name of some supposedly remarkable Rhode Island public figure made into a statue. Then I shamed him for not knowing who James Mattis was, getting him mixed up with James Comey. We talked about the fireworks, police, white supremacy, books, teaching, life during lockdown, friends, love, writing.

It was wonderful to be around Rafa, but because we were outside all day, we were in masks. And I hated being in masks for ten to twelve hours a day. I couldn't see Rafa's smile or hug him. It was almost worse being around my friends and not being able to see or do the most basic human gestures. Masks reminded me of COVID. And whenever we went out to eat, and sat outdoors on restaurant terraces, everywhere had virtual menus. Restaurant managers shot us in the forehead with digital temperature guns, and asked for our names and phone numbers, to contact trace us. All of this felt sad and terrible. There was clearly no escaping the pandemic.

Or work. In Providence, my phone blew up with a crisis. Now I was trapped in my soulless hotel room stuck on conference calls for hours. When I got back to New York City, my overriding feeling was, There is no escape.

* * *

That July, Mike's health took a nosedive after he received blasts of radiation to kill tumors in his back that were impairing his ability to walk. Swallowing became a problem. He lost his sense of taste. He coughed and complained of severe chest, throat, and esophagus pain. Difficulty breathing. GI issues.

"Maybe I caught something," he told me and Ylfa. "Some kind of virus."

Ylfa and I texted each other side-eye emojis.

COVID was exploding in Las Vegas, Nevada a hotspot. A few weeks before, out of loneliness, Mike had gone unmasked to a bar and let a bunch of people hug him. Ylfa screamed at him about that, as did I.

One day I came out and said it to Mike. Said his symptoms flagged to me as COVID. But who could be sure? He refused to get tested because if his COVID results came back positive, doctors would stop treating his cancer, and he'd be toast. He would also be toast, I thought but did not say, if he had COVID on top of stage four cancer.

Then one Sunday morning Ylfa and I woke up to news that Mike was going to the ER. He couldn't swallow and was in agonizing pain. He gave us his niece's number. After we got the news, I staggered around my apartment sobbing. I felt like our little makeshift family had been walking slowly down a steep, dreadful stairway toward death. Then suddenly someone pushed us to the bottom, where we lay in a stunned heap.

I wasn't ready for Mike to die. I panicked, thinking I needed to fly out to see him immediately. But traveling to Vegas in the pandemic was complicated. New York now required everyone traveling to a red-zone state to quarantine for two weeks upon returning home, contact-tracing people and fining them two thousand bucks if they broke their self-declared agreement to cooperate. At the same time, I knew these rules were a sham and cheese. No one was enforcing them.

One of my friends had told me a story about a guy who'd recently flown to COVID-infested Texas to pick up a rescued dog—a story with logic that made no sense to me, but anyway. After fetching the animal and flying back to New York City, the airline told passengers they had to stop at a medical desk upon disembarking at JFK and do the aforementioned things: quarantine, be contact traced. But no one was at the medical desk when the passengers deplaned, so they sailed straight back from COVID-infested Texas into supposedly doing-better New York City.

It was a joke. The numbers, tests, travel restrictions. I made frantic phone calls to friends, soliciting advice.

"Do *not* go to Vegas right now" was the resounding response.

But I wasn't sure I could live with myself if I didn't fly out to see Mike on what was rapidly appearing to be his deathbed. I wasn't afraid of catching COVID. I was exposed to it weekly on the ambulance. But I was worried about infecting him. If there was any chance whatsoever that I could give him the virus, and he died of COVID, I wouldn't be able to forgive myself. Then again, his behavior had been so relaxed in regard to COVID that it wasn't as if I presented the only risk.

I had no idea what to do. Just thinking about going to Vegas accelerated my pulse. The timing could not have been worse.

Recently, my day job had become a nightmare. My phone rang nonstop with clients in some kind of BLM crises. This person at one point called a Black person a racist slur, and someone had recorded the interaction on video and posted it on the Internet, and now said person was receiving death threats. Using an alias, someone had posted a comment on a news article stating we should bring back slavery, and the alias linked to the employee of a school, the school had been advised and interviewed the employee, who denied involvement, and now they wanted to see if I could prove who'd made the racial slur and/or if there was any evidence online that the employee was racist.

Summarily, crisis clients across sectors were experiencing the Great White Awakening, coming to realize racism was historical and real, and my phone became a Baskin-Robbins bucket of BLM-related cries for help, thirty-one flavors of white pain.

Between cops sending me Senate bills to nay, articles about "the myth of racist policing," and affluent white clients waking up to pervasive injustices the Black community had been suffering for hundreds of years, I started for the first time since the pandemic commenced to feel hopeless.

"Jen," Nathan said when I warned him of my rocky emotional state on the way to base. "Are you sure you want to ride today? We can bang out."

I was sure. It was one small thing I could do. Get out of the house. Get on the ambulance. Take my mind off Mike, myself, my job, the warring, heartbroken world. As I drove, I kept whispering the poetic words of Rainer

Maria Rilke to myself: "Let everything happen to you: beauty and terror. / Just keep going. No feeling is final. / Don't let yourself lose me."

By *me* I think he meant God.

As I was gearing up in the crew room, grabbing keys to the truck, radios, and a run sheet, one of our new members staggered through the door with furrowed eyebrows and a shamed look on her pale, round face. Sarah was an EMT and Coast Guard veteran who rode the day tour on Sunday with Ship. We often caught up at base between shifts.

"How was your tour?" I asked, though her face said it all. Her face said Not good.

"We just had a bad run. I froze on scene. I don't know what happened, I just froze. It was terrible."

"Oh, that happened to me when I was new. I was riding with Ship and we went to a pedestrian struck and I froze on scene. In broad daylight. With firefighters and cops and bystanders watching. It was humiliating."

"That's exactly what just happened to me. We had a guy hit by a car and I froze on the street. I was paralyzed. I don't understand why I couldn't move. I've been in the military. It's not like I haven't been through these kinds of scenarios."

"But was this your first trauma job as an EMT?"

"Yeah."

"There you go. You can train all you want and have all the experience in the world, but you haven't seen a job until you've seen a job. It's new to you. Now it's not. Now you've seen trauma, so next time you'll be able to perform, I promise."

Just then Ship walked in and, seeing me, put his arms around my shoulders and said, "The same thing that just happened to you happened to her. She froze on her first trauma, and let me tell you, next trauma job we got, she fucking flew off the ambulance! I wasn't even stopped yet and this bitch was out of the truck collaring the patient!"

"It's true," I said, laughing. "Next time you get that call, just move, move, move. If it's trauma think bleeding control, collar, stretcher. Assess the patient for head, neck, back pain and LOC. Cut their clothes off in the ambulance and look at their injuries. You got this, girl. I promise you it gets better."

"I don't know," Sarah said. "Now I'm doubting myself. I'm doubting if I can do this."

"You can absolutely do this. I respond to a trauma job now and my heart rate doesn't even go up. I've done a hundred ped strucks at this point. I could eat soup on scene. But I haven't seen other things yet. My first shooting I was mildly helpful at best. I didn't freeze. I haven't frozen on scene since that first trauma, but I wasn't going to win any awards for patient care."

"Mildly helpful," Ship said, putting his run sheet away. "I love you."

"I feel so much better knowing this happened to you," Sarah said.

"Oh, yeah. It was a moment of grave humiliation." Pointing at Ship, I said, "He yelled at me afterward."

"I didn't yell at you. I spoke with you."

"He spoke with me. In a loud, scolding voice. I cried."

"She did cry," Ship said. "But then on that next run, my girl performed!"

Sarah laughed. A week later when I saw her again at base, she ran up to me. "Jennifer!" she said. "I did it! It was just like you said! We got the exact same job, guy hit by a car, and I got off the ambulance and did what I was supposed to do!"

"See? You're a hero now. You're a good EMT. You got this."

"You helped me so much. I was honestly thinking of quitting after I froze."

"Nah," I said. "You belong here, girl. You're good."

Nathan arrived for our tour. I was so glad to see him I threw my arms around him and hugged him. He was the perfect partner for this rotten day, so kind and sensitive. On the truck the radio spat up jobs every two minutes. Pedestrian strucks. Sick fever coughs. Arrests. We got sent on a run for a ped struck.

"I think it's a kid," Nathan said as he sped down the street. Then PD radio confirmed a child had been hit by a car.

I gloved up, masked up, and got slammed by a shot of adrenaline after hearing it was a kid. Soon, Nathan parked cattycorner on a block where a woman stood on the sidewalk holding a baby. We were first on scene, because Nathan had kicked the bus into high gear after the detail came over that it was a child.

Thankfully, the baby was unharmed. A driver had hit the child's stroller as he was turning. The stroller shook but the baby had no signs of trauma or cries of distress. The mother was rattled. She didn't want to go to the hospital. She just wanted us to check the child to make sure she was OK and asked us what she should look for in case things changed later on.

In order to RMA a baby, we had to call telemetry and speak with a doctor, since the baby, being a baby, couldn't speak and tell us she was unharmed. Police arrived and provided zero assistance. I saw a Black woman cop and got trapped in bias myself, thinking she'd be better than some white guy. But no.

The cop walked up to the shaken mother and asked what happened and where the driver went in a demanding, patronizing voice. When the mother said she'd spoken to the driver and since her child was OK, told him he could leave, the cop lost it.

"Why'd you do that? You shouldn't have done that. You can't tell him to leave. That makes this a hit and run. We need him for a report. How can we do a report without the driver?"

Nathan tried to interject and get the cop to stop being a cop. I walked away and grabbed the Toughbook off the truck so I could start writing the chart and gathering the needed signatures.

The cop was still in robot mode when I returned, chastising the mother whose baby had just been hit by a car for releasing the driver. The officer was wholly unable to dip into her humanity for one instant, one second, to have compassion or even sympathy for the mother, which infuriated me.

"That cop was an *asshole*," Nathan said after we'd secured the RMA with a doctor's approval, said goodbye to the baby and mother, and cleared the scene.

"Yeah."

I don't know what goes on behind that thin blue line for women cops. But it doesn't always play out well on the street.

Later that same tour, Nathan parked under the shade of a tree and we relaxed. After an hour or so we got thirsty, so he headed to a deli so we could get some cold drinks. As he drove, "If the World Was Ending," came on the radio.

"It's my song!" I said. "Where's my phone?" I scrambled and found it. "I have to make a video of myself singing."

Nathan glanced at me like I was crazy.

I turned the volume up on the radio. Then I started a video and sang my heart out to and for Mike, stopping my phenomenal performance once to tell Nathan the traffic light was green. I sent my beautiful music video from the street to my sweet husband in Las Vegas. Mike loved it. Nathan did, too.

"You killed that song, Jen."

"Thank you. It was for Mike. I practiced in my car."

I hadn't been able to eat much that day. I was too upset about Mike. On the ambulance, I ordered takeout dumplings from Dumplings & Things. Ten minutes, they'd be ready. Nathan and I looked up the block at a long line of people waiting outside CityMD. I figured they were getting COVID tested. But Lexi had told me her friend who worked at the clinic said everyone was coming in for STD tests. Nathan said he'd gone to CityMD a few days before because he'd been feeling tired and unwell. They told him he was dehydrated.

"That's like the first thing they teach you in EMT school," I said. "If you're tired, drink water. You're probably dehydrated."

"Do they? They didn't tell me that."

"Clearly."

Another job came over for a pedestrian struck. Nathan hit the sirens and off we went. Sometimes I thought ordering food was a way to get jobs. Order dinner, and you'll get a run. Very similar to needing to pee. Every time I needed to pee, we got a job.

This next ped struck was a motorcyclist who'd been plowed down by an Uber driver. The bike lay on its side in the street, but the driver was stable. Broken collarbone, probably. Mild concussion. Nothing terribly exciting. He remembered the accident, more or less, but couldn't remember what day of the week it was, or what year. "What about the president?" I asked. The patient mumbled, "Yeah, I know who that fucking asshole is."

Good enough for me.

It took us over an hour to clear the job. The cops took a while getting the information they needed on scene and the hospital was busy when we rolled into triage. The patient was a nice guy whose father used to ride on an ambulance in Hell's Kitchen, so he was super appreciative of EMTs and the work we did—which was rare.

Driving out of the hospital, Nathan stopped as we descended the ER bay ramp to chat with a paramedic he knew, who walked around the ambulance to go speak to Nathan. The two of them talked for a while with the ambulance idling while I worked on the last patient's chart.

We asked the medic why he thought FEMA hadn't deployed us to the hot-zone states yet, given the fact that FEMA had come to New York City and saved our overextended asses when COVID peaked here. The medic said FEMA had fifty trucks in those states, but they hadn't activated New York because we were anticipated to explode with the virus again, too.

We all knew that. We knew the numbers coming from city and state officials were a farce. We still heard the calls for sick fever cough and cardiac arrests. It was only a matter of time before we entered the second wave and went into hot-zone mode again.

"Over six hundred new cases yesterday," the paramedic said.

Dumplings & Things was closed by the time Nathan and the paramedic ended their conversation an hour later.

"Oh man, I'm sorry, Jen," he said as he drove to the restaurant.

"Yeah, you're sorry. You had to talk to that medic for an hour. Between Mike and COVID and protests and work and the call volume picking up, I'm going to end up in the locked psych ward at Kings County. I'm going to admit myself just so I can sleep."

Nathan turned to me. "Jen, you know I live two blocks from Kings County. I can visit you all the time."

I got off the ambulance.

Dumplings & Things was dark inside. A solitary man was in the back, washing dishes. I could see him through a slat of light. I pressed the microphone and he came to the window. I told him I'd ordered steamed dumplings an hour ago. I saw a bag sitting on a shelf, so I figured maybe those were mine.

"They're cold now," the man said.

"I know. I couldn't pick them up until now. It's OK, I'll eat them cold."

"No, I'll make you new ones right now," he said, running to the back. And outside, standing there on the sidewalk I couldn't believe this man's kindness, and how far out of his way he was going for me, a total stranger. He reappeared five minutes later and handed me a fresh batch of hot dumplings. When he gave them to me with a free bottle of water, I nearly wept.

"Thank you so much," I said. "I really appreciate it."

I tipped him every dollar in my wallet.

When I got home that night and showered, I felt so grateful I had spent the evening on the ambulance with Nathan, and helped a few patients, and received enough tenderness from the man in the dumpling restaurant to restore my hope in the world and belief that people, in their humanity, were at root kindhearted and good.

But good feelings in the pandemic expired fast.

Having a critically sick person in your life is like being on a roller-coaster ride in hell. I don't know how else to phrase it.

Next day, Mike was worse. I'd thought we'd already been pushed to the bottom of the stairs, but it turned out we had another flight to fall. He was now vomiting so much he couldn't get off the bathroom floor and thought he was going to die. Ylfa and I braced for the end.

Then on Tuesday, our husband had an unexpected comeback. Life was all about that. It was all about coming back. My Turtle called me giggling and said he felt much better today. He was in his truck, driving around, running errands.

I was relieved he felt better. But I was also exhausted beyond endurance. It seemed every other week Mike called me or Ylfa or Michael Daly and told us this was the end, he was about to die, any minute, it was happening, he could sense it. Then out of the blue his fear diminished, and he'd relax into the reality that he was still alive, and believed he was going to emerge victorious. Ylfa said something poetic and genius about his behavior:

"He's the boy who cried wolf, only there is a wolf."

Duck was so smart. I was so glad I married her. And Turtle.

Nowadays whenever Mike went off the books with his treatment plans, cooking up some scheme to treat himself as a patient, we came down hard on him for refusing to follow doctor's orders. We told him he wasn't being Mike or Turtle, he was being Murtle. He hated it when we called him that. The nickname conjured images of a granny shuffling around in a muumuu and flew in the face of his self-image as swaggering firefighter, an "unbridled stallion in a cage," as he called himself during COVID lockdown, which sent Ylfa and me into fits of laughter so loud and wild our shrieks could have broken windowpanes.

"A lesser man would be dead by now," Mike said of surviving cancer this long. And we reminded him of that often, too. "You're not just anyone, Turtle. A lesser man . . ."

One day on the phone together, the three of us, Mike was in so much pain I bit the bullet and said the thing I never thought I'd say, to cheer him up.

"Turtle, as soon as you get through this, you and me and Duck are going to get in your RV and travel the whole country, just the three of us."

Ylfa texted me. "I can't believe you just said that. The RV!"

"I know! It just came out! It's his ultimate dream! We need to keep the dream alive!"

But we couldn't.

Mid-July, Mike's health took yet another turn for the worse. He had a fever and difficulty breathing and was in tremendous physical pain. He decided to go rogue with his treatment—what else was new—and get radiation to treat his esophagus. He found a doctor to agree. Ylfa and I decided to meet each other in Manhattan to catch our breath and spend time together.

We met at Pat's firehouse.

That afternoon, I arrived at Ladder 3 before Ylfa, bereft to discover the bench plaqued with Pat's name was gone. Where was it? The firefighters must have moved it because of COVID. They didn't want people sitting outside the firehouse, I guessed.

"The bench is gone," I told Ylfa when she rounded the corner and saw for herself.

"Oh, no. That's new. Do you think it's because of COVID?"

I wasn't sure. We walked to the firehouse and stood outside the red door. There was nowhere for us to sit. No bench in memory of Pat.

Oh well.

We found a nice café around the corner and sat outside in a little garden. We drank coffee and talked about Mike. How all we could do was let him know we were here for him, and that he was loved. We reminded each other that Pat loved us and was looking out for his kid brother.

* * *

Toward the end of the month, Mike was having a hard time swallowing. He couldn't eat. Late July he surrendered to going to the hospital and allowed himself to be admitted.

Finally, Ylfa and I thought. Finally, he'll get a COVID test. He got the test alright.

Negative.

We were shocked. Fever, cough, chest pain, and a negative COVID test? It made no sense.

Doctors said the radiation treatments had burned Mike's esophagus. The cancer was also now in his lungs. He was sucking on ice to try to get some fluids down, and on an IV. He named his IV pole Agnes and sent us videos of himself strolling around the hospital ward with his new favorite person, his medicine dispenser.

A day or so later another doctor told him if he couldn't get any nutrition in him his kidneys would fail, and he'd have to do dialysis. Due to the pandemic he was in an isolation room. No visitors allowed.

Isolation just about killed Mike. He was dying of loneliness. He didn't understand why the hospital wouldn't let anyone visit. He didn't want to die alone. The problem was also connected to Pat. Mike knew what happened when Pat or any firefighter got hurt: Everyone turned up at the hospital and waited in line to see them. It was a party of support, a brotherhood, a family, and because of COVID, Mike wasn't getting anything like that. He wasn't getting anything at all.

One morning he called me crying from the hospital. "This is some end-of-life shit. I don't want to die like this. It's horrible. I'm all by myself."

He wept, then we talked about how lonely he felt. I reminded him he was loved. That we were all here, calling, texting, sending him videos and photos.

"I know if I looked at your phone right now it would be nuts with a hundred missed calls and messages."

"You're right. But it's hard to talk because my throat hurts."

"I know you're lonely, honey, but we're all right here with you."

Mike told me he didn't want dialysis. He was going to sign a DNR. He liked talking to me about grim medical stuff since I was an EMT. His EMT Chick.

"First of all," I said, "sign whatever you want. A DNR is a standard medical document. I'd sign a DNR at this point. It doesn't mean anything terribly significant unless you go into arrest. And it doesn't sound like you'll arrest at the moment. Do you feel like you're going to die today?"

"No," Mike said quietly.

"OK then, Turtle. I have the same feeling. I think today you'll stay alive. Let's just take it one day at a time. For today, we're both pretty sure you won't die, right?"

"Right."

"There we go. We'll deal with tomorrow tomorrow."

Mike said if he did start to feel like his kidneys were failing, he didn't want dialysis. He was going to try to convince the hospital to allow him one visitor before he died. He wasn't asking for a lot. He just wanted to see one person. We all knew who that person would be: his new girlfriend, who he'd only known for a few months and met online after getting diagnosed with cancer. We kept our mouths shut about that. Not our business.

"I think I scared Erin, mentioning the DNR," Mike said of his niece. "Will you call and check on her?"

"I'll call her as soon as we hang up. And I'll call her tomorrow, and the next day. I'll check on Erin for the rest of her life, and so will Ylfa. Stop worrying about everyone. Your wives are here. And Paul and Bobby and James and Michael Daly and Gonzo and your family. All of your people. Pat's people. We've got Erin. And we've got you. You just worry about yourself. And even then, let's just stay in the day. OK, Turtle?"

"OK, EMT Chick. I love you."

"I love you so much it hurts."

After we hung up, I called Erin. We spoke for almost two hours. Turned out, we both needed to talk. I adored her. I could see why Mike loved her so much.

That night, Mike's circumstances haunted me. If I was going to die, and I got to see one person before I left the earth, one person only, who would it be? Who was my person?

Next day, I canvassed my friends and asked them the same. Felice said it would be her mother. Tommy, his girlfriend, who he'd also known for a metaphoric ten minutes, but that was his choice. Tommy was like me; he fell in love with everyone fast. "Mother" was hands down most people's answer to this question. But it had to be someone who would bring you comfort.

My mom hated hospitals. Felice did, too. Those were my top two choices. For weeks I thought about this.

I didn't have a person.

Just under a week later, Mike got released from the hospital and sent home. Alive again. He was the boy who cried wolf, and there was a wolf, and it didn't get him. Not yet.

At home, he was only able to eat soft foods. Eggs and soups and milkshakes. But he'd escaped, for now. Since he'd been diagnosed last September, it seemed he'd died a thousand times.

I felt like I had, too.

21

THIS IS SOME END-OF-LIFE SHIT

On the street in August, emergency call volumes remained eerily low. There was a spike in 911 and 311 calls during Hurricane Isaias, but that passed relatively quickly. Most of the 911 calls across the city were for the usual: shootings and stabbings, pedestrians struck by cars and EDPs, intoxes and cardiac arrests, wavelets of sick people complaining of fevers and coughs, the newly infected with COVID and the long-haulers, not to mention patients with chronic health issues now returning to hospitals with cancer, congestive heart failure, and lung disease, among other complaints.

The city was quiet, hushed, as it often got in August, when loads of people fled for nearby beaches and mountains. Media outlets ran stories with headlines like NEW YORK CITY IS DEAD FOREVER. I went to Riis Beach a few times. I wore my new bikinis inspired by *Love Island* and dove headfirst into crashing waves. Pretended I was somewhere else. The ocean renewed me. I felt younger and happier and full of salt and sun when I came home.

And then came a real pandemic surprise from California.

One August day my mother suddenly became a rescuer. My mother, who hated hospitals, sickness, and death.

These last few months, she'd dialed back her presence on Instagram (thank God). And one day, she e-mailed me out of the blue and announced that she was flying to Sequim, Washington.

What?

My sheriff uncle wasn't doing well, her e-mail said. He'd had that heart attack a few months back. Now he was home, and my aunt was having a hard time taking care of him. So off my mother flew to Washington to help out.

The fact that my elderly mother, who was at high risk for getting COVID, was getting on a plane from a hot zone—California—and flying to another hot zone—Washington—to visit my elderly aunt and uncle who were also at risk for dying of COVID struck me silent. I didn't know what to say in reply, except "OK, Mom. Be safe and wear your mask."

Then I stepped away from my phone and reminded myself I was her daughter, not her mother. My therapist reminded me of that, too. That my mom knew the risks of traveling in the pandemic. She was an adult. She could make her own decisions.

I spoke to her two weeks later, when she got back to Bakersfield. She started talking about going up to the mountains, and how well her blueberries were doing, when I interrupted her and said, "Mom, please explain why you just got on a plane."

Things were bad up in Washington, she said. My aunt was a wreck trying to take care of my heart-attack-recovering uncle. Doctors had put him on medication that made him dizzy and unsteady on his feet. My aunt was terrified he would fall down and injure himself, and she was tiny, so she wouldn't be able to pick him up. To borrow Mike's words, this was some end-of-life shit. So my mother put on her cape and flew to Washington to save her sister.

"I love my sisters," my mom said. "I didn't even ask if I could come. I just told her I was coming. They were so grateful I came. I really helped a lot."

For two weeks my mom cooked for my aunt and uncle and gave them emotional support. My other aunt, the retired ER nurse, joined them for a few days in Sequim. My mom was glad she'd gone. Glad she'd helped. Glad she'd seen her sister.

"Family is everything," my mom said.

"Yes, it is."

My mom, the hero. I was my mother's daughter. I was proud of her, that rascally superwoman. Never had I met a woman capable of so much change. The pandemic had brought her to life. It had that capacity, too. It didn't just remove bullshit. It also brought the wonderous to the surface.

Amazing grace. It activated my mom's best qualities. She loved her sister, and she'd raced to be by her side in a pandemic.

My mother, the rescuer. The action figure. Love was an action. I believed this. And I believed in her. But I was unsure of California's powers to wiggle its way out of catastrophic disaster.

Whenever someone asked me if I would ever consider moving back to the Golden State, my answer was always the same:

"Hell, no."

California was one big natural disaster. Earthquakes. Fires. Mudslides. Floods. It was a global-warming fiesta. My opinion was that one day that whole state was going to break off and drop into the shark-infested sea, unless North Korea nuked it first.

Mid-August, fire season commenced in California. My one-armed-and-dangerous (his words) fire contractor pal Jeff Denholm lived in a rural mountain neighborhood above Santa Cruz. The CZU Lightning Complex fires were ripping through his town, scorching the forest. Jeff disregarded evacuation orders and stayed behind to help firefighters battle it out.

Talk about heroism.

Cal Fire's resources were spread thin on massive blazes happening in too many areas. The bulk of big agency teams were staged at high-density urban interfaces. Jeff's rural town was until recently on its own. Having his fire-retardant gel and fire experience, Jeff said, was paying off where it mattered most—at home. His Internet was down and cell service spotty. Northwest winds were picking up and lightning was on its way, too. He was holding strong so far, helping neighbors when he could.

"It's really been awesome seeing the community rallying to help each other prevail," he said.

Another word I loved these days. Prevail.

If all through the summer I'd dreamed of fleeing New York, in August a feeling of pride and embattled affection for the city returned to me like good health. I felt proud to be here. Happy, even. Grateful. As for those who'd left when things got tough—see ya later.

Felice felt the same.

"There's no place I'd rather be," my sister told me one night on the phone. "Where would I move? My people are here. New Yorkers."

Agreed. However, I was feeling a wee bit cooked from being on the street. I made weird mistakes that made me suspect I might not be doing as well as I thought I was.

One August night, I put a pot of water on the stove to boil and turned on the burner and walked away. Minutes later I heard a loud crack. I ran to the kitchen. I'd turned on the wrong burner and broken a beautiful ceramic bowl sitting on top it, which I'd bought in Spain. I did the exact same thing with a different bowl two days later.

Since the pandemic started, I'd gotten three or four parking tickets. Prior to 2020, I hadn't gotten a ticket in my driving life. I kept forgetting I had a car, or forgetting where it was, or what the alternate-side parking rules were, or lastly, what day it was.

Time lost all meaning. High-five to anyone who experienced time as a linear construct in 2020.

After one August tour on the ambulance, I came home and showered as usual. It had been swelteringly hot that day, so my face was wrecked. I dabbed some toner on a cotton ball and swept it across my face, and the cotton was black when I finished. My skin burned like crazy and I wasn't sure why. It was the same toner I'd been using since the pandemic started. The N95 masks tore up my skin, especially after being on the truck. Then I looked at the bottle and realized I'd toned my face with 100 percent pure acetone nail polish remover. I must have burned off three layers of skin.

Then I decided to cut my hair again. I guessed it was one thing I could control? I gave myself layers, but it didn't go as well as I'd hoped it would. Now I looked like I had a mullet. Life was becoming tragicomic. I was laughing a lot, like a scary clown.

This was me, in the pandemic.

"It's everyone in the pandemic," Felice said.

On the phone one night we talked about people trying to pretend everything was cool when they were struggling just to get through these infinite sad days. At one point we discussed God, and what we believed in terms of the world's religions. We talked about the doctrine of the Trinity, and how the Holy Ghost didn't get enough airtime compared to the Father and Son.

"The problem with the Holy Ghost is in the title," Felice said. "People here the word 'ghost' and they think it's something negative. It's like 'defund the police.' It sounds negative, so people can't get behind it."

"Sis, you're a genius. I never get tired of the shit that comes out of your mouth."

I never got tired of what came out of Jon Laster's mouth, either, my comedian friend from the neighborhood. We went for a walk one August day and sat in the park. It was so nice to reunite with friends. Everyone had stopped calling me. My phone never rang. But then Felice reminded me I'd blocked everyone during COVID, so I unblocked them, and my phone rang a little more.

During the protests, Jon dedicated his Instagram feed to posting videos of Black people telling stories about their experiences with police. The videos were tragic and endless. One Black person after another, after another, testifying about what it felt like to be Black in America, pervasively targeted by cops. In the park I told Jon I thought the videos were incredible.

"I just felt like a lot of the people protesting, you know, there's a lot of white people out there, and they've never asked a Black man how it feels to deal with the police. That entire side of the story is missing. I didn't want to do some 'fuck the police' thing. I wanted people to hear from Black men. So I asked them. I told them to give one story about an experience they had with the police, and to say how it made them feel. That was also missing. How it feels to be arrested and targeted by the police."

"Well, I watched a ton of them, and they're amazing. I hope you get a shit-ton of press. You deserve it."

"Yeah, the media's calling," Jon said. "I've gotten a lot of work in the pandemic."

"It's good. They called all me, too. They called EMTs and medics when COVID blew up in the spring. A hundred years ago, when people cared about healthcare workers. My phone's stopped ringing. That's over. They're done with us now."

"It'll end for us, too," Jon said. "Elections are coming up."

"Yeah. Hey, did you get a ton of white people calling you when the BLM protests erupted?"

Jon laughed. "Oh my God. It was crazy. And they all kept saying—wait, what did they say?" He looked up at the trees.

"I see you."

Jon folded in half laughing. "That's it," he said. 'I see you.'"

* * *

Toward the end of August, I started to feel like maybe things were improving. I met this cool guy online. He wasn't a civil servant, for once, so I thought maybe I was making some dating progress. Tommy sure was. He and his girlfriend were blasting into the future and had decided to buy a house together in the Rockaways.

The guy I liked was cool. His name was Quincy. He was tall and did jujitsu, a handsome brown guy who worked at a school for autistic children, loved '90s hip-hop, protested for BLM, called me often, and then one day asked if I wanted to grab coffee. He lived in Harlem.

One afternoon I drove into the city to have my first pandemic date. It took me eons to get into Manhattan. Pandemic traffic was out of control, since no one was taking the subway. We sat outside at a little café. Quincy looked like what I expected, except he had a lot more hair than he did in his pictures. "I know I look like a caveman," he said. "I am a caveman, sort of."

"Perfect. I love cavemen. I've been dating them for decades."

We had a great first date. Although I had to drive a long way. And I paid for our coffees. And cookies. And he kept asking me what I liked to cook.

When I called Felice to debrief about it later, she asked where Quincy was from.

"I don't know," I said. "I didn't ask. He said he had asthma as a kid growing up in Panama, so I'm guessing he's Panamanian."

"But you didn't ask?"

"Look. I'm a white woman, OK? And I date outside my race. And when I dated Jim, the only thing he ever got asked was where he was from. People spoke to him in Spanish. People spoke to him in Arabic. Black people said he looked like his mother, who was white. It was literally the only question that came at him. And it's a time of racial reckoning. And I'm white. So I'm not going on a first date and being like, 'So, I see you're brown. What country are you from?'"

"Got it," Felice said. "But did you like him?"

"I did. He's great. And he texted when I got home. We're going on another date soon. He wants to go for a bike ride. But I'm a little concerned by some of the things he says."

"For example?"

"Like every time he texts, he says, 'What's for dinner?'"

Felice thought this was hysterical.

"That's some 1950s gender shit," I said. "The woman's in the kitchen roasting chicken. And the man's out in the world, making money. What if every time he texted that's what I said?"

"What?"

"Hey, what's up? So nice to hear from you. Where's the money?"

We laughed hard. That August, I was laughing again.

And then one day I stopped.

On August 25, I watched a video of Kyle Rittenhouse, a white seventeen-year-old boy armed with a rifle at a protest in Kenosha, Wisconsin, breeze by cops and kill two people protesting against the police shooting of a Black man, Jacob Blake. The victims were white, a detail widely omitted by news sources, which Felice pointed out to me. The video I saw captured a partial story. The media write-ups, too. That was always the case. But the video also exposed the underlying issue: What happened to white people suspected of crimes in this country differed vastly from what happened to Black people suspected of crimes. This teenager, not old enough to legally consume alcohol in America, who described himself as a militia member, strode by police while armed with a rifle, and removed two people from the earth.

He also strode by Facebook.

Citizens had sent more than four hundred warnings to Facebook about the Kenosha Guard and Boogaloo Bois, right-wing groups using that platform and others to organize against protestors in Wisconsin. Facebook ignored these pre-attack warnings—*over four hundred of them*—contributing to those killings. CEO Mark Zuckerberg publicly apologized for his company's inaction in regard to the Rittenhouse murders. He attributed his company's error to an "operational mistake."

Operational mistake?

And then on Facebook and other social media platforms dozens of alt-right groups celebrated Rittenhouse as a hero. Just like that the bottom dropped out of my career. It was pointless. My job was a joke. I gave up.

I'd been here before, in 2008. I'd cut my teeth as an investigator in the financial-services sector. Doing due diligence on hedge fund managers and venture capitalists for institutional investors like banks, universities, and the Roman Catholic Church. For years I wrote lengthy due diligence reports showcasing red flags sticking out of the heads of a hundred felonious hedge fund managers—all the big boys. The ones who tanked the global markets in 2008 that resulted in people like me being jobless, unable to pay rent.

"How could this happen?" I asked my boss after the markets crashed and he called me to say there was no work. "We did the due diligence, we investigated these guys, the banks saw our reports, they saw the red flags, and they invested anyway?"

"Yes," my boss said. "Some of them chose not to invest after seeing our reports. But most of them invested. They knew the returns were inflated and they didn't care. They ticked the box that said, 'due diligence completed,' and they invested."

I was so shocked I almost lost my lunch. I couldn't find the right word for this behavior. Then it came to me.

Looting.

"You have to get over it," my boss said. "That's just the way the finance world works."

Anyone who knew me, and certainly anyone who'd had the blessed experience of dating me, knew that I was not a woman who ever just "got over it." I changed fields after that. I got back on my feet and got the hell out of finance-sector investigations. Diversified. Broadened. Drilled down on what eventually became my subject-matter expertise. Electronic crimes. MCIs. Crises. I typed "no finance bros" onto my Tinder bio. #StillNotOverIt.

Since then, I thought I liked my career. It was tough, yes. But I was satisfied. Now, in 2020, after the Rittenhouse killings, I didn't know how else to feel aside from defeated, or what else to say that hadn't already been said by smarter people, except perhaps, while we were at it, tearing down walls and renovating the country, Disarm America. Defund Silicon Valley.

Burn it down.

Elections were coming. So was September 11. The commissioner of the Fire Department distributed a letter and posted social media messages discouraging 9/11 veterans and first responders from gathering to commemorate the nineteenth anniversary of the attacks.

Ylfa and Mike and I decided to have a Zoom meeting that day, since cancer and COVID prevented Mike from traveling to New York. Chemo stopped working and he'd been rejected from yet another trial. But his doctor said he could keep receiving treatments anyway. Mike was alive and he had hope. That was all that mattered.

Life and hope.

Then one afternoon he called and said his fever and cough were back. He'd prescribed himself antibiotics, a Z-Pak.

"I guess things can never be simple with me," he said.

Ylfa and I spoke. "I don't know if Mike will die of COVID or cancer," she said.

"I think it's a race at this point. COVID is highly likely with him in and out of the hospital. But the cancer is in his lungs and chest now, so."

For now all we could do was pray and love him from New York.

One tour with Nathan, we sat on the ambulance with the air conditioner blasting and the windows rolled down, talking about how burned out we felt, how ready for a break.

I was going on four years on the street, Nathan was going on five, and both of us seemed a decade older every week. It wasn't just us. Every first responder I knew was fried. Tommy was contemplating retiring from the Fire Department early. Larry was also looking for jobs and wanted to retire from the NYPD. One day I asked Gabriel how he felt now that things had calmed down a bit, after he'd worked all those cardiac arrests that resulted in dead patients followed by the protests. He said he saw a therapist to talk things through and got slapped with the unsurprising diagnosis of anxiety and PTSD. "I feel some sort of way about all this," he said. "The ultimate millennial sentence."

"I have a medical question for you," Mike texted that night after I'd missed his call while Nathan and I were on a job.

"Sorry to miss your call," I said when I got in touch. "I was with a patient at the ER."

"The nerve of the patient!"

"He was drunk and cracked his head open."

"I had this drunk lady that fell down a flight of stairs, scalping herself. She said, 'Get this fucking hat off my head!' It was her scalp, hanging in front of her eyes. Then she looked at me and said, 'I don't want no fucking Mexican touching me!' While I repaired her head I kept saying, 'Sí sí, sí.'"

As far as Mike's query went, he wanted to know if, when I'd been sick and felt I had the Rona, one of my symptoms had been severe fatigue? Like, no matter how much I rested I felt wiped out? And nauseous?

Sí, sí, no.

I told Mike I didn't have GI issues when I'd been sick, but reminded him that Lexi had, after taking a Z-Pak. And that some COVID patients with fevers and coughs had vomiting and diarrhea. I remember this call that came over the radio at the peak of the virus for a man standing on the street complaining of a fever and cough, who was vomiting uncontrollably, which sounded like hell incarnate.

"How long did it last?" Mike asked.

"My Rona that may have not been Rona lasted seven to ten days. Lexi's lasted three weeks with vomiting and GI issues while she took the Z-Pak. What's your SpO2?"

"It's been 94 percent to 95 percent, but I got shit growing in my lungs. I feel better. Thank you. When things get bad, I start burying myself."

Things got bad for me and Nathan later that night.

Around nine o'clock we responded to a red-phone job in Prospect Park. Dispatch said we were looking for a young Black man sitting under a tree who'd injured his foot and couldn't walk.

When we got to the park, we got lost looking for him. This park was made of trees, after all. We saw a tiny white car with doors marked with trees and asked some park ranger people sitting inside the vehicle to lead us to the location where the injured patient reportedly sat. They took us on quite a journey and seemed no better equipped than we were in terms of locating our destination. At one point they led us down a road that dead-ended into a set of stairs. We got out of our vehicles and looked at the park map.

Just then a short, older Black man with gray waist-length dreads came racing down a grassy slope holding a large walking stick in his hand, waving it around and screaming at us in an accent that sounded Caribbean.

"Get the fuck out of here!" he yelled. "This is our land! You don't belong here! Get the fuck out!"

He came closer, shouting that he was going to fill us with bullet holes. I didn't know if he was drunk or mentally ill or just enraged or what was going on.

Quickly I climbed back in the truck. Nathan and the park rangers waved him away, and Nathan returned to the ambulance.

"I'm stressed," I said.

My heart was pounding. I could hear it thumping in my ears. There was music blaring in the park, and a fair share of people wandering around.

Nathan started to back up, but he needed my help since there were a lot of people on bikes and on foot walking behind us, and he couldn't see.

"Jen, I need you to get out and help me back out of here."

"OK. Roll your windows down so we can hear each other."

I got outside and directed him back as the angry man ran up to Nathan's window, waving his cane and screaming that we didn't belong there, and to get the fuck out. Then he started running toward me.

"Stay away from her!" Nathan shouted. "Don't go near my partner! Stand back!"

Quickly he reversed the ambulance and I hopped inside, and we resumed our search for the patient. We said nothing of what had just happened.

Finally we arrived at the right tree and found our patient. The four of us stepped out of our cars and there stood the injured man standing on one leg, one hurt foot hovering above the ground. We helped him inside the ambulance and took a look-see at his ankle, which was swollen and bruised. He needed to go to the hospital.

He didn't want to—he was afraid of the insurance bill—but he was non-ambulatory, and it would be near impossible for an Uber driver to find him inside the dark, crowded park. On the truck we told him we were a volunteer crew, and if he got a bill he couldn't pay or his insurance didn't adequately cover, he could send a financial hardship letter to Park Slope asking for assistance. We couldn't promise anything, but it was an option.

He agreed to go.

At the hospital, a triage nurse shouted at a curtained bed, "You have a brain bleed! Your brain is bleeding!"

I saw Nathan's eyes widen. He poked his head behind the curtain to see who the nurse was diagnosing.

"Jen!" he said. "That's the intox we brought in earlier. He has a brain bleed."

"Yes, I heard that."

"The nurse said it's not a small one, either."

"Fascinating. Let's get our patient onto this bed."

We moved our patient, and he wept when we said goodbye. "Murphy," he said, weeping and taking my hand. "Thank you."

"Why are you crying, sweetheart? Are you OK?"

"I'm just happy. I'm just grateful to be alive and have breath."

I was grateful too. And reeling, apparently.

I didn't know the man shouting at us in Prospect Park had gotten to me. But half an hour or so later, after Nathan and I returned to base and said goodbye, walking back to my car, a deep sadness overtook me. By the time I was halfway home I was sobbing in the car. I called Felice as I drove.

"Hey, sis," she said. "Are you OK?"

I sobbed out what had happened.

"What?" she said in an outraged tone. "Sis, I'm so sorry this happened to you."

"I don't know why I'm so upset. I can't stop crying."

"Um, because you just got attacked by a man who said he wanted to shoot you and you were scared for your life?"

Yeah. That was probably right.

We talked until I was home safe and inside my apartment. I felt so much better after talking to my sister. I loved her so much. I told her that the funny part about all of this was that the man screaming at us looked like a poet we knew from the Nuyorican, and because of his accent I couldn't stop thinking about a conversation Felice and I had just had, often had, about Caribbean Americans being extremely polite, and how they were often viewed as different than Black Americans.

"I couldn't stop laughing inside because the guy had a Caribbean accent and I kept thinking, 'This man did not get the note about immigrant politeness that my sister told me about.'"

Felice laughed. "Apparently not. Beneath all that anger is hurt."

"I don't think this gentleman has reached the hurt layer yet."

"No. And I mean—I want to come for this man now, after he attacked my sister. Who does he think he is, screaming at you and threatening to shoot you while you're in the park trying to help someone, while you're out on the street saving lives?"

"People are angry. I understand. They see us in uniform, and they think we're all the same, it all comes out. All the pain and rage. It's heartbreaking."

"Heartbreaking," Felice said.

Heartbreaking.

* * *

As for Quincy, I never saw him again after that first date. He got hit by a car one afternoon when he was riding his bike in Harlem, so we never went for that ride we'd talked about.

Because pandemic traffic was crazy, and no one was taking the subway, and everyone was riding their bikes, people were getting hit by cars left and right. Some tours it seemed that was the only 911 call coming over the radio, pedestrians and bikers getting hit by cars. I used to ride my bike in New York City, too. But I stopped soon after I became an EMT. It wasn't worth it. Helmets were nice. But in car-versus-bicycle accidents? The bikers did not fare well.

Quincy was pretty banged up after his accident. Concussion and knee pain. But that wasn't why he vanished.

We made plans to see each other one Friday toward the end of August. He asked if we could have coffee again in Harlem, in the morning. I said sure. He was worth a long drive. He called me babe and was cute and consistent and we had the same value system. Loved that. But then that Friday morning he asked if we could move our date to the evening. Sure thing, no problem. And then an hour before our date he texted this shocker:

"Hey, I'm in DC for the March on Washington. My frat brothers scooped me up last minute. I forgot to hit you up earlier. Didn't want to leave you hanging. [Smooch emoji.] Next week?"

I mean, you left the state and you forgot to tell me? And you're telling me now, an hour before we're supposed to meet, when you're already in DC, which is a five-hour drive from New York City? That would be all.

I called Felice. She said, "This reminds me of when Marko went to Colorado without telling you."

"Yes, it's painfully familiar. But Marko ditched me for a concert. At least Quincy cut loose for a good cause."

"He'll be back," Felice said.

She was usually right. We shared the belief that all men came back—always. It was only a matter of time. Nietzsche's eternal return theory. But in this instance, for once, my sister was wrong. I didn't hear from Quincy for months.

The march for racial justice was clearly very long.

When August ended, I was single. I still didn't have a person. But then I got to thinking about how, after my mom masked up and flew to

Washington in a pandemic to help her sister, maybe it was time for me to change my mind about her capabilities as a rescuer. Maybe if I got sick or something bad happened to me, some end-of-life shit, and I wound up in the hospital and got to see one person, maybe my mom could be that for me after all.

22

DREAM TOURS

Depressing news hit the fatigued New York City EMS community at the end of August 2020.

A review of the year's ambulance response times for fiscal 2020, which ended in June, found that FDNY ambulances took an average of ten minutes and nineteen seconds from emergency operators receiving a call to EMTs and paramedics arriving on scene—almost a minute longer than 2019.

One minute meant lost lives. In EMS, as you now know, response times mean everything. The slower our response time, the more of you who are going to die. Those are the sad facts.

The slowdown in ambulance response times in New York City was attributed to three things. First, the unprecedented 911 call volume that spring, during the peak of COVID-19. Second, the thousands of EMTs and paramedics who got sick and went out of service with the virus, saved by FEMA trucks who rushed to the city to rescue us. And third, the ever-present dilemma of the "worried well" tying up first responders on runs for nonemergencies.

With 911 call volumes down and our chiefs free, a new class of EMTs was oriented at Park Slope. One Sunday afternoon at base I went upstairs to use the bathroom and heard laughter drifting from the classroom. Must be the new heroes, I thought.

As I walked by, I heard my screamed name and saw her standing in uniform—my street bride, my Nina, my Tour 3 volunteer EMT pride and joy, my baby love partner who I hadn't seen since in over five months, not since the pandemic struck and she'd gone off the truck and been trapped at home. I nearly keeled over with joy.

Nina gave me the biggest hug. I blinked, and she was in my arms. She was a hugger now.

"My beautiful wife!" I said. "I miss you so much!"

"I miss you, too! Wow, you cut your hair."

"Yeah, that was a bad idea."

"No, it looks good. Jennifer, you're so pretty."

"No, you're so pretty. The pandemic made you prettier."

"Jennifer!" Ship called from inside the classroom. "Come in here!"

I ignored him. "When do we bake again?" I asked Nina.

"We must bake immediately. We need Sweets in the Streets. I can literally come over any time. Tell me when you're free."

"It's a pandemic. I'm home constantly. I'm open seven days a week. I'm 7-Eleven."

Happy wives, happy lives!

One August night not long after I reunited with Nina, Pat came to me in a dream.

Ylfa and I were standing side by side, and he appeared above us as a face, his face, the size of a cloud. Very godlike. We said, "Oh, there's Pat!" Then he shapeshifted into his human self. He looked the same as he did when he was alive. And he stood in front of me and looked straight in my eyes and we hugged. And then he went to Ylfa and he hugged her for a very long time. They were still hugging when my dream ended.

I was very reassured in the dream that it was real. Pat was here. He came back. My sense was that he came home to get Mike.

Mike was not in the dream at all.

Four or five days later—time made no sense anymore, so who knew—Nina said she was downstairs, outside my building.

Quickly I put on my floppy white baker's hat and cheap rose-colored hexagonal sunglasses I'd bought us ages back, when we'd decided to be Darcey and Stacey for Halloween, blonde feisty twin sisters from *90 Day Fiancé* who drove matching white cars and had matching fake everything: lips, cheeks, breasts. They had their own reality show on

TLC now called *Darcey & Stacey*. Very important show. We still had to look for blonde wigs.

"Oh my God, Jennifer!" Nina said when I flung the lobby door open.

"Do you love it? I have your matching sunglasses and hat upstairs. Sweets in the Streets!"

That evening, we baked chocolate chip cookies. They were tough and unphotogenic, unworthy of the 'Gram. We didn't care. For hours we sat on my couch and ate our terrible product and watched TLC. I showed Nina the beautiful new leaf on my bird of paradise tree, which had emerged during the pandemic. Unlike its mother, my tree really did turn a new leaf.

"What's the status with you going back to school?" I asked Nina.

She gave me that look she gives me when no progress has been made, then said, "Class starts next week."

"And? Are you registered?"

"Jennifer," she said, stuffing her mouth with a cookie. "These are delicious."

Nina's parents said she could go back on the ambulance, so we picked up a tour together the following week. Finally, we'd be back on the street.

But first, I was on this Saturday with Austin. It was our last time riding together before she left for grad school in Boston. Little did I know this would be one of the best nights I'd ever have as a first responder, a greatest-ever tour.

That Saturday, Austin drove the truck, as she loved to do, and taught our observer, an eager new EMT who sat in the back with a radio and run sheet in his lap. Austin loved to teach. She was very good at it, so I left it to her.

It was one of those nights that gave me everything I needed as a first responder who didn't care for medicine, and left Austin starved for what she most cherished, serious jobs.

Our MVA with injuries turned out to be a fender bender with no patients. But I was delighted because on scene we got to see one of our favorite FDNY units. The guys came up to our truck and, hanging on our window, explained the job was a non-job, a 90, no patient found. But they'd had a "good run" earlier. A serious trauma job, where a man washing windows had fallen through glass and ripped his entire leg open.

"Sounds lovely," I said in horror.

Sounded hideous, but I could tell Austin was jealous. She nearly ate the radio with her face minutes later when we got sent to an uncontrolled bleeder in the projects on Third Avenue and Baltic. She bolted to the job, which elicited no passion in me.

"Wifey, I've had an uncontrolled bleeder," I said as she barreled down the streets. "Been there. Not fun. Extremely not-fun call type. Our observer is going to be drenched in blood."

"It will be good for him, wifey! He needs experience!"

We rolled up to the projects and met up with some cops, one bald white guy and his Black guy partner. They told us a Black male had been stabbed and run off.

We followed thc path of his blood to an apartment on the first floor, where a sheltered family said their brother had been stabbed and run off and the guy who'd done it had run off, too, and said he was coming back. I stood with Austin and our mute observer in the hallway while the cops talked to the upset family inside the open-doored apartment.

"Ask him where he was stabbed!" I yelled.

"The arm!" they shouted.

Austin looked disappointed.

The guy was gone, he was in the wind, and we went with the cops back outside to see if he'd returned.

"Hey, I remember you," the bald cop said as we looked for the patient. "I haven't seen you in a while. I'm the one who put the tourniquet on that guy who got shot."

"Oh, hey. You did a great job with that one. You saved that guy's life. He was a jerk."

"Yeah, and it got worse at the hospital after you left. He was cursing at the doctor."

"How you been? You holding up OK?"

"I'm good. I just got back from vacation. And I'm in EMT school. I'm taking classes at night, they're all online."

"Oh, that's great! You can ride with us when you finish."

"Really? They'd let me do that?"

"Sure. We're all volunteers. We have another cop who rides with us as an EMT. He's in nursing school. Or he was. I don't know if he had to drop out after the protests, when you guys got pulled into mandatory overtime."

Just then we saw an FDNY ambulance that had pulled up late. The back doors were open and near them stood two Black men, one big-boned and dark, one light and wiry, both wearing sweaty white T-shirts soaked with blood. The wiry gentleman was unharmed. He was just bloody from helping. It happened. No one knew that happened better than me. The other guy had a deep, dime-sized stab wound above his elbow, which the municipal EMTs were preparing to treat.

"Hey, what's up?" one of the EMTs said, a white muscular guy I liked a lot. "I haven't seen you in a while. How you been?"

"I've been good. I'm usually on Sundays. What day is today?"

"Saturday."

"Well, that explains it. Can I open that for you?"

He handed me a packet of trauma bandaging and I opened it for him while his partner with long, black ponytailed hair opened a bottle of water to wash the patient's wound.

"How bad does it hurt?" I asked the patient. "On a scale of one to ten, with ten being the worst?"

"I can't feel anything because I'm drunk."

"Oh, that's good, because it's a pretty deep cut. You need stitches."

"Oh man. I don't want to go to the hospital."

Our observer watched and helped the FDNY EMTs wash the wound. It wasn't that interesting-looking, in terms of trauma. It was a pretty deep knife cut, so at least our observer got to see some yellow-and-white goop that was probably subcutaneous tissue or something with a medical name. No bone or uncontrolled bleeding, though, so Austin stood back shaking her truck keys in her hand, looking antsy.

When the wound was adequately sterilized and wrapped the white FDNY EMT and I gave each other a blue-gloved fist bump and said, "Good seeing you," and I shut their truck doors.

"That wasn't an uncontrolled bleed," Austin said as soon as we were back on the ambulance, creeping out of the projects.

"No, that was an injury minor. Sorry, wifey, we tried. But isn't it great that cop who saved my shooting victim is going to be an EMT?"

"Wifey, now we need to go on a good run," Austin said.

"I enjoyed that stab. Not much blood, got to catch up with PD and FDNY, patient was cooperative, I give it an A."

But Austin was bored.

I knew she was desperate hours later when the sky darkened, and she looked excited to respond to a job for a sick patient. Sick jobs were way beneath the waterline of her desire for complex emergencies. But tonight was my night, I was just getting rolling, and the next run turned out to be one of the wildest delights of my street life.

Three or five or seven minutes later, Austin turned down a dark, quiet, tree-lined street and told dispatch we were 84 with PD. Our trio slid off the truck. I kept forgetting we had an observer.

On the sidewalk, an elderly white man stood beside a car in the company of two police officers, a white brunette woman and her white male partner.

We strolled up to the cops and the elderly man, who was wearing a surgical mask that matched the color of his pale blue eyes.

"This is Harold," the woman cop said. "We found him sitting in someone's car."

"Hi, Harold," I said. And then to the cop, "What do you mean?"

"Some woman left her car unlocked, and when she went to get inside it, Harold was sitting in the driver's seat. I think he has dementia."

"Oh, I love this story. Who leaves their car unlocked in New York City? Harold," I said, shining my penlight in his eyeballs to see if his pupils were OK. They were fine. Austin ruled out stroke, asking Harold to squeeze her hands and raise his arms and, pulling his mask down briefly, asking him to give her a big smile. He aced all our tests; negative for stroke. Then he coughed a big wet cough and smiled. I could tell he was smiling even though I couldn't see his mouth, because his eyes crinkled.

"Harold, you're very industrious, sitting in that woman's car," I said. "Were you going to go for a little drive?"

No response.

Suddenly a tall, older bystander with a thick Brooklyn accent came up to us with his hands clasped behind his back. "The driver was a bitch," he said. "Some white lady who couldn't get out of here fast enough. She found Harold sitting in her car and we called 911 and all she wanted to know was if he could get out of her car so she could leave. She didn't care about Harold."

"I see. Well, we care about you, Harold. What's your last name, my love?"

No answer. Just those beautiful crinkled eyes.

Harold looked a lot like my grandfather. Same gentleness. Same build. Probably the same affliction, Alzheimer's disease. People with Alzheimer's wandered.

"When's your birthday?"

No response.

"We can't get him to say anything," the cop said. "I want to see if he's missing. I need to check and see if we have any missing elderly in our system. Let's take a picture of him, since he can't tell us his last name."

"Sounds good."

I stood next to Harold and pulled down his mask and said, "Smile," and Harold smiled while the cop took our picture.

Austin said, "Let's get him on the ambulance, wifey."

We walked Harold to the ambulance. He wasn't too fast on his feet, and we had to help him up the step to get onto the truck. We put him on the stretcher and buckled him up. He crossed his feet at the ankles. He was dressed head to toe in a red athletic track suit, like a hitman. Great outfit. Austin and the observer took his vitals and ran his sugar while I played peekaboo with Harold, poking my head in and out of the back doors while he smiled and coughed. Vitals were normal, as was his sugar. He was perfectly fine, except for that cough.

"I found him!" the cop said, shouting out Harold's full name. "He's a missing elderly. He's been missing since seven o'clock."

All at once we looked at our watches. It was quarter after eight.

"How old is he?" I asked.

"Eighty-six. He was last seen in Coney Island. There's a Level 1 mobilization on him."

"Oh Harold! You're missing! The cops are all looking for you! And you made it so far in an hour. How'd you do that? Did you take the bus?"

Harold smiled and coughed. My guess was he took a bus from Coney Island to Park Slope. So creative.

The woman cop said, "I'm going to call my sergeant and tell him to send a unit from Coney Island to pick him up. We just have to wait for them."

"Wifey," Austin said. "What should I tell dispatch?"

"He's not sick. It's not hot out, and it's not cold. He was sitting in a car. He's only been gone an hour. This isn't a medical emergency. The emergency is that he's missing. He has a cough, so he might have the Rona. But if he doesn't and he's this old, I don't want to expose it to him in the hospital. He needs to go home."

"What do I tell dispatch while we wait for Coney Island PD?"

I shrugged. "Tell them it's a PD matter only, and we're blocked in."

She updated dispatch.

While we waited, the bystander lingered with us and chatted. People were lonely. He said he'd heard Alzheimer's patients often wandered to the place where they were originally from. I'd never heard that theory before, but it made sense.

My grandfather used to wander, too. He'd walk out the front door of his house, and my grandma would have to go all over the neighborhood looking for him. Once, she found him outside, wandering behind the house, strolling around the orange trees. "What are you doing out here in the orange trees?" she asked when she finally found him. He smiled and said, "There's something out here."

I think he was referring to something eternal and sacred, something invisible calling him out to the orange trees. After a few years on the street, I agreed with my grandpa. I thought there was something out here.

While we waited twenty, thirty minutes, Austin grew impatient. She got out some disinfectant wipes and began cleaning the ambulance—*while Harold was still inside it.* I knew what this meant. She was itching to leave. Go on another job. We could have easily told Harold to wait in the police officers' car and cleared the scene. But there was no way I was leaving my newfound missing friend squished in the back of an RMP. He was so happy on our stretcher.

I did feel bad for Austin, though. Once again, she'd responded to a job and the gift of the emergency she'd ordered online didn't measure up when it arrived in the mail.

Personally, I was ecstatic we'd found Harold. We'd found a missing person! How often did that happen? Not often, I didn't think. I couldn't stop playing hide-and-seek with him and the ambulance door to make his eyes crinkle. Apparently, he'd last been seen in the care of his home health aide. Whoever they were, they'd be looking for a new job tomorrow.

At last the cops from Coney Island arrived, two stocky white guys who looked like they owned wrap-around sunglasses. They congratulated all of us for finding a missing person.

They were unmasked, I observed.

We unloaded Harold from our stretcher, then eased him onto his feet and helped him into the back of the RMP. I was so sad to see him squashed in the cop car. His knees hit the back of the seat divider. His legs were almost as long as mine.

"He has a cough," I told the cops. "Possible Rona. Do you guys have masks? I'd drive with masks on and the windows down."

"No," they said. "Do you have any extra masks for us?"

Austin went to the truck, came back, and handed them surgical masks. They put them on.

At this time, sometimes cops weren't masked because they didn't have any PPE left and were surviving on donations, and not a lot of donations were flowing their way, so we gave them masks. Sometimes it was because they'd already had the Rona and they had antibodies and felt safe, so they weren't overly worried. Sometimes it was a tough-guy thing. Sometimes they believed COVID was an overblown hoax. But in New York City, where everyone on the street had direct contact with mass death and saw the bodies, that was pretty rare.

Firefighters were often unmasked these days, too. But due to the relentless hero narrative, no one dared yell at firefighters for not wearing masks, or even noticed. I found that somewhat amazing. People were so blinded by the power of those red suspenders they couldn't see anything but a superhero. The Fire Department is a master class in branding.

Whatever first responders believed, politics fell apart on the street, when you were a cop in a pandemic who had to transport a guy with a wet cough in the back of your RMP.

Everyone's an anti-masker until Harold gets in their car.

"Have a good night!" I said to the cops as they pulled away with my friend. And waving through the window, blowing him kisses, "Bye, Harold! Miss you already! Get home safe!"

"Wifey," Austin said when we got back on the truck. "That was a PD matter only. Now we need to go on a real medical job."

"How can you not be happy after spending an hour with Harold? That job was heaven, wifey. Nathan would have dragged that job out for two hours. Nina, too. She would've loved it."

"Wifey, we're different."

"So different. I don't understand you. I've married my opposite."

The tour just kept getting better for me, and worse for Austin.

I thought my wifey would be pleased when, hours later, we responded to an EDP-C. Austin was in the back of the truck teaching our observer when the job came over and Citizen alerted me that a man was behaving violently not far from where we were posted. I told dispatch we were 63.

Austin hopped in the driver's seat and raced to the address near Prospect Park, though perhaps "raced" was the wrong verb, since for EDP-Cs we didn't use lights or sirens. Psych patients presented a flight risk, so for these calls we rolled up dark.

When we got to the job location with PD, a tall, thin Asian cop with glasses said the patient had fled on foot and was running around attacking people. Panicked bystanders walking by our ambulance shouted, "He went that way! That way! That way!"

"What does he look like?" I asked the cops.

"Male, Black," they said.

Great description, everyone who called 911. Very refined. Really narrows it down.

Free advice for people calling 911 to report a possible crime in progress: Look at the person head to foot. How are they built? Tall? Stocky? Muscular? Approximate their age. Note their hair. Goatee? Bald? Sideburns? Color? Length? Move on to complexion. Light? Sunburned? Dark? Freckled? Clothing. What are they wearing? Colors are helpful. Red shirt? Black plants? Pink shoes? Distinguishing features. Tattoos, scars.

And please, please, please, New Yorkers, on behalf of everyone on the street—please stop calling 911 for the "smell of marijuana."

The cops got in their car and another RMP arrived. We followed them around the block, searching for the reportedly violent man. Someone said he'd gone into the park. Just then, a Black man in a pink gingham dress shirt walking a dog came out of the park.

Shaking my head I said to Austin, "This is a bad time to be that guy. This is when shit goes south, and every Black man fits the description."

"True, wifey, true," Austin said.

When we got to another residential block more bystanders on bicycle and foot pointed to another street and sent us on a wild goose chase. I kept calling dispatch to update the address. At this point I'd updated the address three times. We passed by a parked FDNY unit and a bald white guy rolled down his window and said, "Did you find him yet?"

I said, "No, PD is looking. He's on foot. We're following PD."

Laughing, he said, "This guy came up to us and yelled at us. He was like, 'Why aren't you guys doing anything? Why are you just sitting there?' And I said, 'We're EMTs, we're not cops. We're not going to get off the truck and run around looking for someone who's violent.' And they go, "Why not? Just throw a net over him! Catch him!' I was like, 'What? Throw a net? What the fuck are you talking about? We don't throw nets on people.'"

Immediately my mind went to Nathan, that night when he threw a sheet over our lice-infested, drug-addicted patient. "My partner threw a sheet on someone once," I told the EMTs. "It wasn't to catch them; it was to contain some bugs. But he straight up threw a sheet over a patient and burritod her."

"Burrito is one thing," the EMT said. "We burrito people with bugs all the time. But a net? Throw a net on someone? Where do people come up with this shit?"

"TV. They get it from TV. We're gonna follow PD."

"10-4, we'll roll behind you."

We crawled around the block with the FDNY ambulance in tow and stopped midway down the street, where four cops were standing on the sidewalk. We got out.

"You found the patient?" I asked the Asian cop. He was breathless and sweaty. "Yeah, he's here."

I told the FDNY EMTs and the five of us loped toward a brownstone.

On the stoop sat a calm, large brown boy whose eyes looked to the side when I spoke to him.

"He's special needs," his mother said. She was weeping.

I nodded. "Autism?"

"Yes. And he's violent. I don't know what to do. We can't control him when he gets angry. He beat us up," she said, pointing to the boy's sister. Then she leaned over to me and whispered, "He's so strong. He tried to kill us."

"I understand. How old is he?"

"He's twenty-five."

Twenty-five, but as was common with people with autism, he presented like a child. He was quiet at the moment, cheerful even. But his family was destroyed. His mother and sister paced the sidewalk and explained he'd been living in a residential facility, but they missed him, so they'd brought him home. But they couldn't control him. He was too violent. They were sore and bruised and bereft. "He can't stay here tonight," his mother said. "We can't do this."

Just then a Black conditions boss walked up, and she spoke with the mother, listening to the situation and nodding her understanding head.

"I have an autistic child," the boss said, "so I get it. I know what's happening, and I know how hard this is. But we can be smart here. Let me run an idea by you. What we can do is call paramedics and have them come and sedate."

"What does that mean?" the mother said frantically. "I don't understand."

"They'll give him medicine that makes him drowsy," I said.

"That's right," said the boss. "He'll go to sleep. That way, the cops won't have to try to control him if he gets violent again."

"You can trust her," I told the mother. "She knows what it's like. It's the gentler way."

"It's gentler," the conditions boss said. "Otherwise when we try to get him on the ambulance, if he gets violent, the cops will have to control him. This is the gentler way."

The mother agreed to sedation and conditions called for medics. Then the mother explained to me that her son was on the highest dose of medication he could take, and it wasn't working. Meanwhile the cops were hanging out with the patient. His name was Seth. They were being sweet with him, talking about video games and cartoons. I was proud to see them acting so compassionately, and grateful the conditions boss knew what it was like to be the mother of an autistic child who had fits of violence and that she had called for paramedics to help. Everyone on scene was doing their part, and it was awe-inspiring to witness and be part of the emergency.

"This is so hard," the mother said to me. "He keeps banging his head against the wall. He bangs it so hard, it's so violent, he has to have a head injury by now. I can't watch him do that to himself and I can't stop him. I'm not strong enough, I tried. My whole body hurts from trying to get him to stop being violent tonight. I'm going to be sore tomorrow. I'll have bruises."

"It's common for people with autism to do that," I assured her. "He's not trying to hurt himself. He's trying to calm down. He's overstimulated, and he's trying to soothe himself and get his brain to slow down."

The conditions boss said, "He's in sensory overload when that happens. My son does that, too."

"You have no idea how hard this is," his sister said. "We love him so much. But we can't handle him. We don't want him to go away, but we can't have him here. It's too much."

"I do understand. My brother did that when I was growing up. He used to bash his head against the headboard to try to knock himself out. It's awful to listen to. It's horrible. It's the saddest sound on earth."

"It's so sad," the mother said. "We're heartbroken."

"I know you are. But you're doing such a great job. You're doing the right thing tonight, and we're all here to help you. You're doing your best."

Soon, a third ambulance pulled up. When I turned, I saw two FDNY rescue medics walking toward us. Immediately I recognized one of the medics was Chase—the rescue medic I'd worked a dozen jobs with over the years, who'd been on the back of my truck that night I knocked three or four mirrors off cars. I hadn't seen him in months, not since the pandemic started, and seeing him on the street now I was dizzy with joy that he was alive. I didn't even know that was a fear I had inside me, that first responders I worked with on the street were dead. But on the sidewalk, I realized as relief flooded my system that this whole time, all these months, I'd been carrying a secret terror that EMTs and medics we worked with had died.

"The heroes are here!" I cheered.

"Hey!" Chase said, smiling. "Where've you been? Long time. Good to see you."

The conditions boss gave Chase the story, and he walked over to Seth and introduced himself to the patient. "Hey, buddy. What's your name?"

"Seth."

"Nice to meet you, Seth. I'm Chase."

I made my voice high and angelic. "Seth, sweetie, Chase is a paramedic. And we're going to go with him onto the ambulance now, so he can help you. Just follow us, OK? We'll all walk there together."

"OK," Seth said, standing up and following us to the ambulance.

As we walked, I said to Chase, "How've you been? I haven't seen you in ages."

"Yeah, I'm OK. How've you been?"

"Little busy."

Seth climbed onto the ambulance and Chase followed him inside. Before we left, I hung on the back of the FDNY truck and took in the scene. Chase sitting on the stretcher, face-to-face with Seth, placing a band around his arm to prep for an IV. Seth was relaxed, and in good hands.

"We should go now," Chase said to the boss. "While he's calm." Then he looked at the cops and said, "One of you is coming with me."

Perhaps it's worth pausing here for a moment on the medic's request for police accompaniment on the ambulance. Who restrains this patient if he gets violent again en route to the ER so the paramedic can insert a needle into his arm, find a vein, and sedate, without the medic getting assaulted by the patient? I've had civilian friends look at me with a straight face and say I should do it. You want EMTs to restrain violent patients? EMTs, who make between $0 and $14 an hour, wear no ballistics vests, and only get two hours of training in responding to EDPs and volatile patients? I took a Krav Maga class once, but I wasn't that good at it.

Words and physical restraint. Unfortunately, those are your options for getting violent patients—and we have a lot of them in New York City—to comply with EMS treatment and transport without EMTs medics getting hurt. Cops and hospital security guards hold patients down for medics to sedate and control the patient on the ambulance and in the ER in instances where they try to assault EMTs. Words don't work on these calls if the patient is in an altered, violent state.

You can train all you want to talk down someone in a crisis. I'm a crisis communicator. But if your homeless, drunk, schizophrenic patient is hallucinating and thinks you're the devil trying to kill him, so he tries to kill you right back, or he's a violent criminal on angel dust spitting in your face, or he's autistic and having a fit of aggression so violent that he tried to kill his own mother and she called 911 begging for help—best of luck.

The Asian cop climbed on the rescue medics' truck.

"Bye, Seth," I said, waving to him from the street.

"Bye," he said, waving back.

Walking back to our truck, I wished I could have gone to the hospital with the rescue medics. But our work was done, Seth was in capable hands, and the family was relieved, if only for the night. Their heartbreak would linger, as would mine, as would everyone's. But the wonder lingered with me, too. A sense of awe and amazement at what was offered so freely on the street by a family of kind and capable first responders.

Another RMP rolled up when the job was finished. I told the cops it was all good, they weren't needed. They could go. They said, "sounds good."

Before leaving, one of the cops, a petite blonde woman with dimpled cheeks I often saw on the street, looked at me and said, "I said to myself as soon as I saw you on scene, 'Oh, good, she's here. Everything's going to be OK.'"

I couldn't believe she felt that way about me.

That's how I used to feel when I was new, when I saw seasoned first responders like Laverne on scene, one of my sheroes. I stood frozen in the street.

And then a miracle.

From a void of dust and darkness deep inside me, the collapsed towers rose, shook off their dust, and returned to their standing position. Stood tall, shoulder to shoulder, indestructible twins, solid and intact. Just like that everyone dead came back. Pat came back. He was alive and right there in the Brooklyn street. I saw him, alive again. I saw his smiling face in the window of his fire truck, red and perfect and uncrushed, rolling slowly up Lafayette Street as I walked toward the yoga school where we prayed and meditated together, side by side, his arm out the truck window, waving to me from the officer's side of the rig, his voice over the PA, laughing and shouting, "Jennifer! Jennifer! It's me!"

It was me.

Because of him.

I made the road. I drew the map.

Finally, I happened.

* * *

It really was magic, this night. An evening of unspeakable tenderness I would never forget. Everyone so brave and kind. Everyone saving one another. Mutual aid. I wished everyone in America would become a first responder.

Austin was miserable. The night for her had been a total failure. We'd done no medicine whatsoever, so the observer was bored. But it didn't matter to me. I didn't even like medicine.

Of all my years on the street, this tour was by far my favorite. EMS was a job, or a hobby—whatever it was for me at this point—it was an occupation that robbed you blind and stole all of your emotional money. Then one unexpected night it replenished it in full. The street turned people like me, garden-variety people, into courageous rescuers. Magicians capable of facing an emergency with joy and courage.

Austin had her favorite jobs and I had mine. Either way, we were uniquely capable of cauterizing the world's wounds, emotional or medical, traumatic or familial. We were there. And to be there was such a privilege and a salve. It was magic.

It really did save me, I think. All those nights riding on the ambulance.

When I vlogged about the night and sent my video to Mike, he told me he couldn't love me more. When I sent it to Tommy, he said he hadn't had a night like that in years, for as long as he could remember. And Nina, she understood my bliss exactly. Finally, our next tour, she got her dream job, too: an EDP with a knife.

But it wasn't quite what she'd hoped it would be.

One Saturday the first week of September, Nina and I returned to the street. Reunited at last. We could not have been happier. Being together again on the truck, it almost seemed like COVID had never happened. Nina had been off since the end of March. I asked if it had helped, taking time off. If she felt less burned out than she'd felt before.

"No, not at all," she said. "I'm right where I left off."

I guessed there was no way to uncook yourself after the street had done its number on you.

It was a cool, beautiful night. We spent hours talking and catching up. We went to 7-Eleven and bought our favorite snacks. Cracked jokes. Went on jobs that resulted in no patients. Things were calm until around ten o'clock, when we responded to a run for an "unknown." Unknown was unknown. We didn't know anything.

We got on scene and saw four RMPs and eight cops on the street, and a parked FDNY ambulance with two EMTs. Rolling up we were like, Damn, what happened here? We got out and asked one of the FDNY EMTs what the deal was. He told us the call came over 911 as "man in his underwear wielding a machete."

Intriguing.

In New York City, knives of a certain blade length were considered "dangerous" or "deadly," and were illegal outside the home.

Scanning the scene, I saw a young white guy I guessed was in his twenties sitting on the stoop of a brownstone in his underwear, screaming at the cops. The cops were all different races and genders. They looked miserable. An Asian NYPD lieutenant stood to the side, speaking in a hushed voice to an elderly woman who was visibly upset and unsteady on her feet. The patient's grandma. She looked worried and sad.

Before I approached the hostile patient, I asked the elderly woman if her grandson had a mental health diagnosis. Yes, she said. Anxiety. And drinking. When he drank, he got angry. I asked if he ever expressed a desire to hurt himself or others. Not others, she said. But himself, Yes. When he was drunk, he was suicidal. Had he been drinking tonight? Yes. A lot.

I approached the patient sitting in his underwear on the stoop. I could smell alcohol on him from six feet away. He was still shouting at cops because there were so many of them.

I interrupted his rant and said, "Hi, sir, I'm not a cop," then turned around so he could see my uniform said EMT on the back. He gave me his attention and asked me about the cops. How come, he wanted to know, when his car got broken into last year and he called 911, nobody showed up. But tonight, when he was standing outside his own house cutting some grass, there were a million cops at his door.

"It's the machete," I said. "The machete is what really makes the difference here."

I did not say, *And the fact that you're drunk. And in your underwear. And screaming.*

Now, remember, this patient was white. Lived on a very nice block in Carroll Gardens, in a beautiful brownstone I could never in this lifetime afford. It had a yard in the front, with some raggedy grass he was apparently trying to cut—with a machete. Part of me thought, Damn. I feel bad for you. You're about to get slapped with a fine in front of your own house. That sucks.

But I don't care how white you are, all the whiteness in the world is not going to help you when you're drunk and wielding a machete outside in your underwear in New York City. I saw the weapon. With a blade that could easily relieve you of your limbs or head with one double-handed chop. This was Brooklyn. This wasn't Kansas. This wasn't a beach in Punta Cana, where you can open up a coconut with a machete.

I was a white woman, so I got away with all sorts of things because I was white. In my youth I could have been arrested for a plethora of misbehaviors: jumping a turnstile, riding my bike on the sidewalk, public intoxication, smell of marijuana, failing to use my turn signal, speeding. And yet I'd never received a single ticket from any police officer in any city in any country where I'd ever lived in my entire life. But even as a white woman, I couldn't just walk outside my house in Brooklyn and start shooting the petals off flowers with a 9mm. That would not go over well here.

So at first, I felt bad for the patient. Because clearly this was a psychiatric emergency, but he was also bombed, so it was a combo deal. I tried to be direct and asked if he suffered from anxiety, like his grandmother had told me. He said no. I asked if he'd been drinking, and how much. He said no, and nothing. So we were in fiction.

I love fiction, so I was at home. Then I asked if he'd ever wanted to kill himself and he got cute and said everyone thought about hurting themselves sometimes. True, but not everyone was outside in their skivvies with a machete. I told the patient his grandmother was concerned and had given me this information.

Then the guy started yelling at me. He got vicious. He screamed at me on the street for I don't know, ten minutes. So much for being a seasoned crisis communicator. This job was a massive fail. The FDNY EMTs came up to us and asked if they could leave, because clearly this call was going to take well over an hour, and one of them, a woman, was working a night tour on a private hospital ambulance that started soon. Municipal EMTs often worked multiple jobs to survive, since their salary was so low. We said, Sure thing, off you go, have a safe tour.

After this intermission the patient resumed screaming at me. Then his grandmother hobbled over and tried to help, and he turned on her. He called her a stupid fucking bitch and other colorful names for several minutes. That's when my empathy for the patient vanished. I was on Grandma's side now. No one yells at Grandma!

Next up to bat on the verbal wrath front was the Asian NYPD lieutenant. The patient faced the officer and screamed some racist profanities at him. So now my heart went out to the Asian guy as the call turned into a hate crime.

I couldn't keep up with my feelings. I felt like I'd been punched in the face, then someone came along and stabbed me in the heart, then, while I was doubled over in pain, a driver barreled down the street and ran me over with a car. That was EMS, in a nutshell. That was why we killed ourselves ten times more often than everyday people. That was not on any of the sexy posters used to lure people into this remarkable profession.

Not long after the racial profanities hit the air one of the cops quietly told me to step back. In one silent swoop four officers walked up to the patient, lifted him easily to his feet, put him in handcuffs, walked him to the ambulance, sat him on the bench, and fastened his seatbelt.

I sped lights-and-sirens to an ER where the security guards looked like bouncers. This was not a patient we could take to a general 911-receiving facility where the security guards were very nice, slender gentlemen in the geriatric age range.

A white male cop the patient liked, probably because he remained silent on scene, rode on the back of the ambulance with Nina. The patient screamed the entire ride. The cop's partner, who was supposed to be following our ambulance, got lost en route and caught up with us midway to the ER. Finally, we got to the hospital, but there was no parking, so I had to circle the block in search of a spot. Meanwhile all the ERs required codes to get inside, and each code was different. I was so fried from being screamed at nonstop for an hour I couldn't remember the code to get in, so while Nina and the cops and patient were already in the hospital, I stood outside punching the code box like a dumbass.

Beep beep beep, no. Beep beep beep, no. Beep beep beep, oh, thank God.

"I'm looking for my patient," I said to the security guard. "Violent white guy."

The guard clasped his wrists together as if they were handcuffed and raised his arms and said, "Did he look like this?"

"That would be him."

In the ER, the patient had more to say to me. He demanded to know how much this ambulance ride would cost, because he wanted me to pay for it. He also wanted to know why we'd driven him so far away from his house instead of taking him to the hospital right around the corner. I told him because that hospital was busy tonight.

"Your partner said you brought me here because I was being aggressive."

"Yes," I said. "And also because of that."

"Aggressive!" he shouted, raising his handcuffed wrists above his head. "Do I look aggressive right now? Murphy. Murphy. Murphy. Murphy. Do I look aggressive?"

I felt obliterated.

After a while Nina and I exited the hospital just as a pair of cops from the job arrived with the patient's grandma. She looked so tired. I felt horrible for her, that this was her life.

I went up to see if she was OK, and to tell her that her grandson was safe inside, speaking with doctors.

She was worried for him. She said there were security cameras in front of her house, and she wanted the police to look at the footage so her grandson wouldn't get arrested. I wasn't current on the city's machete-carrying consequences, but I was pretty sure he was just going to get fined. Anyway, she said he really was just outside trimming the grass. The weeds were branchy and hard to cut, which was why he had the machete, and he didn't mean anyone any harm. She said it didn't help that when the police arrived out of nowhere and told her grandson to drop the weapon, it took him over a minute to do what they said. So that wasn't good. But she wanted to make sure doctors understood the whole story, so her grandson wouldn't get in trouble.

"I understand," I said. "You can tell the nurses inside. They'll listen to you. But here's the thing. The police didn't just drop out of the sky to swarm your grandson. Bystanders called 911 because they saw him and got scared, so a dispatcher sent the police. And here's how the call came in: 'man standing outside in his underwear wielding a machete.'"

"Oh," she said, nodding in glum understanding. "When you hear that, the story writes itself."

The story wrote itself. The first responder also wrote the story.

"Well," I said to Nina as we headed miserably back to base. "You finally got your dream job, an EDP with a knife."

"I hated it," she said. "That was horrible."

"Horrible."

I didn't know what more to think or feel about all this. It was so complex and dynamic on the street, the way these calls played out. And EMS was perhaps the least-understood medical profession that existed. That was my lasting feeling after that night: People didn't get it. People didn't understand. They had no idea.

How did we fix this? Where did we even start?

The reality:

A mental health crisis plagues New York City, and 911 calls for people experiencing a psychiatric emergency have skyrocketed over the years, doubling from 97,000 calls to 911 in 2009 to around 180,000 calls in 2018.

The city's response to this crisis has been *disastrous.*

ThriveNYC, founded by Chirlane McCray, the city's first lady, is a broad-bucket mental health organization with an annual budget of $250 million. It's comprised of numerous mental health initiatives for "all New Yorkers." But Thrive has been critiqued by experts on all sides of the mental-wellness debate as a massive waste of financial resources with elusive metrics and programs that have neglected the city's highest-need mentally ill citizens. Thrive has done next to nothing for individuals in crisis who flood the 911 system as well as our hospitals, jails, homeless shelters, and drug treatment centers.

In 2016, Thrive formed mobile crisis co-response teams of novice psychologists, cops, and social workers to assist people in a mental health emergency. But it never connected its mobile crisis teams to the 911 system. And it couldn't retain its staff. *New York* magazine reported that 63 percent of its Mental Health Service Corps left their assignments in the first year. And 30 percent quit before working with the organization for two years. Even the DOH noted Thrive had difficulty recruiting and retaining its workforce. Like EMTs, social workers are low-paid, overburdened professionals. Thrive relies on them to execute its vague goals—but it can't retain them.

Should I go on?

Thrive established a call center for people in a mental health crisis. And yet, "More New Yorkers dialed 911 to report a person in the midst of a mental health crisis last year—179,000 calls—than at any point in more than a decade," a March 22, 2019, *New York Times* article detailing Thrive's shortcomings reported. The news piece noted critical failures in the call center: Thrive didn't track patient outcomes for how many callers got treatment, and it linked callers to response teams that were often too slow to address the needs of people in a true emergency. Instead of waiting, those who urgently needed help called 911.

These individuals are our patients. They are the neglected ones.

So are we. EMTs and paramedics remain an invisible class on the street, left out of important conversations about medical emergencies to which we respond.

Thrive's laundry list of offerings has a big, squishy heart aimed to help average New Yorkers feel less frowny, but as Fred Siegel of the Manhattan Institute said to one of the mayor's senior advisors: "The problem is not sad people."

The problem in New York City is the astonishing 911 call volume involving people in a mental health crisis, who EMTs and cops treat and transport constantly, and who the city has roundly and categorically failed. While the majority of these emergencies are resolved without incident, those resulting in deadly police force have been well documented. Those resulting in violence against EMTs and paramedics have been completely undocumented. How to better assist vulnerable individuals, reduce police brutality, *and keep EMTs and paramedics safe*, is an excruciating pain point in New York City.

All the new and best thinking about psychiatric emergencies revolves around how to reduce or eliminate the presence of law enforcement on these calls. That's the right next step. The mentally ill are sixteen times more likely to die from lethal police force than other citizens. Most police departments support this change as well. As mentioned, cops don't like these runs, and many of them aren't adequately trained to handle them. Neither are EMTs. Many states, light-years ahead of New York, have seen great success using new models. California. Some cities in Texas. Eugene, Oregon has an impressive program.

But New York City is not Eugene, Oregon. Or LA. Or Houston, where mobile health units resulted in a significant reduction in 911 calls, whereas our call volume for EDPs doubled.

Our EMS system in New York City is badly broken. And instead of acknowledging that, stepping back, and reimagining the system, the city keeps patching it with ineffective pseudo-solutions concocted by politicians who have no experience on the street, where the city's mental health disaster plays out at the expense of vulnerable patients and overworked first responders. Particularly EMS workers, who the city refuses to pay a livable wage.

In 2020, in response to defund-the-police campaigns and fatal police encounters with the mentally ill, the mayor and the city's first lady, who heads Thrive, announced a plan to launch a pilot program in two neighborhoods that would replace cops with social workers for some 911 calls for mental health emergencies. Sounds good, right?

But the program doesn't reduce the crushing number of 911 calls for EDPs. It's not citywide, so EMTs in all but two neighborhoods will continue to co-respond to the bulk of these emergencies with cops, therefore it doesn't in any foreseeable future reduce the presence of law enforcement on mental health calls. It doesn't provide our patients with alternatives to hospitals or jails, so EMTs and cops will continue to take people to ERs that don't want them and jails where many of them do not belong. It doesn't give citywide EMTs or paramedics who are already on the street responding to these calls any training. It once again relies on social workers it has a track record of being unable to retain. And most perilously, it almost certainly increases the risk of patient violence toward EMS workers, which is already high.

"This is a highly dangerous situation for our EMTs and paramedics," Oren Barzilay with the union representing FDNY EMTs told CBS New York, adding that he would not allow his members to respond to these calls without cops. "On a daily basis, our members get assaulted as is, with the police present."

How did we fix this? Where did we even start?

Maybe we started with the stories. With the experiences of first responders.

No one listened to us. No one invited us to the table. People always skipped that part.

Nina got her dream job at last. But it sure wasn't what she'd hoped it would be.

Neither was my mother's dream, of owning a cabin in the mountains where she spent her childhood, and I spent mine. Toward the end of August, a wildfire had started in the Sequoia Forest, too. The SQF Complex fire was taking a lot of the beautiful trees where I grew up. My mom was evacuated and was safe in Bakersfield, awaiting news. This wasn't our first wildfire rodeo. Last year she'd been evacuated as well, for another forest fire. It was just part of life in California now. Once or twice a year, everything went up in flames.

23

THE WILD ROVER

In September I pulled myself off the ambulance and went out of service. I was in need of a break, and not a small one. I didn't know when I'd ride again as an EMT. I didn't even know if I'd stay in New York City or move away. I was too bereaved to think straight or make any major decisions. Or minor decisions. I struggled to decide what to eat for dinner.

Then something strange happened.

For the first time in nineteen years, I woke up happy on 9/11. The happiness did not belong to me; it was borrowed. It belonged to Pat. That Friday morning I could feel his joy undeniably. But I couldn't understand it. *You're so happy,* I said to him in my apartment that morning. *What's going on?*

I always felt Pat strongly on this day—we all did—his presence and gratitude that we were coming together to tell stories that brought him back to life. But I wouldn't describe his energy as happy. And 2020, of all years? With Mike sick and dying in Vegas during a contagion that prevented him from being here? That wiped out September 11 memorial services?

I was baffled. And happy. I couldn't deny it and I couldn't wait to get into the city. To see Ylfa and Bobby and Paul. The three of us were meeting outside Pat's firehouse. It would be closed because of COVID, but who cared. We needed to be there. Be together. That was all that mattered.

Because of the virus I hadn't seen anyone in days, or maybe it was weeks, I couldn't remember. My memory was shot. And time was surreal, almost hallucinogenic. Time was a Salvador Dalí clock melting over tree branches, furniture spotted with insects, a sleeping face on the desert floor.

* * *

As I was heading out of my neighborhood, into the city, I drove past the street housing Ladder 111, and noticed it was blocked off. Outside, dress-blued firefighters in surgical masks were scrambling around, assembling a huge, white tent.

I couldn't believe what I was seeing. They weren't supposed to be doing anything. Firehouses were reportedly closed, veteran first responders told to stay home due to COVID, due to the fact that they had health conditions from 9/11 that made them vulnerable to the virus striking them dead. But when was the last time a New York City firefighter followed a rule?

"Heroes!" I screamed, banging the steering wheel. They found the guts to disobey the rules. Fuck it, they must have said. They were creating space for us. The families, veterans, complex grievers. The ones for whom not a day went that by that we forgot. Not one day. The whole world had moved on but not us. We were still stuck in those voids. Still waiting. Still digging. Dropping like flies. We were not surviving this event. It was the terror that kept on terrorizing.

And so this morning as I drove over the bridge, leaving Brooklyn and 2020 and COVID behind me, making my reentry into Manhattan, 2001, and 9/11, I thought about those firefighters setting up a tent in Brooklyn, and I felt they were the kindest, bravest, most spiritual people on the planet.

In the car my perspective on their actions widened like the river beneath me, and I thought more broadly, historically, of how vital it was for us—all of us, everyone bereaved by symbols of death and violence and injustice—to reclaim symbols of agony. Take them back, reappropriate them, or burn them down. The agonized get to decide.

When people tell you they're in pain—believe them.

The firefighters had done that today. Taken the ghastly white tent and transformed it from a sign of mass death—from the relentless flood of sick bodies riddled with COVID to the unsurvivable disembodiment of 9/11—and they'd spun out of that twinned horror a new light.

If only for today, the white tent was a sanctuary. A church. A sacred place for us to gather and pray.

* * *

In Manhattan I parked near Pat's firehouse and trudged up the blocks, fifteen minutes before the time when the first plane struck, when New York City was untouched by tragedy and Pat was still alive. I had a little hope that maybe his firehouse would be open, too.

As I turned down Thirteenth Street the half-masted flag of my heart unfurled when I saw Ladder 3's fire truck parked outside, lights flashing, garage door wide open, masked firefighters standing in distanced clusters in the street.

It was happening here, too. And I believed it was happening, and my chances of surviving skyrocketed.

Heroes.

Pat's bench was back.

The firefighters had taken the banners of the fallen from inside the house and strung them above the red garage door. The wind was strong and constant, lifting the bannered men, lifting me. And there across the street, Ylfa and Bobby and Paul, all of us here for Pat. Gonzo, too. He was here, wearing jeans and a turquoise shirt instead of his uniform this year. I ran up to my friends and hugged them hard. "I had to be here," Gonzo said when we embraced. We all did. This was home. I'd expected nothing. And look at all this, for us.

"Sister," Ylfa said, her eyes lit up like those of a little girl. She took my hand and pulled me toward her. She pointed across the street, at a firefighter on a ladder, adjusting Pat's smiling face. The firefighter was leaning, reaching over, carefully straightening the banner, adjusting it as if he were helping a man with his bowtie.

"Look at Pat," Ylfa said. "His banner keeps getting twisted and flipping, so they keep having to adjust it. He's the only one who keeps doing that. He's getting so much attention."

"He loves it. He's so happy today."

"Right? I felt that way, too. We're all here for him, maybe that's why."

"But we're always here for him. Why would he be happy this year more than any other?"

"I don't know. But do you feel the wind? How strong it is?"

"The wind."

* * *

When it was time, we crossed the street. The firefighters came outside and fell into formation for the first moment of silence.

We lived and died in these moments. At 8:46, the North Tower was struck. After a moment, bagpipes. "Amazing Grace." That's when I usually lost it. And yet this year, no tears. Heaviness, yes. Pain in my chest. Somnolence. But no tears. Was it possible EMDR had helped? I never thought this day would get better. Not in my lifetime. And yet this morning, a new happiness. *Pat.*

Somewhere between the second and third moment, 9:03 and 9:37, when the South Tower and pentagon were struck, Pat's sister, Carolyn, and her husband walked up the block wearing masks.

"We couldn't miss it!" Carolyn said, smiling under her mask. "We had to be here. We took the train."

Amazing grace.

We hugged and caught up. Hi, sweetie. Hi, love. How are you? Have you talked to Mike? We're texting him right now. We're sending him pictures and videos. It's so good we're all together. And they're doing it. It's so great, right?

Then we turned, and there on the sidewalk were three disabled bicyclists with leg prosthetics and tiny American flags on their bikes, all of them double- or single-leg amputees. They rolled up and stopped in front of Ladder 3's fire truck.

"Vietnam!" they said, shouting out their years.

My hand went to my heart.

Paul said, "I'm Vietnam!" He dashed up to the men, shook their hands, told them his year.

Welcome home. Welcome home. Welcome home.

The firefighters ran inside and came back with bottles of Gatorade. They handed them to the Vietnam vets and surrounded them. We took their picture with the firefighters encircling them, and as we did—and you could not make this up—the wind tore the clouds apart and sunlight shined down on them.

It was magic, this day. It was Irish. It was Pat. I had no words to capture it.

They call it the unspeakable for a reason.

After a moment the bikers floated away, their flags snapping in the wind, and we cheered them down the street. I swam in and out of conversation and silence, endless texts and videos and photographs zipping across the country to Mike.

"I'm with you today," he told me, Ylfa, and Paul.

"You're with us," I said. "And we're with you."

"Hey, send some more pictures."

Paul sent him the photograph of the Vietnam vets.

"I need to be there," Mike said.

Paul said, "You are. I carried you in my heart."

A woman came up to the firehouse holding a bouquet of pink and white and green flowers. Prayerfully she set them down on Pat's bench, then she lumbered away.

"Do you know who that was?" I asked Bobby. "Did you see that woman?"

"Never seen her before. She may have been someone one of the guys saved. At Pat's wake a lot of them came. People no one knew. They came to the wake and said Pat had rescued them."

He rescued me, too.

Outside the firehouse, Carolyn and I talked about the state of the world. A priest appeared in a mask and we nodded to acknowledge him. We spoke about being Catholic and not going to Mass. Carolyn said she was thinking of returning. She prayed, as did I, but neither of us went to church. She said she felt that's what the world needed most right now, prayer.

I couldn't agree more.

We spoke about Mike. I told her Ylfa and I had been in constant touch with him.

"You know he calls you his wives," Carolyn said.

"Yes, we know. We encourage it."

We spoke about Pat. Carolyn said she had no idea who he was until his funeral. "I thought my brother was a firefighter. I didn't know he was—"

"—The Firefighter."

"Exactly."

"I didn't know, either. I had no idea. His funeral changed my life."

"Pat kept his life separate. No one knew until he died who he really was."

We spoke about how many people he touched. How the stories about him kept pouring in from all directions. How they kept him alive. How many of them were unexplainable.

"Listen to this one," I said. "A few years ago I spoke at a conference, and I mentioned losing a firefighter friend in 9/11. I didn't mention Pat's name. Out of nowhere a man in military dress came up to me and said, 'Was your friend Patrick Brown?'"

"I have chills," Carolyn said. "I have chills all over my legs."

"Me too. I told the man yes, I was talking about Patrick Brown. He asked me if I knew about the four S's. I had no idea what he was talking about. He said he knew Pat, and that Pat talked all the time about practicing the four S's: Service involving Sacrifice done in Silence equals Serenity. I asked Bobby and Ylfa and Paul if they'd ever heard Pat talk about the four S's, and they all said no. No one had ever heard of this. I turned to talk to someone else and when I turned back around the man was gone. I'd never seen him before, and I've never seen him since. I have no idea who he was. Full military dress."

"My whole body is covered in chills," Carolyn said.

We made it through the last three moments and bagpipes, 9:59, the South Tower's collapse, 10:07, the crash of Flight 93 in Shanksville, 10:28, the North Tower's collapse, when Pat was taken.

This year because of COVID there was no firehouse Mass, no wooden chairs lined up for us to sit. But the priest was going to read the names and bless the plaques. We stood at the edge of the firehouse, between inside and outside, this world and the next, and listened to the reading of the names. Then we watched the priest bless the plaques with holy water.

I felt blessed, too.

After the priest whispered his blessing, we lingered outside for a while. Gonzo was in good humor. He was buzzing around, talking to everyone, smiling, laughing, shaking hands, in high spirits. So nice to be around him and see him in this mood. He deserved every bit of laughter and joy the world had left. He was one of the only remaining men at Ladder 3 who came to the firehouse every year, and he'd done such a good job staying close to Mike, not forgetting him, not leaving Pat's brother behind.

Soon, the bagpiper was leaving. I wanted to tell him the mysterious and amazing story from last year, about hearing the bagpipes in the shower when my phone was off. I went up to him and we hugged and laughed about seeing each other in the middle of an emergency he was working some time ago.

"I have an Irish story about your bagpipes from Pat. Do you have time for it?"

"Of course. I want to hear it."

Before I could get the story out, an extremely important and spiritual story from the other side, an Irish magic story from and about Pat, Gonzo came up to the bagpiper and whispered something in his year, and the two of them laughed.

"Gonzo!" I said. "What did you just say?"

"Jennifer, I'm sorry—it was a joke. He knows I was joking. I told him, 'Hey, Jennifer just asked me if you're wearing any underwear under your kilt.'"

I pushed Gonzo and we hugged and slapped each other's backs. "You're out of control today. I'm trying to tell a fucking spiritual story and you're cracking dirty jokes."

"I couldn't help it!"

"Yeah, you guys can never help it."

I told Gonzo to get lost and told the bagpiper the story.

"So keep playing your music," I said. "Pat loves it. It's important to him."

"Thank you for telling me this, it means a lot. I will."

After a moment or two, Gonzo looked at all of us gathered there for Pat and said, "Guys? We going down?"

We looked at each other and scrambled to make a decision. Was the memorial even open? We didn't know. It wasn't supposed to be. They said it was closed. We'd find out. Were we going down? We were going down. But how? Impossible to find parking down there. The train. None of us had taken the subway since the pandemic hit. We were fine with it. We had masks. And the train was probably the cleanest place in New York City.

Gonzo said, "Where'd everybody park?"

I had to feed the parking meter before we left. Gonzo told me to run and do it now, before we all went down. He said they would wait for me. He said go.

As he walked forward and I walked backward, away from Pat's firehouse, bench, flowers, freshly blessed plaque, burning candles, Carolyn, Ylfa, Bobby, Paul, my family, and as I was walking a sudden fear overtook me that I would hold everyone up waiting for me, or worse—they would leave without me.

"Don't leave me," I pleaded with Gonzo.

"We won't leave you."

"It's my biggest fear."

"We won't leave you."

The subway was beautiful.

"I've never seen the subway so clean in my life," Gonzo said.

We got off the train and rose out of the station near Ten House. A fire truck was parked outside, the garage door open, flags waving. There was only a dozen or so people scattered in the blocked-off street as we walked to the memorial, but it was happening. It was open for families and veterans, like always. We checked into the tent for family members and pinned our little blue ribbons on our shirts.

Silently we trudged toward Pat's name.

There he was, etched in black, sun-warmed marble. One by one, we approached the altar of reflecting pools and spoke to him. I ran my fingertips over his beautiful name. Thanked him and told him I loved him. And we were here. And Mike was here.

That's when it struck me, why he was happy.

Pat was happy because Mike was coming home. Soon he would get to see his brother. They'd be together. Mike's nearing death was Pat's happiness. Message received. I blew out a breath and stepped back.

Carolyn set Pat's laminated photo in one of the cracks, near a little American flag, and I wept.

Then I caught my breath and listened to the names being read over the loudspeaker. Not by family members in person this year, due to COVID, but recordings of family members. It didn't matter. The names of the fallen were called. And we were here to listen. To acknowledge the world's loss.

There were uniformed servicepeople wandering around in silent clusters. Maybe a hundred people scattered about. Nothing compared to the usual crowd. Police officers. Soldiers. Firefighters young and old. Then a sight that surprised me, a flock of pilots and flight attendants. *Of course.* I hadn't seen them here before, but of course. The planes. American Airlines.

Ylfa came up to me with a startled look on her face. "I thought I just saw Mike."

"Oh no. Down here? That's a bad sign."

"This guy, it was the way he walked. I swear—I thought it was Mike."

"Pat's here. I think that's why he's happy. The only thing different this year is that Mike is dying. Which means he gets to see his brother soon."

"I hadn't thought about it like that. It makes sense. I think you're right."

Eventually we wandered out of the memorial and back to the train. Gonzo went up to the subway attendant and, pointing at me and Bobby, said, "I'm a firefighter, and I got one firefighter and one EMT with me."

I guessed I was the EMT.

Back on Thirteenth Street, we hugged him goodbye. Ylfa and Bobby and Paul and I decided to have lunch together. But Gonzo had to get back to New Jersey to go to another ceremony in the town where he lived.

"I love you," he told Ylfa as they hugged goodbye.

"Do you love me, too?" I asked him.

"Yes, Jen," he said, hugging me. "I love you, too."

After Gonzo left, Paul met up with me and Ylfa and Bobby for lunch, and the four of us sat outside in a garden at a little café near the firehouse. We sat for hours. Talking. Telling stories about Pat. Ylfa and Paul mostly listened. I couldn't shut up.

I sat across from Bobby, which was a big mistake. Bobby was a volunteer firefighter created by Pat, and I was a volunteer EMT created by Pat, and as two Pat-created first responders, we took a nosedive into stories from the street. Me and Bobby, we drowned poor Ylfa and Paul in our insane and uproarious tales from the ambulance and fire truck, respectively.

We discussed the mayoral suggestion of putting social workers on the trucks with us instead of cops, which we both felt was dangerous for first responders, and said a lot about suits at city hall being treacherously out of touch with how much violence we received on the street.

We talked about the disastrous state of policing. Bobby thought cops should have more psych evaluations. That all it used to ask them on the test was how they felt about the color pink. Then I went into a monologue about how many questions about mothers were on the psych test for police. How the test was like, "Do you love your mother? Do you ever think of her? Do you have dreams with your mother in them? When you're angry do you think it's OK to hurt people? When you're standing on a cliff do you think of jumping off? Are you scared of sharp, pointy objects? Do you love your mother? Do you ever dream of it, of fucking her?"

Bobby tipped his head back in laughter. Ylfa said it was like watching ping-pong, listening to us go back and forth. Then after a few minutes we told Bobby the story of Mike getting sober. He hadn't heard it yet, not the whole thing.

"So courageous of him to get sober," Bobby said.

"How long do you think he has?" I asked. "I feel like he doesn't have long."

As soon as I said it, I wished I hadn't. I wished I could take it back. I didn't want to speak it to life. The street taught me that words could do that. Words could make things happen.

Everyone stared at their knees. A moment of silence.

And then Paul, superstitiously, "I try not to say stuff like that."

Bobby said, "He's very sick."

"He's very sick," Ylfa said. "And Pat's here."

Later, after Bobby and Paul left, Ylfa and I sat in the garden, just the two of us. We called Mike. FaceTimed him so we could see each other. His cousin Jay had gone to Vegas to spend the day with him so he wouldn't be alone. Finally he answered. The second he saw us he dropped his head and wept. He was shaking with tears, crying harder than I'd ever seen him cry.

He looked so sick. His face was huge and bloated, his skin so pale he was almost gray, and what hair he had left was white and swept off his moonlike face.

"I'm sorry," Mike said, raising his head after some time.

And we said, "No, no, no. Don't apologize."

He tried to get off the phone because he couldn't stop crying. "OK, guys."

Ylfa said, "We don't have to go yet, Turtle. Stay with us a little longer. Stay with your wives. We love you so much. And it's OK to cry. It's good to let it out."

He cried more, and we held him in our hands.

What a changed man. From the guy I met at Ladder 3 two years back who didn't shed a tear at the firehouse on September 11, to this beautiful, sober, feeling soul. It was miraculous to witness. I was so proud of him. Bobby was right. What courage, to get sober on your deathbed. To be awake for life, in all its beauty and torment. It was heroic. That's what Mike was. A hero.

"I just miss you guys so much," he said, catching his breath. "I want to be with you in New York. I miss Pat. And I don't feel good."

"We know sweetheart," I said. "It's so hard. We love you so much and this isn't fair."

"No, it's not," Mike said.

Ylfa said, "You were here with us all day. And Pat was here. We were all here together."

"Yes, we were," Mike said.

"And Timmy Brown was out there promoting your book," I said. "Everyone is going to know your story. Have you talked to Gonzo and Mike Daly? Everyone is with you."

"I talk to you guys more than I talk to anyone," Mike said.

Ylfa said, "That's good. We're your wives."

"And we're going to get married," I said. "You're our husband. And you're Shackleton's father. And we're all going to live together in New York. And go on trips in your RV."

"Next year we'll all be together, and I'll be cancer-free," Mike said.

And we said, "Yes."

Fiction. Because reality was too much for us to bear, ultimately.

That evening, at dusk, when the last scraps of pale pink-and-yellow daylight were still clinging on, about to plunge into darkness, Mike sent us a message with a revelation.

The day he got sober—December 14—was the day they found Pat's body.

He didn't realize that until today.

None of us did.

"My heart is so full," I told him and Ylfa. "I don't know what I would do without you two. You're my dream come true of a family. More than I could have ever asked for."

"I was thinking the same thing," Mike said. "I was remembering after escaping the ER, the film festival, our dinner, I was standing on the other side of the subway platform and watching both of you laughing and carrying on. And my heart felt the same. So full of love, so full of joy, and my soul so blessed to have you in my life. I will never stop feeling that way."

"I love you both so much it makes me cry," Ylfa said.

* * *

Later that evening, when I was home, I stumbled upon the most resplendent sight. A video from the sundown ceremony at Ground Zero.

Illuminated in light, with the rising blue towers of light behind them, the blue lights that almost got canceled because of COVID, but went up in the end, there at Ground Zero, a swaying crowd of firefighters and soldiers, cops and civilians, masked and unmasked people with green plastic cups raised, singing the most fabled Irish folk song, "The Wild Rover," the song so often sung in times of war.

In my apartment I released the Irish alehouse ballad from my lungs and the wonderous, doomed sailing ship described in the song's aboutness rollicked in my blood, its masts snapped in my breath, the enormous cargo of whores and bricks and packets of bones slammed down my throat, the wild, precious crew died in my chest, and I guessed I was the sole survivor of the Wild Rover, the narrator with no one left alive to contradict my tale.

And hearing the song, I felt carried and responsible all at once for the freight of stories I was meant to tell. I felt Pat's strength in my teeth and skull and hair until it spilled out of my eyes as I listened to the song over and over, twirling around my apartment in wild gratitude for my sacred, disastrous life.

That night I sent the video of the soldiers singing to Marko, who'd gone to war four times. Who'd lost so much. "I know you will understand this. Thank you for fighting for us."

"I do understand," he said. "I've heard it many times. You sharing how New York heals with me is profound. I fought because I believed in something greater than the American experiment. And I'm very scared. I don't fight anymore, I teach others to fight, which makes me feel even more guilty."

"Possibly we'll have a civil war. I don't fight, I save lives. And I think love will win. I have no evidence of this aside from days like today that show me love will win. And that there is something greater than this life and what we can see. The spirit lives on. I am sure of it. And I am Irish."

"Love will win," Marko said. "No civil war. Just two sides making strides to understand each other. Love will win, otherwise I'll break. I can't take this country I love and sacrifice so much for dividing itself. We are all Americans. We are in this together. But emotions take over, and decency subsides."

"We can hold all the stories from all sides. I will, at least. I will hold all the stories. It matters so much. Nothing could matter more."

"You always knew the truth, even when it was ugly. You have that gift."

"It's also a curse."

A memory. In September 2001, within hours after the attacks, stores ran out of flags. Americans of all races, nations of birth, and political affiliations ran out of their houses and bought flags. By the end of September, the oldest and largest flag factory in the country had tripled production. It called laid-off workers back to produce flags, extended work shifts by two hours, and added Saturday to the work week.

In a time of crisis, Americans worked overtime to produce flags, enough to satisfy the country's voracious need for unity. Nothing was more important. Nothing is more important. Nothing will ever be more important.

We can hold all the stories.

We can keep digging. We have it in us. If we keep digging, we will find buried deep inside ourselves a golden treasure of care for other people. Even those we disagree with. Especially them. They need our love and prayers, too. We are really no more than a heartbeat and breath to catch and release our spirits.

And then a new day: 9/12.

One of the most beautiful days on the calendar.

There I was. The sky blue and the weather holding. Saturday morning. Parched from lack of sleep and dehydrated from losing so many tears, still drunk on the day before's magic. I felt brave. Strong. Resilient. Loved. Part of something greater than myself and up for whatever inferno life threw at me next. Second wave, civil war, cancer, death.

Mike was too sick to speak on the phone. "I'm not well today," he messaged us. "Hopefully I'll get better."

Pat was close.

Everyone goes home.

Ylfa went for a walk that evening in Central Park and gave a red rose to Pat's tree. If Pat had survived 9/11, he probably would have married Ylfa. If Mike hadn't been too sick to make it back to New York, we probably would have married him yesterday. Walking home from the park, Ylfa saw a rose on the ground, so she picked it up. She sensed it was from Pat. She'd given him a flower, and he returned it.

Then she passed by a wedding. The bride and groom were wearing black.

My grandmother taught me to believe in ghosts.

Years ago, Ylfa told me that Pat doesn't like it when we call him a ghost. Don't say you fell in love with a ghost, he told her. Just say you fell in love with me.

That same day, 9/12, one of my clients reached out to me in crisis. The burning world continued ripping people apart. The details of the disaster didn't matter. Someone needed help. And this was what I told them; told myself; am telling you:

"This part of your crisis is about withstanding enormous amounts of agony. It's part of every crisis. Keep doing what you're doing. Turn inward. Ask yourself difficult questions. Ask your friends to tell you the truth about your behavior that you may not be seeing if you have self-doubt. Talk openly to everyone who loves you. Write letters you don't send. ('If you're explaining, you're losing.' Who said that, Reagan? I heard it from a lawyer defending victims of a mass shooting.) Stand tall. Maintain prayerful silence. Ask for help. Take walks. Stay close to your beloveds. Write your story. This is your work right now. I know this crisis is destroying you. But I promise you'll be OK.

"Today is 9/12. Which for me, who lived in the disaster zone and lost a firefighter brother figure on 9/11, a guy who inspired me to become a first responder, and whose firefighter-turned-ER-doctor brother is one of my dearest friends, and is currently dying an agonizing World Trade Center–related cancer death caused by digging the pile looking for his brother—today, 9/12, is one of the most beautiful days on the calendar.

"Much of the talk in the Crisis Counseling Unit of the FDNY after 9/11 was about encouraging surviving first responders to find 9/12. Just get to 9/12, they said. Move forward. Forgetting is not an option. The long-term consequences are painful and often fatal. But there is a future beyond that god-awful day. And while I know this crisis is still unfolding for you, and it keeps coming up, it will pass. You are going to find your 9/12. And I am going to help you. And so are all the people who love and support you. And there will be singing."

The next day, Ylfa and I managed to get Mike on the phone hours before he returned again to the ER, and asked if he had any final messages, things he wanted to convey to the world before he joined Pat, since we both felt his time here was coming to an end.

"Is there anything you want people to know, Turtle? Is there anything you need to tell your wives, or that you want us to do?"

"Pray and meditate," Mike said.

My hero. Pat's brother. My brother. My shared spiritual husband. Mike's words were the ones I'd whisper to myself over and over all through the waiting fall, when there was nothing left to do but pray and meditate.

I kept saying it to myself the next week, when my mother called to say she lost the cabin. The wildfire took it. It took all the cabins in the little hamlets in the Sequoia National Forest and burned them to the ground. The fire was still uncontained, devouring the ancient trees.

I grew up in those mountains. That forest was my church. My childhood. My mother's childhood. And all of it was gone.

And I said it to myself the following week, in the evening, when I walked a few short blocks to Clara's house to gather outside on her stoop with Natalie and Felice for the last time. Clara's landlord had sold her building and forced her family out, and now she and the kids were headed to Martha's Vineyard to stay in her aunt's house, let the kids run wild at the sea. She was the main reason I moved to this neighborhood, to be near her, and now she was leaving. So many tear-streaked nights and close-contact saves in her apartment, elaborate dinners at Clara's table and holidays spent together, screaming with laughter. It was our shelter, this place. We sat on the stoop for hours, the four of us, listening to music thrumming from a car speaker across the street, and then we said goodbye to Clara, and to our sisterhood, now disbanding.

"It's the end of an era," Felice said.

Pray and meditate. Nothing in this world was fixed. Everything could go at any minute. And it did it go. It was still going. Everything went except God.

Pray and meditate. Pray and meditate. Pray and meditate.

* * *

The last time I rode on the ambulance was September 29.

"Wanna pick up a tour tonight?" Nathan texted me that Tuesday afternoon. "My favorite partner?"

I said, "I'm not your favorite partner, but OK."

It was a quiet, rainy night. On the ambulance the radio had very little to say. COVID was upticking in Kings County and in Queens. We figured it was quiet on the street because people were inside, installed in front of their TVs, gearing up to watch the first debate between then President Trump and former vice president Joe Biden.

For hours Nathan and I sat on the ambulance in the tinkering rain. Out of the blue I got a text from Larry, who I hadn't heard from in some time. I wasn't sure if we'd recovered yet, or ever would, from our political blowouts over the protests. Nick and I hadn't talked since he sent me those e-mails back in June. I hoped he was healthy and safe. I prayed for him. I hadn't reached out to him. Not yet. I guessed I wasn't ready.

"I haven't spoken to you in a while," Larry said. "How are you? I miss you, Jen."

I missed him, too.

I told him I was on the truck with Nathan. He said to swing by the precinct to say hi, and I said we would. But then we got dispatched to an "unknown," so we went to that. Lexi texted. Her unit was also on scene. I hadn't seen her since the protests. She'd been asking me to pick up tours and I kept putting her off. I had no desire to ride. The only way to get me on the truck these nights was to ask me at the last minute, apparently.

Surprise me.

The job was an intox inside a deli. We walked in, and found a drunk homeless man paralyzed from the waist down on the floor. He'd purposefully slid out of his wheelchair and sank onto his knees, then lay on the ground, according to the store manager. He was now laid out on the floor, mumbling but otherwise nonverbal. A bottle of liquor sat at the foot of his wheelchair. The four of us first responders sheeted him and then lifted him onto our stretcher, and then wheeled him outside and loaded him into the back of our ambulance.

"Thanks, guys," Lexi said before Nathan and I headed to the hospital. And then to me, "Nice to see you, Ginger. How've you been?"

"I don't know," I said. "Not great."

The hospital was busy. An elderly Asian man stretchered in the triage line with a nasal canula snaked up his nose let out a dry, hacking cough I recognized as coronavirus.

Here we go again, I thought. Wave II. And so it begins.

After we cleared the hospital Nathan and I swung by Larry's precinct to say hello. When he came outside I shrieked and hoorayed, and he turned to a cop standing outside, and said, "You hear that? She loves me!"

"He's the worst of the worst!" I screamed.

Larry leaned on my open window and the three of us caught up. He was still on desk duty because his lung was damaged from COVID, so the doctor wouldn't clear him to be on the street.

"How is it out there?" he asked us.

"Pretty dead," I said. "But COVID's back. The hospital's busy again and patients have the cough." Then I asked Larry if he was going to watch the debates.

"I can't wait," he said in an animated voice. "I'm going to watch it on my phone. Trump's gonna destroy him."

"Well, he's destroyed all of us, so I don't see why this would be any different." Then I gave him a hard, serious look and said, in a tone of somber gravity, "It's not a hoax."

"It's not a hoax," he said.

An hour or so later, Nathan and I watched the presidential debate on the ambulance. We streamed it on our phones from different news channels, so the bickering, name calling, and interruptive verbal assaults came in overlapping soundbites, in duplicate, which made it unbearable to watch, like two yapping dogs. It was like watching my grandfather get beaten up on TV.

What was the point? Neither of the candidates supported universal healthcare. Neither was going to say a word about the environment, wildfires swallowing California whole, burning my childhood forest to the ground.

Marko texted. We'd spoken on the phone a week back, for the first time in years, and caught up. He was not getting a PhD in the weaponization of data. He didn't get the promotion that would have made his education free. He was deciding what to do next, when he retired.

"You better be pulling your hair out watching the debate like a good citizen," he said tonight.

"I'm watching it on the ambulance with the ERs packed with COVID patients," I told him.

"Holy shit. That is the most 2020 thing I've read."

Pray and meditate, Mike said.

24

NEW YORK CITY IS UNDEAD FOREVER

Three days after the presidential debate, on Friday morning, October 2, the president announced that he and the first lady had tested positive for COVID.

This was not a murder mystery.

That same evening he was admitted to Walter Reed for difficulty breathing.

The Internet exploded.

"This feels like Ronald Reagan getting AIDS," Dan Savage said on Twitter. Dan Savage, the queer sex column king of the *Village Voice*, the free newspaper of old New York.

Bold. But truer words were never tweeted.

People dispatched so many death threats upon the president on Twitter that the platform tweeted a statement: "tweets that wish or hope for death, serious bodily harm or fatal disease against *anyone* are not allowed and will need to be removed. this does not automatically mean suspension."

Facebook went lighter with its policy on hate speech, as it so often and fatally did, distinguishing between the rights of public and private citizens. On that platform, you could say you hoped the president died as long as you didn't tag him in your post or purposefully expose him to "calls for death, serious disease, epidemic disease, or disability."

As usual, Silicon Valley arrived late to the murder scene, social media jerry-rigged to the point of being farcical. Women, queer, trans, Black, Indigenous, and people of color had for years been receiving death threats on Facebook and Twitter, which these companies largely elected to do nothing about. Four hundred threat warnings against Kyle Rittenhouse.

As far as the hospitalized president went, I wasn't among those wishing death upon him. The disasters of 9/11 and COVID had softened me, as disasters always did. By now I had reached a place of speechless defeat.

If only in my mind, I rejected the timeline of events as it pertained to the president getting sick. I'd seen enough COVID patients to know they didn't test positive and wind up hospitalized the same day. It took the virus three to five days to ransack the body and advance to the point of respiratory compromise.

And no COVID patients went to the ER as a "precautionary measure." The president didn't want to be at Walter Reed, surrounded by injured military veterans he publicly called "suckers," doing a media stunt to show he was doing great by signing his name on a blank sheet of paper. The timeline of him testing positive to hospitalization was fiction, half the White House was now infected with COVID, and over 200,000 American citizens were dead, and counting.

This was my country. And it disgusted me. I was a first responder during COVID. I saw the sick and dying. I saw the body bags, the sheeted corpses, the refrigerator trucks that people were loaded inside, and I considered myself a patriot, so I felt I had the right to my revulsion.

We thought we would lose Mike in September, when Pat and Mike's wife Janet died. But he stuck around, kind of.

Toward the end of September and well into October, he stopped communicating with all of us in New York. Including his family. Including me and Ylfa. We called him. Straight to voicemail. Sent him photos. No reply. Texts. Almost nothing back. Sometimes, but rarely, "I love you." We were in regular touch with his niece Erin, who he lived with. She said he was in a lot of pain. Ylfa and I assumed he was too sick and depressed to speak.

One day Paul called me for news. "You haven't heard from him, either? I just talked to Bobby and he said Mike's not answering his calls, and I'm getting his voicemail. But I figured at least he was still talking to his wives."

"No," I said. "Wives are also out. Everyone's out. No one's getting through."

Mike had been such a huge part of my life, and suddenly, he was gone. He was alive, but in the silence of his disappearance I started to grieve him as if he were dead. I couldn't sleep. I couldn't stop crying. I grew terrified I wouldn't get to see him again or even say goodbye. I'd never felt so tormented. At one point I sobbed for six days straight, all day and night, as if grief were my vocation.

My friends grew worried about me. They called and texted constantly.

"Talk to me," Tommy said. "Are you OK? You're going through fucking hell."

"Mike is the saddest show on earth. My mom is bereaved from losing the cabin. One of my closest friends just moved away. It's too much. I don't see the point of life at the moment."

"It's a lot, but it's not too much. The point of life is to keep going. To push through and reap all the benefits of the hard work and challenging decisions you've made. You've literally saved lives and continue to do so. Mine included, whether you like to think that or not. You're a beautiful, sexy, talented, and smart woman, and I'm here for you."

"I love you so much. You're going to have to scrape me off the floor when Mike dies. Just put that in your calendar now."

"I will. I promise I'll be there for you."

"You're always there. 'There' is very broad. But you're always there."

"Can you get away? Take a break?"

"I don't know. Work is busy. Mike calls me on my landline, and I'm afraid if I leave town, I'll miss his call. I'm not on the ambulance right now. I haven't been on the street in weeks. I have nothing to give."

"Stay off the ambulance," Tommy said. "Try to get away."

Another day Felice texted to say she was in my neighborhood, and she could stop by to hang out if I was around. I told her I was definitely around and wanted to see her. But then she texted when I was writing and had my phone silenced, so I missed her texts. When I called her, she was already in an Uber, heading back to her apartment.

"I can come back," she said. "Should I turn around?"

"No, I don't want you to turn around, it's OK."

"Are you sure?"

"Yeah."

But the second we got off the phone tears raced down my cheeks. I texted Felice. "Sis, I can't stop crying."

"I'll be there in ten minutes."

And she was here. We sat outside together in a little garden and for an hour Felice listened to me talk and weep.

Tommy was right. I needed to stay out of service. Au revoir, flashing lights, sirens, partners, patients, street. I needed to take a break. Leave town.

Felice was looking at places we could go away together. One morning one of my girlfriends called who knew I was desperate to get out of the city. She and her husband had unexpectedly purchased a house in Vermont. They'd rented a house upstate on Airbnb before they'd bought it, in the Catskills. And now, because they'd bought a new house, they were no longer going to use the Airbnb. They offered it to me as a gift. They asked if I wanted to go for a week, two weeks, a month.

These people. My friends. They were taking such good care of me. My girlfriend who offered me the Airbnb upstate was one of the people who sewed me masks that spring, when PPE was running low. Her husband, an innovator and businessman, had partnered with other companies and began manufacturing ventilators and other critical medical supplies. They were first responders, too. My rescuers.

"Sis," I said when I rang Felice. "We have a house."

I sent her pictures. The place was beautiful. Four bedrooms. Big windows. Trees and grass. We invited Natalie. She'd recently lost her beloved aunt and was reeling. Natalie was in. We decided to go for a week. Two weeks, if we wanted.

"Just the thought of sitting around, just being with you both," Natalie said. "Just the thought of it."

Happiness. No, not happiness. Pandemic happiness.

A day later, a delivery man buzzed my apartment. I hadn't ordered any groceries or anything. I looked at the security camera and there stood a man bearing a huge bouquet of flowers.

Flowers? For me? From who?

I flew downstairs and ripped them out of the delivery man's arms and screeched with joy just as another woman who lived in the building came into the lobby. "Yes, girl!" she said. "Flowers!"

Flowers! I held them like a baby in my arms and fumbled through the tissue for a note. Found it. They were from the crisis client I'd helped on 9/12. The type on the cream-colored card said, FOR THE FIRST RESPONDER . . . AND FOR ALLOWING US ALL TO RESPOND. DEEPEST THANKS.

My heart. I clutched it. I thought it was going to burst in my chest. I flew upstairs, taking the steps two at a time, and lifted my babies out of their chic paper dress.

Wow, dahlias. In an exquisite circular vase like one I'd never seen, the long green stems swirled up one side, the purple-mahogany flowers careened over the lip. Breathtaking. These babies were expensive. I knew my flowers. I was a Plant Lady. I took a photograph of them and thanked my client.

"These are the most beautiful flowers on this (dead, worthless) earth, and the little note was perfect. I'm profoundly moved. Thank you so much. You didn't have to but I'm so glad you did. I wanted to be a florist as a girl, so this touches my most ancient inner self. They may be the most beautiful flowers I've ever received."

"Yours is the most beautiful advice I have ever received. And if advice were flowers, the world would be so colorful. And if flowers were advice then we (maybe) would be wise."

I loved my clients. My job. Felice. I sent her the picture of them, too, and said, "How come you never send me flowers?"

She called me that evening and spoke to me in a stern voice. "I asked you, thirty times, what I could give you or do for you after you brought me not one, but two birthday cakes, because it meant so much to me, and you said you didn't want anything. You just wanted me to stay healthy and alive."

"I was wrong," said, laughing. "I also want flowers."

"I have no words."

"I'm teasing. And you already saved me, that day you turned around in the Uber and came back to see me. Sis, I didn't know how badly I needed these flowers. I didn't understand why you cried when I brought you a cake. But now I understand."

"That cake saved my life."

"I see that now. That's what these flowers did. This is really showing me the importance of Sweets in the Streets."

That night before bed I told everyone I knew to stop whatever they were doing and send flowers or a cake to someone they cared about. It was a pandemic. It was important. Small loving gestures were all we had left in the long-gone world.

A few days later Ylfa suggested we get together in the city. We went for a walk in Central Park and visited Pat's tree. We sat on a blanket in the grass beside it and made up a funny song about being two wives, recorded it, and sent it off to Mike.

No reply.

After the park, we sat outside a sushi restaurant and lunched. We reached out to Erin for news. She told us Mike was depressed and had some bad days, but he always had his phone, he just ignored it. She didn't know why he was ignoring everyone. She said he didn't want to believe the treatments had stopped working, and the cancer was devouring him. If he didn't talk about it, then it wasn't happening. That was her theory. She said at the moment, he was in his room, watching *The Goonies*.

I dropped my chopsticks and looked at Ylfa. "*The Goonies*?" He's not talking to us or anyone else he loves because he's in his room watching *The Goonies*? I'm staggering around sobbing and he's watching *THE GOONIES*?"

"He's being Murtle," Ylfa said.

We lost it laughing. In one cinematic word I went from crying to falling off my chair.

Only Mike.

"Pat," Ylfa and I said to the heavens. "Get control of your brother."

Something about the absurdity of that word, *Goonies*, loosened a boulder of sorrow inside me. I stopped crying over Mike, knowing that he was alive. My tear ducts were drier than Bakersfield. Then one day, after a month of not hearing from him at all, finally, my phone rang.

"Turtle!" I said. "You called me! I love you and miss you so much."

"Hey, EMT Chick," he said in a soft voice. "I love you and miss you, too."

We talked for half an hour. His voice was punctuated with coughs and deep, sighing breaths. When I asked if he'd dropped off the face of the earth because he was sick or depressed, he said both. He was short of breath, so it was difficult to speak. He didn't like taking his pain meds, so he refused to take them. Then the pain blazed back, and he took more pills than he needed, gobs of them. Most days, all he did was sleep. He couldn't eat. To walk from his bed to the kitchen was a great task.

He didn't want to talk to anyone because he didn't want to talk about being sick. Because talking about it made it real. He thought if maybe he stopped talking, and just holed up at home, none of this would be happening. But lately he'd been so sick he was giving up hope.

"That's OK," I said. "You don't have to have any hope right now. Why would you in this situation? It's so depressing. But I have hope, and Duck has hope, so your wives can hold all the hope for you. You can borrow our hope and live on that when you run out. We'll keep all the hope for you."

"Wow," Mike said. "Thank you so much. Yes, you guys will hold all the hope for me. You're so smart, EMT Chick."

"This is basic sobriety I'm feeding you. This is shit you learn in your first year. I survived on Pat's faith when I had cancer. He told me I'd be OK, and I believed him."

"I want to be back in New York with you and Ylfa."

"We want that too, my love."

Then Mike perked up, let a long, dry cough rip, and said he wanted to give me a plan for my future.

"Oh, perfect. I love it when my husband tells me what to do. Let me get a pen, so I can write it down."

A moment later, pen in hand, Mike gave me a three-part plan for my life, and what I was going to do next. His plan for me was as follows: 1) Marry a wealthy doctor, meaning him; 2) finish this book about being a first responder, and then go on a nationwide book tour in his RV, with him and Ylfa, my husband and wife; and 3) not become a paramedic.

"No? You don't think I should become a medic?"

"No. You're too smart for that."

"I can barely do basic math."

"You're too smart for it, and you'll get burned out. You're burned out already. And after three or four years working as a medic, you'll be so burned out from the job you'll be heartless. That's what happens. You won't care about any of your patients. And then you aren't of use to anyone. So what you're going to do is become a therapist."

"A therapist."

"Yes. You're really good at helping people, especially people like me, people with PTSD, so I think that's what you should do. You'll have to go back to school and get another degree, but you can do that. And you can work with first responders. You can treat all the wives of divorced firefighters. You'd be so great at it. You've helped me more than anyone with all this stuff."

"Oh, Turtle," I said. "I love number one and two, but I'm not so sure about three. I don't need a title or another degree. And I like helping people for free."

"Will you consider it, at least?"

"Yes. I will consider anything my husband suggests."

These late October weeks, in place of tears and texts and phone calls with Mike, I registered something new. Something extremely bizarre. Nowadays, I laughed hard and constantly, sometimes hysterically, often inappropriately, at everything and over nothing. The smallest thing and grimmest news shook me into thunderstorms of laughter. I rained tears. I howled.

It wasn't joy pouring out of me, I understood. It was similar to the cackle I'd heard in the locked psych ERs, radiating from the mouths of emotionally distressed people. Clinically, mentally, I was probably an EDP at this point. I was an EMT, not a doctor, so I wasn't in the business of diagnosing people. But I suspected that if I were an emergency call type, I'd come over the radio as an EDP. "White woman behaving suspiciously." "White woman howling. Perp has a mullet."

One day I told Tommy what Mike had suggested, and he had quite a lot of feedback about my husband's idea of me becoming a therapist for first responders—firefighters and cops.

"You'd be the best, yet also the worst," Tommy said. "The best for obvious reasons, and the worst for obvious reasons."

"I'd be pregnant with all of my clients' children."

"One hundred percent."

One hundred percent. Lol.

Tommy was pondering what to do when he retired and wanted my thoughts. He said he'd love to write. He'd always fantasized about writing some type of memoir or life story. He just wasn't confident that it would be interesting enough, nor did he trust his ability to buckle down and do it, write it all out.

"Petal, you're truly a beautiful and very talented writer. And I'm not just saying that."

"Wow. You just blew my mind. Thank you. I've never heard that nor thought that."

I suggested he check out the NYU Veterans Writing Workshop, where, strangely, I'd found a writing home. I told him it was for veterans only, and free. He said he wanted to check it out. I messaged my ex-Marine employee/writer/friend I'd met there years back to see if the workshop was still meeting this fall.

"Yep," he said.

"In real life or Zoom?"

"Zoom. I just forwarded you the e-mail and link."

"Perfect. Thanks, pal. Bro."

"No prob, bro."

Bro. Lol.

My fits of laughter just kept thundering on through October.

When I read news that Europe was reporting record numbers of COVID-19 cases and the continent braced for the pandemic to intensify through the locked-down winter, I laughed.

When Italy recorded 16,079 new cases in 24 hours and local governors called for new lockdowns, I laughed.

When France's president said he foresaw the crisis extending through next summer, 2021;

When news outlets said which stocks to buy right now during COVID Wave III and I didn't know we'd surpassed Wave II and we were now supposedly on an entirely new wave;

When the United States reported the second-highest day of new COVID-19 cases, 83,718;

When Dr. Fauci said then President Trump hadn't attended a COVID meeting in weeks;

When a doctor in a New Jersey hospital said COVID Wave II had started;

When first responders in New York told me the call volume was picking up and the COVID patients they were seeing right now were much younger;

When two vaccines failed;

When the ERs got crowded again in New York City;

When the sound of ambulance sirens pierced the air;

Lol. Lol. Lol.

And then shit got even surrealer.

Felice and I headed upstate on Friday, Columbus Day weekend. My therapist suggested, after I mentioned to her that Mike was back in the ER and that I was delirious, hadn't slept in three days, hadn't eaten much, and was alternating between crying and laughing manically, that I not get behind the wheel. Solid advice. Felice loved to drive, so I figured it was a win-win.

My sister agreed. "No problem," she said.

We packed half our houses thinking we'd stay upstate as long as we could, one or two weeks. On the street outside Felice's place, I handed her my car keys and warned her that pandemic driving in New York City was not like regular driving in New York City, which was already nuts. Pandemic driving was much worse. Road ragers were ragier. There were no rules. Traffic quadrupled, since no one was taking the train, and everyone seemed to have bought a car.

Felice said she understood, but I had a feeling she didn't quite know what I was talking about. Pandemic driving was very similar to operating a vehicle in an emergency. The emergency was the world, the overlapping pandemics. I loved driving the ambulance now. It was fun as hell to blast lights-and-sirens around town, ignoring rules everyone else had to follow. I loved being lawless. But it wasn't for everyone, as Felice soon found out.

My sister looked so cute driving my car. She sat up straight with her glasses on, looking studiously ahead. She was driving very cautiously, very slowly. She reminded me of my grandma.

"You drive with two hands," I said, chuckling.

"That's how I was taught. With my hands at ten and two."

"I haven't seen anyone drive like that since I became an EMT. I can't drive with two hands anymore, only one. Left hand on the wheel, right hand on the gear shift as if it's the sirens."

"I'm not an EMT," Felice said. "And your driving—"

Felice had gotten angry at me over the summer because I drove us to our friend's house on City Island, and I blew a few red lights. I didn't really *blow* them. I was careful-ish. I took them like stop signs, like I did on the ambulance. You know what a red light means to a first responder? Nothing. Felice didn't like that.

In Brooklyn, we hit pandemic traffic. And holiday weekend traffic. Back-to-back honking vehicles on every street and highway we inched across. It took us an hour and a half just to get from her house near Flatbush across Brooklyn to Hamilton Parkway. By the time we got over there I already had to pee.

"Just tell me in advance when you need to stop and I'll pull over somewhere," Felice said.

"I can't give you advanced notice because my bladder's fucked up. I have to pee, and I think I can hold it an hour, but then all of a sudden I have to go immediately."

Felice gasped. "Do you think it's because of that surgery?"

"I don't know. Probably. My bladder was never the same after that catheter."

Onward we went. More traffic.

"Be aggressive!" I said when she hesitated to enter a lane. "Just go fast and get out there, sis. Use the horn. Honk if you need to. Just go. OK, go. Go now. Change lanes. Now get in the left lane. Get in the fast lane. Just cut those assholes off. They've got Jersey plates. Assholes. This is New York City, jerks. Go home and learn how to drive."

Felice sighed then sucked her teeth. She seemed stressed. I sensed I might have something to do with it. I tried to shut up.

Didn't work. My brain was the spinning rainbow of death on a Macintosh computer. My brain was soup. I just wanted to talk and talk and talk. But I couldn't remember the most basic things. While I was trying to be quiet the phrase "the dark arts" came into my mind, and for the life of me I couldn't remember what the dark arts were. For a second I wondered if it was my profession. Were detectives in the dark arts? Was I a dark artist?

"When people refer to themselves as working in the dark arts, what are they referring to again? Is it what I do?"

Behind the wheel, staring straight ahead, Felice lost it. She shrieked with laughter. Tears streamed down her cheeks.

"Stop laughing at me! You're going to make me pee!"

So then she started making this loud crazy hooting sound, stifling laughter, she sounded like an owl on drugs.

"Stop it! Stop making that ridiculous sound! What is that sound, what are you doing? That's even worse than laughter, you hooting like that."

Finally she caught her breath and explained that the dark arts was not detective work. "It refers to the occult," she said. "To magic."

"OK, thanks. Now I have to pee. Turn right here."

She pulled off Hamilton Parkway and I directed her to Park Slope's ambulance base, around the corner, so I could run inside and use the bathroom. She seemed kind of relieved when I got out of the car. May not have been true. Just an observation.

A lost-looking dude was standing outside the ambulance garage. He tried to ask me something, but I rushed past him and said I'd be back. Minor urinary emergency, what else was new. When I returned five or so minutes later, the guy said he was looking for someone to help him out. He'd filled out an application to volunteer as an EMT, but he hadn't heard back from anybody.

"How long ago was that?" I asked.

"About a month."

"Oh yeah, no. It's going to be a while before they get back to you. It took me like three months to start riding here. Six months, actually."

"No."

"Yeah. And they just finished a new orientation class, so I'm sure they're not ready to do another one just yet. But they'll get back to you. You just have to wait."

"It takes that long?"

"It's an all-volunteer org. The chiefs are EMTs and work full-time. Everyone's working two hundred jobs and trying to get new people through orientation and on the street before the Rona Wave II, so everyone's super busy. They'll get back to you."

He said thanks, and I ran back to Felice. I ran past my own car. I didn't even see it.

"Um, sis?" Felice yelled as I zipped by.

After I got back in my RAV4 Adventure and Felice pulled into the street, she stopped at a red light. My car's beeper fired when someone walked across the headlights. Felice was looking all around for what was beeping. I reached over the steering wheel and switched it off.

"The beeper's super sensitive. It beeps at everything. The beeper is a woman who orgasms from being winked at."

She gave me a look.

Then she turned right on a red light accidentally, which was illegal in New York City. And this goateed guy in a truck pulled up in front of us and unleashed about three minutes of pure unbridled rage on her. We just sat there and looked at him. Then he drove off and Felice blew out a big breath.

"It's the pandemic," I said after he drove off. "Pandemic driving is crazy."

A few minutes later I told Felice maybe I would get a dog, seeing that Ylfa and Mike and I were supposed get one and name him Shackleton, but it didn't seem like that was going to happen.

Felice giggled. "You? With a dog?"

"What's so funny? I can take care of things. My plants are *thriving.* And I was a nanny for several years after 9/11, when I couldn't find work. And I happened to be very good at it. I took care of a small child."

"A dog is not a child."

"Right because it's an animal, so therefore it's easier."

"OK. Get a dog. I can't wait until it starts shitting all over your rug and eating your plants."

"You know, sis. Not every thought needs to be expressed."

Then Felice missed a turn on the map, and getting back on track, we got stuck in a traffic jam. Suddenly a fleet of rough-looking dudes filled the block and barricaded the street with trucks. They were passing boxes of food to one another and filling their truck beds with it. Several of them were extremely attractive.

"Are they Hells Angels?" Felice said.

"I don't know. I feel like Hell's Angels are mostly white. These guys are Black and white and brown. I can't figure it out. But I love them. They're addressing food insecurity. That's hot. Look at that one."

One of the men came up to our car and asked if we needed food. Felice said, "No, thank you."

"Who are they?" I said.

"One of their shirts says 'The Punishers. Most Wanted.'"

I got out my phone. "Let me look them up." A moment later I told Felice what I'd discovered. "The Punishers Law Enforcement Motorcycle Club is a brotherhood of law enforcement officers." I looked up and said, "They're cops. And they're feeding starving people. I'll marry them all."

Felice shook her head at me.

After two and a half hours, we were still in the city. In Manhattan, near Thirty-Fourth Street. We were supposed to be upstate by now, and then some. The entire drive to the house was only two hours.

Manhattan was gutted. A ghost town. The only people outside were people driving cars. Empty sidewalks. Boarded up windows. Closed stores. Homeless people wandering around. It was some grade-A organic wartime shit. Weeks before, downtown, I'd seen block-long lines of people standing outside a soup kitchen. The Russian breadline. I asked Felice if she'd read that piece that went viral, NEW YORK CITY IS DEAD FOREVER.

"No, but I read Jerry Seinfeld's rebuttal. He roasted it."

"He should roast it. The guy who wrote that definitely lives in Manhattan."

"Absolutely. I think I read that he owns a comedy club?"

"Yeah, he's a finance guy. Those are the people who killed New York City. They forced us out and turned Manhattan into a giant shopping mall. And now he's sad he can't go to *The Nutcracker* on Christmas and buy his Patagonia vest at Neiman Marcus. That guy's never been to Brooklyn in his life."

"Brooklyn's alive and well. My neighborhood's lively. Everything's open. People are in the street. Outside eating dinner, having drinks. Music playing all the time."

"Same thing in my neighborhood. And Queens and the Bronx. People are all coming together. There's a real feeling of community. That's New York. That's why I moved here. Not to go to Barneys. Shootings are up, but that's every neighborhood now. That's the entire country. And that's also New York City. Welcome back, everyone. Manhattan's dead, but that's because all the rich people left. And they should leave. And they should stay gone. They ruined New York. They killed it twenty years ago."

"I mean, remember downtown Manhattan in the nineties? Artists and all these different kinds of people? I loved it back then. I used to drive all the way from Mount Vernon just to go to the Nuyorican. And I saw all the veteran poets. I thought they were so cool."

"I did, too. I used to be able to afford to live here, until it got outrageously expensive and I got drop-kicked to Brooklyn. But I'm glad I did. I love Brooklyn. Manhattan needed to die. It got torched during the protests. People lit that shit up like Fourth of July. And of course it was sad to see all the destruction. But people were dying of COVID and protesting for social justice, so I wasn't sobbing over it. Corporate America's done a real number on you if you're crying when a brick flies through the window of Chase Manhattan Bank."

"I remember after 9/11, everyone said New York would never be the same again. It's forever changed. I was like, is it? And look what happened. We recovered from that. It took a few years, but we recovered. We recovered so well that now people forget it ever happened. They're like, 9/11? What's that?"

"Exactly. And we'll recover from this. It's going to take a decade, but we'll bounce back. New York City is undead forever. But I still can't wait to get out of here for a few weeks."

Five hours after we left Brooklyn, we finally saw our exit coming up on the thruway. It was nighttime now. We'd already stopped to eat, use the bathroom, and switch seats, so now I was driving. When we turned off the highway a sudden darkness enveloped us.

"We're in the country now," I said, and turned on my brights. Then I turned down a road. Then another. I turned on my brights and then realized they were already on. I said, "I didn't think it could get any darker." Then after a pause, "What if the road we're on just keeps getting narrower and darker."

Felice chuckled.

Then we turned down a darker, narrower road.

I was so happy to finally arrive upstate I nearly kissed the wet, green ground. But almost immediately, the trip turned into a horror movie—a pandemic horror movie.

We got our stuff out of the car and looked at the house. Fine. Great house. Beautiful. But strange. There were a bunch of dead animal heads mounted to the wall. So I was like, "Taxidermy! Love it. Americana." But Felice was all, "Um, I don't love it." Then I looked around and there were photographs of sad white people nailed to the walls. They were creepy as fuck. "I'm not into these things," I said. And Felice said, "I love the sad white people."

Three of the sad whites were hanging above the bed in the master bedroom, so I rapidly gifted the biggest room to Felice, because I wasn't closing my eyes in a bed beneath those creepers. "Really?" she said. "I can have the big room?" She sure could.

I slept like shit, and I was desperate for sleep. My room had twin beds, and my big clown feet hung off the edges. The sheets were rough and cheap. I froze in the night. So I woke up more exhausted than I'd been when we'd arrived. I made coffee and tried to work out where to set up my office, a problem I discovered I had the previous night the second we walked in.

This house. Let me tell you something. No human beings ever lived here. It was a museum. A mausoleum. Every table was wobbly. There were weird carved statues and fur rugs thrown all about. The light was dim and terrible, so there was nowhere to sit and read. Every other wall had a dead animal slaughtered on it, and I was so tall I kept bumping my head into decapitated moose. I was a reader, and I could tell right away these people never turned a page of a book. Finally, I smooshed my desk against a wall and moved things around and set up the enormous computer screen and bazillion books I'd dragged up here from Brooklyn, so I could work and write. I thought I'd won this home-office battle. But no.

The wall had a window, and while I was writing and working, these masked, white, quacking flocks of people on a trail kept looking through the window at me. While I was sitting there in my pajamas, thinking I was alone. So clearly, we were on public land and this was a nature reserve or some such shit. I didn't enjoy being gawked at while I was trying to accomplish something magnificent on the page. So that was unpleasant.

And then the real horror started.

All that stuff before, the five-and-a-half-hour drive from Armageddon to the Catskills, only to be greeted by taxidermy, sad white people, terrible beds, zero solitude, and no place to work or read or write—that was only the trailer.

Bugs. They were everywhere, we soon discovered. Fat brown bugs the size of cockroaches. When I found the first one, I didn't know what it was, so I just captured it in a paper towel and trashed it. But then I found another. Then another. And here comes another one.

The property owner swung by later that morning, unannounced, and I told him about the situation. I didn't know the gravity of it yet. And I explained to him I wasn't a city woman, not really. I grew up in the mountains in a cabin that was very indoor/outdoor. Bears came to our door. Wasps bult homes inside. I considered myself a bug person. But even for me, this was a bit much.

"They're probably stink bugs," he said nonchalantly. "We'll bring you a vacuum later. We'll leave it outside."

"Thanks," I said. I'd never heard of stink bugs before, so I didn't understand what was happening. When I closed the door and looked at Felice, I was like, "A vacuum? He wants us to vacuum the bugs? How? A bug goes across my window in my bedroom, so I come down here, get the vacuum, lug it upstairs, plug it in, and then I lift it and vacuum the wall? Bug's gone by then, sis. Bug's in Hawaii. This makes zero sense, a vacuum."

Felice didn't respond, because she was crying laughing.

* * *

This house was comedy—tragicomedy. I tried to take a nap later. Just as I fell asleep, a bug choppered across my bedroom sounding like a flying chainsaw and I screamed in terror.

Felice called. "Sis. Are you OK? I heard you scream."

She was in her room. I was in my room, shaking like I'd just stepped on an IED. I wasn't sure if I still had a body. Was I dead? No. I was huddled in the corner with my back against the bedroom door, staring at the big, fat, brown bug that was now on my pillowcase, in the divot where my sleeping head just lay.

"No, I am not OK! A bug just woke me up! It was fucking terrifying! I was just falling asleep! I haven't slept in three fucking days! I feel like I just got blown up! Now it's on my pillow! This is some biblical shit, sis. This is the setup of a horror flick. This is Stephen King meets Franz Kafka, that scene in *Magnolia* when the sky opens up and rains frogs. We're in the apocalypse! We have to get out of this house!"

Then we calmed down. I didn't know how. We tried to cope. Denial was the river that ran through us. We'd worked so hard to get here. We'd driven five hours, in pandemic traffic, and brought all our stuff. Natalie had been through hell losing her aunt, and she was supposed to come up the next day. We really needed a break. So we tried. We thought maybe we were overreacting. Being too urban. Too fussy. I liked bugs, so I had some doubts. But we tried to relax and hang tight.

We went about our day. I went for a walk, alone, in the trees, and called my mom. She was doing a little better. Being in shock helped. I told her I was upstate, and maybe I should buy a house for us, since our cabin and forest burned down.

"No major decisions right now," she said.

"Mom! That's what I tell people in crisis! No major decisions while the ground is opening up beneath you. Wait until the disaster passes and things level out. Unless you need to change things that are killing you and you've been avoiding, and the crisis is forcing your hand. In that case, use the crisis and take action."

For all of you feet-draggers out there in pandemicland, this free crisis counsel is for you: Get the divorce, soldiers. Leave New York. Buy the house. Get sober. Have the baby. Come out of the closet. Marry her. It's time. It's been time. Quit stalling. As art by Peter Beard that used to hang in a gallery window in SoHo once read: TIME IS ALWAYS NOW.

Felice and I went for a drive. We got sandwiches. Sat outside. She said her biggest fears in the country were being murdered and bears. I wasn't scared of anything, until more time progressed. That night we lay on our stomachs, side by side on Felice's bed, which didn't have bugs in it—yet—with our legs crossed at the ankles, watching *Love After Lockup*.

After one of the dentally challenged reality show stars came onscreen, I said to Felice, since we'd both noticed in the Zoom world that our bottom teeth bothered us—mine were a little crooked and hers had a gap—I said as one of the characters spoke, "Some people are at peace with having a missing tooth."

Felice giggled and pulled her bottom lip down. "See?"

"Oh don't fix that. It's charming. Don't waste your money."

I pulled my lip down. "Look. It's crooked."

"I can't even see that. That doesn't need to be fixed."

"Ask our dentist anyway. See what she says."

Later that night, when I was in my room and Felice in hers, she sent me some funny (she thought) Twitter hashtag, #UnflatteringCatPhotoChallenge. I didn't quite see the humor yet. I thought this was a little off-brand for us. Next morning when we woke up, I said, "Help me understand the cat tweet."

Her eyes lit up like it was her birthday. "We never get to see cats like this! This is what cats are really up to when they're at home! People never show this, their cats always look cute. But these cats are crazy. Finally, thanks to the pandemic, the truth comes out about cats."

So that explained it.

Somehow, we made it about forty-eight hours. We left Monday morning. Told Natalie not to come upstate. Said it was not safe here. There was an infestation. This was war. Bugs against sisterhood. Bugs won. Bugs were the hill we died on. Take the house, bugs.

They were in our beds. Kitchen. Bathroom. A bug fell out of a mirror and landed on Felice's toothbrush. We screamed night and day. It was like living in a house with bombs. We were accruing significant trauma.

We had to get back to the city. We were never leaving New York again. Never ever. Big mistake to try to escape New York in a pandemic. Bugs try to climb in our luggage and freeload a ride home and fuck with New York

City? Bugs are going to die. Don't mess with New Yorkers, bugs. Piss us off, we'll bomb your village. We loved New York City, me and Felice. Greatest city in the world. We'd kiss the filthy asphalt in Times Square when we got home. We'd dive headfirst into the overflowing trash cans.

And yes, shootings were up, who cared. Violent crime rising, fine by us. NYPD gearing up for protests no matter who won the election, been there done that, sort of. Trash cans on fire, broken store windows boarded up, riot-geared cops and mostly peaceful protestors, but also, a good deal of violence, bricks and bottles flying, explosives outside hospitals where COVID patients lay sick and dying, gasping for air, seen it before. Saw the spring and summer shows. COVID World War Wave I. Got on stage. Played a role in it. Clap, clap, clap.

"We love you," Felice and I told Natalie. "But gotta get the fuck outta here. We have to come home. Sorry, Nat."

She was OK with it. She wasn't feeling well. She'd been around a kid with a fever. Now she was feeling sick.

This pandemic.

It wasn't all death and bugs. The sacred also met us upstate.

One night, we drove to get pizza. A song came on thanks to my Spotify playlist. No one knew this song. But Felice and I did, and we loved it. "It's our song!" she said. It was called "Lost Stars," and in it, Adam Levine sang his heart out, with lyrics about drunkenness and dust, fantasies and grief, and not letting your sorrows crush your dreams since we were only luminous specks in this galaxy of stars.

Felice turned the volume all the way up, and she sang the hell out of our song while I drove down a dark, narrow road. And there in the car with my singing sister, the person I loved more than anyone on this planet, my first first responder, I wept with gratitude for her presence and aliveness, and our friendship, through all life's tortures and victories.

I was so relieved by this moment. It rescued me. It was salvational, like one of the defibrillators we used on the street, to shock a dead heart back to life.

We weren't comedians, I thought when we got home. We needed a new word to describe us.

Tragicomedians.

25

AFTERMATHEMATICS

A week or so after I got back and recovered from my bug PTSD, Nina came over to discuss our strategy for the only thing left that mattered: Halloween.

For the first time since we met, we didn't feel like riding on the ambulance that coming night, or any night. Apparently, we were not alone in this feeling.

Park Slope's schedule was empty as of late. Nearly every e-mail that came from the chiefs was an e-mail pleading for people to pick up tours. One Sunday in October, no trucks went out at all. I guessed everyone was cooked? The new people were on the busses now, but they weren't driver trained yet, and there was no one to train them. And all of us veterans—I hesitate to call myself that—all of us who'd been on the street for a while, particularly in 2020, were nuked.

Instead of riding, Nina planned to come over and bake. We invited Chad and Nathan to our two-person pandemic Halloween party. Chad said he was going to come by, but we suspected he'd cancel. Nathan was undecided, as usual. We figured we would probably celebrate the greatest holiday on the calendar just the two of us, like the love song. Nina's boyfriend was going to be on the ambulance that night. So we planned to hop in my RAV and drive to our battalion and give the people what they wanted—or didn't want: holiday baked goods from Sweets in the Streets.

As for our Halloween costumes, we needed something pretty powerful for 2020, seeing that it had been quite a year. Our old idea, Darcey and Stacey, the twin sisters from *90 Day Fiancé*, wouldn't cut it. After some consideration, we decided to be tactical bakers. We didn't know there was such a thing, but boy was there.

When Nina discovered the existence of tactical aprons, we bought two. They were designed for "creative outdoor chefs" with a mission "to contain and control all grilling tools." "Perfect for storing condiments, grilling utensils, salt/pepper, and your phone." They were gunmetal black and looked like something Teutonic knights might wear, with tons of pouches, side straps, and a removable Velcro patch. The patch they came with said CHEF. But we were not chefs. We were tactical bakers. So we bought patches that said BUT DID YOU DIE? and RUB SOME DIRT ON IT, EVERYTHING STOPS BLEEDING EVENTUALLY.

After the costumes arrived in a week or so, we had a dress rehearsal at my house and tried on the aprons and baker's hats. I fell on the floor and rolled around on my living room rug clutching my stomach. We agreed this was, by far, the best Halloween costume we had ever chosen.

Thank you, 2020, for allowing us to become tactical bakers. This was pandemic Halloween perfection. Now we were ready to ride, off the street and in my kitchen.

A week later, I lay on the couch and clicked around Netflix. I came upon a documentary the video-on-demand service said was a 98 percent match for me. I knew, perhaps more than most people, the algorithm knew me quite well. Technology was deeply acquainted with my desires, so I gave it a try.

The documentary was called *American Murder: The Family Next Door.* It was a true-crime show about Chris Watts, a seemingly solid family man who found a girlfriend, had an extramarital affair, then one morning woke up and murdered his pregnant wife and two daughters.

It was the only thing I'd viewed since the pandemic erupted that I watched all the way through, without stopping or taking breaks. The closing title cards on the documentary gave statistics I was vaguely aware of but were thereafter seared in my brain:

"In America three women are killed by their current or ex-partner every day. Parents who murder their children and partner are most often men. This crime is virtually always premeditated."

It helped me, seeing the documentary. I appreciated the families who allowed it to be made. Watching it, I understood there was no understanding in cases like this, just as Rafael had told me when I talked to him about Heather so many years back. It went into the unknowable pile.

But whenever I encountered the unspeakable—murder-suicide, cancer, 9/11, COVID-19—I needed to hear the stories again and again. I needed to hear them from a thousand different storytellers. I suspected I would need to hear them for the rest of my life. No understanding was reached. But I was still seeking it.

A life of seeking seemed like a pretty good one, to me.

As far as economics went, New York City was still in the flusher. COVID eliminated community events and fundraisers that generated income for volunteer EMS organizations. The disaster also added the extra costs of buying PPE, and with dwindling funds, made it hard to keep ambulances running in good condition. EMS agencies across the city, especially volunteer crews, were having trouble staying operational. The Bed-Stuy Vollies were presently closed. In a mostly Black neighborhood hit hard by COVID, at the start of flu season and winter.

The losses kept coming. A retired veteran firefighter named Jim Wind from Ladder 3 died unexpectedly in early October. He chauffeured the truck when Pat was captain. He was one of Pat's guys.

As for me, one of Pat's girls, and my future as a first responder? And how I was feeling about all this?

Oh, you know. I'd been better.

I wasn't suicidal or anything. But I wasn't exactly bursting with rainbows. As Gabriel said after he tried to save all of his COVID patients and they died, I felt some sort of way about all this. I can't say I was terribly excited about being a first responder at the moment. Or an investigator.

My EMT card expired last spring, during the peak. But due to the state being short of helpers, they automatically extended us expiring first responders for a year. Park Slope handled our recert paperwork. I finished all my Continuing Medical Education classes last winter, before COVID hit, aside from one required course no one could find online, about transporting pediatric patients. That was a quintessential EMS scenario: "This course is required. Also, it's not offered anywhere on earth."

There was a CME coming up about transporting babies this weekend, which one of our chiefs e-mailed us about. I wasn't feeling up for the class.

I also wasn't sure how Chief Beck was going to feel down the line about me running my mouth in this book, or if he'd even want me to ride on the ambulances as an EMT.

Volunteer EMT.

Same thing, work-wise. I wasn't sure anyone on *the force* was going to be calling me anytime soon, or ever again, to see if I had any (free) intel. Or my billionaire clients. Or my family. My resounding thought about the possibility that I might lose a lot after writing this, and maybe even get some death threats, was, *That's fine.*

I bet the house here. I said a lot of things about a lot of powerful institutions and people.

Was it worth it?

Hell yeah.

In times of crisis, you have to bet the house. You have to take a step back and ask yourself if the house is even worth saving. If it's not, you have to burn it down.

I followed higher laws. Irish laws. I took my lead from Pat.

Two weeks before he died, Pat told Paul three things:

1) He was in love (with Ylfa); 2) he was practicing yoga; and 3) he was going to risk his career calling out the Fire Department's radios.

At the time, the Fire Department used notoriously shitty Motorola Saber IIIs that made it nearly impossible for firefighters and officers to communicate with each other during emergencies. The World Trade Center attacks brought Pat's foreshadowed radio nightmare to life. More than one hundred firefighters stayed in the North Tower, having never received the radioed order for them to evacuate before it collapsed. Some firefighters heard the evacuation order, others didn't.

"Talk about the radios!" Eileen Tallon screamed on day two of the 9/11 Commission hearings in 2004. Her son, a young rookie firefighter, died needlessly in the North Tower.

We have to risk our careers to talk about the radios. We have to bet the house to talk about the uncounted dead, and how bad it was on the street during COVID. We have to tell the difficult stories, the stories no one wants to hear. We have to keep telling them over and over and over. We have to, or people will die.

And we might, too.

* * *

A reflection. One day in the dust-choked streets of downtown New York City after September 11, I saw this guy wearing a T-shirt that said ART SAVES LIVES.

I hated his shirt, and I hated him for wearing it. I thought it was insulting. Art did not save lives. First responders saved lives. And they died doing it. Pat died. My feeling at the time was that art, music, writing, business, finance, technology—all of it was pointless. It was fluff. Bullshit frosting on the important cake. I felt the only serious work was the work of saving lives, the work done by first responders. Every other vocation was silly.

But now, in 2020, almost twenty years later, I understood the message on the gentleman's T-shirt, and I agreed. I thought writing this book, creating something structured and artful out of all this tragedy, having a place to tell painful stories, writing it all down, probably saved my life. It was like Medic Nate said in EMT school. It never happened unless you wrote it down.

It happened. I wrote it down.

I remembered what Nathan Englander had said about my tendency to kill all of my characters, and thought about the Coen Brothers, and *Fargo*.

I kept the woodchipper. ALL the woodchippers.

And ALL the Jennifers. Writer Jennifer and First Responder Jennifer, Big Backstory Jennifer and Paris Jennifer, Elegant Jennifer and Street Jennifer, Crisis Manager Jennifer and Plant Lady Jennifer.

I designed my life in the spirit of Pat, but I also did what he did: I architected my worlds like a railroad apartment with rooms separated by partitioned walls. I kept my life separate, even from myself. I was friends with such a diverse bunch of people I didn't think they'd really enjoy spending quality time together if we all gathered. I often had the passing thought that if there were a civil war, my Instagram followers, all four of them, would probably murder each other.

But in the pandemic, all the walls I'd thrown up over the years to separate different parts of my life and my personality came crashing down. I thought that was a good thing.

On the street you often hear first responders brag about their ability to compartmentalize. "I can compartmentalize" is by far one of the things most often said. Most of the time, first responders are talking about their ability to not bring the horrors they see on the street home to their families. Not to bring up the car crash at the dinner table. Frequently, they're also talking about their ability to sleep at night without being bothered by the fact that they're cheating on their wives, who they hate, and who hate them right back. "I can compartmentalize," they say.

But can they? Could I? Could any of us? And should we?

Because here's what I learned through it all. In the end, in death, all the walls come down. Someone goes on the news and breaks your anonymity, which you worked your entire life to keep private. The person you think is insane comes flying out of the woodwork and publicly claims you. People you barely know start grieving you on the Internet while your true friends suffer the loss of your presence quietly and alone. That was a fact I swallowed hard in 2020. And if that was a fact, why not just let the walls fall down now? Knock them down. Force the door and destroy them. Call the Fire Department—they love breaking shit. They'll do it.

After COVID, compartmentalized, railroad-style Jennifer was loft-living Jennifer. Everything was out in the open. That felt good. A little scary, but good. What was I hiding from anyway? Myself?

I planted lots of flowers in this graveyard of a book. Diversionary stories about my cramazing love life and Halloween and brilliant friends, along with several book and song recommendations, as well as things to say or do if you find yourself in an emergency and have to meet one of us first responders on the worst day of your life. "Don't just bring me the problem," Nick used to say back when we were coworkers. "Bring me the solution."

Solutions.

I didn't do this to distract from the essential story I wanted to tell, about being a first responder. I did it as a kindness. Books have always been, for me, a form of rescue. In my girlhood books saved me. The information I found inside them. The things people said to make me feel less alone. Books were my first-on-scene first responders.

And tone-wise, I devoured Hanya Yanagihara's groundbreaking trauma-porn book, *A Little Life*, which came out a few years back and rocked the literary community. I read that monster, which, as its marketers said, "goes into some of the darkest places fiction has ever travelled," in two sittings. But that wasn't my storytelling style. I didn't want my listeners or readers to be brutalized by my stories, like all of us were on the street last spring. It was unbearable for us, ultimately. For some, it was unsurvivable.

Plus, it felt truer to allow space for jokes and beauty and quietness. At service funerals we never just stood around weeping. We also laughed and joked and sang.

That being said, I do admit there is more urine in this story than I ever could have ever anticipated. I guess I marked my territory.

The paper I wrote on was once a tree.

As for what I've been up to as of late, I've been off the ambulance for over a month now, since that rainy night tour in September, when I'd watched the presidential debates. That really took it out of me. I lost something that night, though I wasn't sure what.

Hope, maybe.

Nathan was still on the street occasionally, riding with young "No Note for the Gunshot Wound" Barry. Chad was in the wind, no longer an EMT. Aaron worked for the Fire Department now, and most of his Instagram posts were of his cute newborn baby. Lexi was technically a nurse now, she'd finished her schooling, but she was still working as an EMT. Nina was donezo. Austin was in Boston, working transport. Gabriel was on the truck but cooked and heavily salted.

For now, I just wanted to lie low. Rest. Catch my breath. I didn't know if I'd go back on the ambulance. I was undecided.

"Do your best," dispatchers told us last spring when COVID peaked, and we had no paramedics available to ventilate our suffocating patients in the field, and we couldn't get ambulances to people fast enough to save them, and the counted and uncounted dead were pronounced after twenty minutes of CPR, or in triage lines of hospitals that had no beds, then stuffed in body bags, then loaded into refrigerator trucks.

I did my best.

I hoped talking about what happened was OK, and that maybe something I said helped someone, somewhere. I wasn't a career first responder or an established author or anything. This is my first memoir. I studied and wrote fiction because real life was bullshit. Real life was too hard, in terms of telling the story straight. I'd never written nonfiction before this. After I signed my publishing contract I Googled "How to write a memoir."

I felt bad about getting an agent and then a publisher for this book during the pandemic. But it was nice to have some joyful news. Over the summer, when I told Ellery about getting an agent and selling a book, he said I shouldn't feel bad at all. He called me and screamed, "People celebrated during slavery! Get over your white guilt and throw your hands in the air!"

So I did that.

And I felt so blessed to be a writer. To have gotten a chance to give some of my friends at the NYU Vets Writing Workshop what they said they'd been waiting for—a chick to write the next great book about war.

My friends from workshop were really proud of me. All of my first responder family was. Everyone was so excited and supportive and helpful. They wanted people to hear all of our stories. When I told Luna people were finally going to get to meet us, and hear about our lives on the street, she cried.

People really had forgotten us. We worked so hard, and so thanklessly, for so little, for nothing, and we'd been invisible. And for a moment in time, we were seen.

I thought Pat was proud, too, because whenever I wrote passages about him in this book, my whole body broke out in goosebumps. And Mike, he loved writers. He couldn't wait for people to hear about our spiritual marriage, and to see how hard it was, 9/11 Act 2. Over the summer he sent me an e-mail and requested I use Pat's real name in my book. "Pat spent his life making other lives better and even now continues to do that," Mike said. "A long-forgotten saying came out of post-9/11: 'Doing a Pat Brown,' meaning a selfless and kind act. The kind Pat would do. Stories of Pat continue to inspire and will do so in your book. And Paddy Brown's will—it will continue to be done."

Mike asked the same for himself. "Please use my real name and any story, good or bad, about me. Over the past year I have grown significantly as a person, and you are the main reason that happened. It would be an honor to be in your book, and do not sugarcoat anything."

These guys. I love them so much. My heroes. They shouldered their way into my story to such an extent that Ylfa laughingly referred to my book as "their book."

"I like that," Michael Daly said. And another time, "Pat doesn't like being dead."

No, he doesn't. For us, he is alive.

God bless Pat and Mike Brown, the fallen and still falling.

I didn't know if what I wrote was great. But it was something.

Mama tried.

Mama also thought that in addition to lawyering up and entering the witness protection program after writing this, I should alert my coworkers that I was potentially going to be a future disaster. One day I rang one of my crisis colleagues, a woman I treasured who worked at a gold-standard crisis management firm, the best in New York.

"I just want to give you a heads-up that I might become a crisis when my book comes out," I said.

My colleague didn't miss a beat. "No problem, Jennifer. We'll manage your crisis."

So that was good, in case I went out with a bang. To conjure Audre Lorde, "I'm going to go out like a fucking meteor!"

26

UNIMAGINABLE LOSS

Late October, Mike was still alive. But barely. His cousin's wife, Judie, said he wasn't eating. He'd lost a lot of weight. He was gray. She said he looked like a different person. Like Luis Alvarez, the cancer-riddled detective who'd testified with Jon Stewart to an empty Congress to try to get funding for 9/11 first responders. So these were his last weeks, it seemed.

Mike was refusing to see family or let anyone from New York come visit. He knew if people got on a plane, it meant he was dying. So if people didn't fly out to Vegas, to him that meant his life wouldn't end.

"What about Ylfa and Jennifer?" Judie asked him.

"Well," he said. "I'd like to see them."

When Judie told me this, I didn't know what to do. There was no way Ylfa could go, since she took care of elderly people for a living, and if she flew to Vegas and back to New York, she'd have to quarantine on both sides and lose a month of work. It tortured her not to be able to go. It tortured me, too. If I went, my presence communicated to Mike that he was a dead man.

There were no good choices for us two wives. Fly to Vegas to see Mike, or stay behind in New York?

After many tortured, tear-filled nights, Ylfa decided to stay in New York, which I and everyone else agreed was the right thing to do. We all had the feeling that Pat would want her to stay here. COVID was alive and well; the only way we were going to stop this thing was to wear masks, stay put, and care for others.

Besides, we all knew Mike loved Ylfa and felt the strength of her love back, no matter the distance. She was always his number one. We were co-wives, so there was no hierarchy in our spiritual marriage. Ylfa and I referred to each other as "Wife 1A," and so did Mike. Whenever he ignored one of my suggestions (commands), that's what I would say to him, tossing him to Ylfa: "Have you spoken to Wife 1A about this?" Together, we were Wife 1AA. So we could really shoulder this hellacious monster together, as sister-wives.

I didn't know what to do. I sought spiritual counsel. I called Michael Daly, my priest, the man who was supposed to marry the three of us, and wept. Then I asked for spiritual advice.

"Spiritual advice? From me?"

"You're my priest. You wrote the book on Mychal Judge—literally. So I need you to channel him and give me some spiritual advice."

He paused, then cleared his throat and spoke in a voice weighted with spirit.

"Life," he said, "is for the living."

Langston Hughes.

"And Mike doesn't want you to fly out to say goodbye. He wants you to tell him he's going to be OK. And you can't."

I blew out a breath.

"And the only way we're ever going to stop this virus is if we stop spreading it around."

"Wow," I said. "You really do come from holy lineage. That was really good. I'll pray and meditate about it. I'll talk to Pat."

Two days later, I had my answer.

I decided to go. The Vegas crew initially said they thought it was a good idea for me to surprise Mike, rather than tell him I was coming. If I told him, he might panic and say no, since my presence would essentially mean I was there to pronounce him dead. So that was the plan. Show up on his doorstep like FedEx.

Surprise.

My only prayer was that I would get to see him again, if that was fated, and he would get to see me, if that was what he needed and wanted. This wasn't about what I wanted. It was about Mike. And Pat. Doing my sacred duty.

My priest must have sensed what I was going to do before I knew it myself. Priests could be like that. They have those weird spiritual feelers, like Martians. The good ones do, at least.

Father Michael called, and before he could say a word, I blurted out that I was going to Vegas ASAP, flying in two or three days, showing up unannounced to see my husband.

He was completely unsurprised by this breaking news.

"That's why there's two wives," he said. "One wife goes, and one stays."

Then he gave me a magnificent idea.

He advised me to wear my Park Slope EMT uniform when I went to see Mike. To tell him I didn't come all the way from New York City to Vegas in a pandemic because he was dying. I came because I was trying to break the world record for the longest volunteer ambulance transport in history—2,522 miles—and my next call would be to Guinness World Records. I agreed this was a most excellent idea and committed to doing it.

"Don't let him vote! Don't remind him it's the election!"

I roared laughing. Like his friend Mychal Judge, Michael Daly could make you laugh in the darkest moments, when laughter was sacrament, all that was left.

"He's going to be so shocked to see me walk into his house in my EMT uniform he'll drop dead. Then I'll be the one who accidentally killed Mike Brown."

"Perfect," my priest said.

So that was the latest plan.

That same afternoon I called Paul and told him I was heading west.

"I'll go with you," he said quickly. "I'll follow your lead."

"My lead? Now I'm the leader?"

"We don't do this stuff alone, honey. I'll go with you."

What a guy. No wonder Pat loved him.

It was all too much. It was impossible, 9/11 dovetailing with COVID.

I couldn't say I was looking forward to seeing Mike on his deathbed. He was in and out of the hospital at the moment, waiting for a company to deliver home oxygen. A day after I decided to surprise him, the doctors told him the cancer was now in his kidneys. He knew what that meant. My husband was a doctor.

Finally, he accepted his fate. Mike told his cousin people in New York could fly out to see him now, to say goodbye.

I'd already decided to go. But I didn't know if I should tell him. Again I spoke with his family in Vegas. Together we decided to keep my arrival a surprise. That day, I bought a one-way ticket to Vegas that left in forty-eight hours. Wednesday morning out of JFK. Due to COVID, Delta offered free passes for people who needed to adjust their tickets, just in case the plan changed.

I pulled my EMT uniform out of my closet. I decided I'd pack it. But now that Mike knew he was dying, the bottom fell out of the surprise. I'd been told our husband was being a real handful to his nurses. He kept ripping off his oxygen mask and morphine patch. That happened to patients sometimes. When you can't take in enough oxygen, and you're loaded with narcotics, and in ten-out-of-ten pain, and terrified of dying, it makes you crazed.

As Mike once said to me many months back, "Dying is hard."

That night, packing to fly to Vegas, I was deranged with grief and rage, wild with it. I had never known rage so bright. I was not by disposition a hateful woman. I felt this rage was not entirely my own. I sensed it belonged to Pat. And I was so adrenalized with it I could have lifted a car and lit up Times Square. Pat was not happy about being murdered on 9/11, or his brother dying of World Trade Center–related cancer, and neither was I. Fuck this country, this city, the Fire Department, I thought. Or Pat thought. I didn't know which feelings or thoughts were my own anymore, which were coming from deep inside me or the other side, a thin place between this world and the next, New York and Ireland, the now and the eternal. Either way there's your song, Snoop. And it's not over until the Irish lady sings.

The way we treat each other in this country is a monstrous disgrace.

We deny death in America. Deny sickness. Deny disease. Militarize illness as if it's a war and stigmatize asking for help. No one wants to deal with the hard fact that life ends. This is possibly the only thing at this historical moment we can agree on: life ends. It is sacred and it is finite.

As far as we know, this one precious life is all we have. It starts, and it ends. But no one wants to witness the ending. It's too ugly. Violent. Slow.

So they push it out of sight. They push it onto the street, onto civil servants. They push it onto first responders.

Why, in a country where people shoot each other to death regularly, doesn't everyone know how to stop bleeding and apply a tourniquet?

Why don't people know how to do CPR? Thirty and two. There, now you're trained.

It takes anywhere from a few hours to one week to learn basic skills to save a human life.

One week—if that.

No one has time? When your child's heart stops, you want to wait for us to arrive in an ambulance, lights and sirens? No interest in learning how to do CPR yourself? Or bleeding control?

Why?

Don't have a calling? You do now. I'm calling you. Now you've been called.

Mandatory civil service. That was my feeling this October as a solution.

Mandatory civil service for everyone who calls themselves American.

"How are you?" Tommy asked the next morning. "I saw a photo of something posted on Instagram saying pray for Mike and my heart sank. Any updates?"

"I'm not good. He's dying. I'm flying out first thing Wednesday morning. I'm a wreck. His family is flying in from New York."

"Good for you for sticking by his side. And by doing so you are also honoring Pat, and he would be so pleased with you."

"This is going to destroy me."

"Don't let it. Don't allow it to. You're stronger than the task ahead of you. By a long shot."

"I'm losing my mind with rage and grief. It's a nightmare."

"Or an honor."

"I feel that, too. I feel blessed. It's an honor. It's sacred. And it's my duty. It's for Pat. And Mike is one of my best friends. He's family. And I'll be with him until the end. I just pray he lasts another day so I can see him. Even though I know seeing him will destroy me."

"I know you're up for it, and I know Pat will appreciate it."

"Pat is alive and well. I'm channeling his anger. Pat was an angry guy. He once rammed a fireman's head into a wall hand dryer because the guy wouldn't stop teasing him about liking Broadway musicals. Pat liked them because his mom loved them, and she died while he was in Vietnam. So he almost killed a firefighter. AND HE IS MY FUCKING GUY! He's the reason I became who I am."

"I LOVE IT! Plenty of guys need their heads bashed in once in a while. Oddly enough, I did that when I came home from Iraq. I was getting teased for having had 'the last year off of work and hanging at the beach in the Middle East.' I had enough and snapped. Never happened again."

"Exactly. People get pushed and pushed and pushed. And then it's like, OK. You piss me off, I'll bomb your village."

"It's so true!"

"Thanks, solider. Love you. I'll text you from Vegas. I just pray I get there in time."

"Love you back. You're not alone and I believe in you. Walk tall. Stay strong!"

This was agony. It was a nightmare. I couldn't bear it.

I hated the way these first responders were treated.

They were deserted.

That's what no one wants to say but that's what happened.

They were deserted.

Every time my phone rang today, I thought Mike was dead, and I didn't get there in time.

I needed to bring a book with me to Vegas; it felt as necessary as air. What book do you bring to visit your friend who's dying of cancer? *The Book of Mychal*, by Michael Daly. It practically jumped off my bookshelf. Of course.

Things change fast in emergencies. And that's what Mike became the next day.

His family didn't know if he would still be alive by the time I got to Vegas, fourteen hours from this moment. He was anxious at home because he was dying in the same bed his wife died in, of the same thing. He turned his phone off. He kept trying to get out of bed, and falling, because he was so weak. He asked to see his sister. She was in the air now.

Judie called me. She said tell Paul not to buy his ticket as she didn't think he would still be alive on Monday, which was the earliest Paul could come. She said they wanted to tell Mike I was coming. They thought it would calm him down. Help him feel less anxious.

"Tell him," I said. "Tell him I'm on my way. Tell him I'll be there in the morning. I don't want him to wait for me if he needs to go sooner. Do whatever calms him down. Whatever he needs. You guys are on scene, so you're seeing it. I trust you. Do whatever you need to do."

"What if he says no? I don't think he will, but what if he says no?"

"That's fine. This isn't about me, it's about Mike. He gets to choose. We'll do whatever he wants. You can tell him I'm coming, I'm on my way, and I'll stay as long as he wants, or I'll stay here and won't come at all, or something in between. Whatever he wants."

We are out of practice in the West with caring for the sick and dying. We are bad at it. We must do better. If you remember nothing else of what I've told you, I beg you to remember this:

The dying should get what they want. Do not make it about you. It is *their* death. Grant the sick and dying their every last wish. If you can't be there for them in person at the end, as was so often the case for family members during COVID, or if they wish for privacy in their final moments, when they are in the throes of death, talk to them in prayer and meditation. Sing to them. Tell them your messages. The door between this world and the next is open.

Everything is heard. Every message is received. Your presence is felt.

Tell them they are not alone. That you are with them in spirit, and you will be with them until the end. Tell them their fallen friends and family members are with them, too. Name them. Let them know they are being divinely protected.

Tell them you love them and thank them for loving you. Tell them they did everything perfectly. They made the best choices they could in accordance with their own soul, and they were perfect choices. Let them know you're proud of them. They do not have to have any regrets. Their fate was assigned, their number was called, and they are dying a sacred death.

Tell them they are going home. And that we are all going home, and you will soon join them and be together again. Assure them that while you're separated, you can still communicate with one another. The walls between worlds are thin. They can talk to you whenever they want, and you will talk to them in prayer and meditation and song. You will keep telling their stories. You will tell them over and over, to each other and to the world, in as many ways as you can. You will honor them and keep them alive forever.

Understand that your loved one could not have done anything differently. They made the best choices they could for their own soul. Forgive them absolutely, and yourself, absolutely, for any judgments you may have held about their treatments or final moments. They did a perfect job.

So did you.

Let go of your guilt, judgment, anger, and shame toward yourself, and anyone else you might hold with resentment in your mind and heart, about your relationship with them. Each of you did your best, and you did a perfect job. Like them, you are to have no regrets. Your loved one had their own path. Respect their path and do not diminish it by assuming you know better and think things could have been different. Be forever kind to one another, as each of us carries deeply personal agonies from losing people we love. We are all we have. Let your anger fall away and remember that sickness and death are not wars to be won or lost, they are a natural part of life, and we are all going home. When we do, we will see our lost friends.

All people hear voices. Only emotionally distressed people hear voices others do not hear. For me, these messages are from the voices of 9/11. Captain Patrick Brown and Chaplain Mychal Judge.

All today I cried and prayed.

Pat, if Mike needs to see me, and I'm supposed to see Mike, then make it happen. If not, if you need to take him before I get there, and you don't want me to see him, I trust you. Whatever you want. I really want to see him, but I trust you.

This evening, Judie called.

He would like to see me.

Here I come, my sweet husband.

* * *

Tonight, I was packing and sobbing. I hated my uniform. I didn't want to look at it, let alone pack it or wear it to Vegas to see Mike. If I showed up with my uniform it meant I was an EMT and Mike was my patient and he was dying.

Last breaths, last words.
In person, or in spirit.
Sacred witness.
I was called.

ACKNOWLEDGMENTS

My first and eternal gratitude is to Captain Patrick Brown and Dr. Michael Everett Brown, heroes and brothers, who spent their lives helping others, and ultimately sacrificed their lives in love and service. You are forever alive in my heart. Thank you.

I'm indebted to the extraordinary patients in New York City whose medical emergencies I relay in this memoir, and to all of those at Park Slope Volunteer Ambulance Corps who took such good care of the community, particularly during the COVID-19 pandemic. I owe a special debt to the group of first responders who directly or indirectly contributed to this book, especially those who entrusted me with their stories. You have my endless gratitude and respect. In particular, I must acknowledge my partners, Mendy Habibian, Kasia Tylawski, Dalas Zeichner, and Kristina "The Pole" Shmulik, as they have been my profoundest allies and teachers. Thank you also to those at Ladder 3 who have created a place of remembrance for Pat, and now, Mike.

I was blessed to have a literary dream team that worked miracles to bring this book into the world and served as a sanctuary in times of strife. I'm especially thankful to Ned Leavitt who believed in me, offered vital editorial feedback, and generously introduced me to my wonderful agent, James Levine, who moved mountains to make this book happen and never gave up on me. Lindsay Edgecombe and Courtney Paganelli at Levine Greenberg Rostan Literary Agency provided brilliant notes that allowed my story to be brought forth. Thank you to my gifted editor, Jessica Case, for her wise, protective editorial hand and vision that ultimately shaped this book into what I most hoped it would be. I'm grateful to everyone at Pegasus Books who so thoughtfully and eagerly worked on this project, from copyediting to publicity.

I owe so much to friends and writers who read versions of this book and offered support: Josh Levine, Dan Murphy, Karen Shepard, Bobby Burke, Omri Bezalel, and Yael Hacohen. Thanks especially to Michael Daly who calmed my nerves and helped me find the courage to tell the stories I most needed to tell, and who always looked out for me during the pandemic. I'm grateful to my writers group that has cheered me on for years: Felice Belle, Misa Dayson, Steve Gray, Ben Snyder, Christopher Fox, and Thyra Heder. Many people at NYU, especially the NYU Veterans Writing Workshop, devoted their creative talents to helping me find my voice.

I'm deeply thankful to my friends and loved ones who took such good care of me this agonizing year, and many others: Natalie Edwards, Robyn Twomey, Rachel Knowles, Bridget Goodbody, Anna Morgan-Mullane, Paul Colliton, Larry Scheingold, Dan Witz, Lynn Margileth, Ellery Washington, Jermaine Spradley, and my therapist, Anne Stern. My beautiful mother, Sheila Eynaud, offered unconditional love and always believed in me. Thanks, mom.

Finally, this book would not have been possible without Ylfa Edelstein, who carried me through it all, rescued me in innumerable ways, and whose faith in me helped bring this book into the world. I couldn't have gotten through this crushing year without you, sister. You're Irish now. And we will see our lost beloveds on the other side.